# WOMEN
## *under the*
# KNIFE

D1345214

HUTCHINSON RADIUS

*By the same author*

THE INTELLIGENT PERSON'S GUIDE TO MODERN MEDICINE
A CHILD IS BORN
CICELY: THE STORY OF A DOCTOR
MOTHERS: THEIR POWER AND INFLUENCE
THE MORBID STREAK: DESTRUCTIVE ASPECTS OF THE PERSONALITY
WHY WOMEN FAIL
INVENTING MOTHERHOOD: THE CONSEQUENCES OF AN IDEAL
A DOCTOR'S STORY

# WOMEN
## *under the*
# KNIFE

*A History of Surgery*

---

# ANN DALLY

## HUTCHINSON RADIUS
### LONDON SYDNEY AUCKLAND JOHANNESBURG

04770182

This edition first published in 1991 by
Hutchinson Radius

Random Century Group Ltd
20 Vauxhall Bridge Road, London SW1V 2SA

Random Century Australia (Pty) Ltd
20 Alfred Street, Milsons Point, Sydney, NSW 2061, Australia

Random Century New Zealand Ltd
PO Box 40–086, Glenfield, Auckland 10, New Zealand

Random Century South Africa (Pty) Ltd
PO Box 337, Bergvlei, 2012, South Africa

British Cataloguing in Publication Data
Dally, Ann
    Women under the knife: a history of surgery.
    1. Medicine. Surgery, history
    I. Title
    617.09

ISBN 0–09–174508-X

Photoset in Sabon by Speedset Ltd, Ellesmere Port
Printed and bound in Great Britain by
Butler and Tanner Ltd, Frome, Somerset

# CONTENTS

# LIST OF ILLUSTRATIONS

*To*
ANNE KELLEHER
*with thanks*

# PREFACE AND ACKNOWLEDGMENTS

I am a practising doctor and psychiatrist. A previous book of mine (*Inventing Motherhood: the consequences of an ideal*) had historical aspects, but this is the first real history book I have written. I hope that readers, especially scholars, will be tolerant of imperfections. It has been exciting to write and has taught me much. I was surprised, and of course delighted, when the manuscript was praised by several distinguished historians, but I am aware that others may not be so generous. I began *Women under the Knife* more than five years ago from a desire sometimes to escape from daily medical practice in a stressful field. Research time was snatched with difficulty. Gradually the book took over part of my life and gave me a desire to explore further in the 'new' social history of medicine, which, I was surprised to find, is one of the most exciting and expanding fields in both arts and sciences. At present, medicine and the way it is practised are increasingly questioned and criticised, not least for the attitudes of many doctors and medical institutions and the way they behave. One might think that psychiatrists would attempt to ameliorate this, or at least study it, but in many ways psychiatry is the worst and the most criticised of all the medical specialties, disappointingly stagnant at present, though expanding in self-importance. Many people both inside and outside the medical profession are confused or misled: not only the future but also the present and past are unclear. I doubt whether the necessary reappraisal of medicine and its services can be done adequately without a new understanding from an historical and sociological point of view. The old history of medicine, devoted to charting progress and glory, tends to make things worse. Medicine needs to absorb its own new history as much as it needs a cure for cancer, and perhaps needs to do this before it can find that cure.

Obstetrics and gynaecology have become an important part of women's struggle for recognition as human beings with choice and access to opportunities. Nowhere is the fight for 'control of the body' more involved than here. I don't believe you can really understand what is happening in this area today without knowing something about how it all arose. Sadly, this knowledge is often lacking and much of what is oft-repeated is misleading. Some medical historians lack understanding both of women and of medicine as it is or was practised, or else they concentrate on the ideas about health and disease that were prevalent at the time about which they are writing. Some take for granted many of the things that feminists and others question. Some feminist writers are also ignorant about practical medicine and its procedures or are imbued with the idea that it can all be explained as the 'oppression' of women by men. I was inspired to write this book when I found that excellent pioneer writers were getting so much of it factually wrong and were being misled into spoiling their powerful arguments and deeds by invalid statements.

One of the many pleasures of the research for this book has come from contact with historians and other scholars. Seminars and private discussions, often on subjects far removed from this book, have intrigued and influenced me and I hope have given depth to my amateur historical outlook.

In a book intended for the general reader but also written with scholars in mind, footnotes and references have created problems. I have tried to make it easy for readers to check statements without deterring those who simply wish to read. The book covers a long period in a field with more sources than one could read in a lifetime. Many of the primary sources have been quoted by others in secondary works. I have checked and used a number of these, sometimes asking different questions from their authors and coming to different conclusions. Older histories, and those written by doctors, practising or retired, tend to regard medicine as part of the march of progress and medical history as a celebration of the profession, nevertheless they often give information useful to someone who wishes to appraise the situation from a different point of view. These works are all listed in the bibliography and I have tried to ensure that readers will be able to find the original sources without difficulty, even if they are not listed in my text. The older works include those of Ricci, Castiglione, Cianfrani, Jameson, Morton and Garrison, Munro Kerr. In particular, I acknowledge the works of Harvey Graham. This was the pseudonym of the late Dr Harvey Flack, a great medical writer. Under his editorial guidance, more years ago than I care to remember, I served an unofficial apprenticeship (or baptism of fire) in medical writing, working for the British Medical Association's contribution to popular medicine, the journal *Family Doctor*. His books on the history of surgery and midwifery were uncritical in the modern sense (as one would expect from the time they were written) and they have been attacked by feminist writers, but they were meticulously researched and annotated and I know from experience that he was open-minded and original in outlook with a passionate interest in trying to understand what was going on. The restaurant in Charlotte Street, Bloomsbury, where he used to expound his ideas to me still exists and I think of him whenever I pass it. It is sad that, although all his original sources are listed in the first edition of his *Eternal Eve*, 1950, he was persuaded to omit them from the second edition, 1960. I appeal to librarians, if it is not too late, not to throw out the first edition in favour of the second.

Among modern writers I am particularly grateful to the following, to whom I acknowledge my debt and apologise to any inadvertently omitted. Their relevant work is listed in the bibliography which should help find any references required: Flavia Alaya, Joan Austoker, Ben Barker-Benfield, Patricia Branca, Vern Bullough and Martha Voght, Jill Conway, Pietro Corsi and Paul Weindling, Francois Crouzet, Lenore Davidoff, Sara Delamont and Lorna Duffin, Anne Digby, Jean Donnison, Jacques Donzelot, Carol Dyhouse, Barbara Ehrenreich and Deirdre English, Elizabeth Fee, Karl Figlio, the late Michel Foucault, Elizabeth Fox-Genovese, E. Freidson, Ludmilla Jordanova, the Kaisers, Sheila Kitzinger, Lawrence Longo, Irvine Loudon, Ornella Moscucci, Ann Oakley, Roy and Dorothy Porter, S.J. Reiser, Ruth Richardson, Gunter Risse, the Rosenbergs, Edward Shorter, Elaine Showalter, Richard Shryock, Henry Sigerist, George Stocking and Lawrence Stone.

Searching for illustrations has been fun and frustrating for both me and my publisher. Much visual material showing surgery is available but little of it concerns women, although we know that they were most commonly the recipients. It seems that, except in specifically 'female' situations, such as childbirth, it was not part of the image of Woman that she should be so portrayed. An interesting insight into modern life came when I discovered that several librarians who work with the material had not noticed this.

I thank Anne Kelleher for drawing my attention to feminist material about surgery that led me to write this book and also the many experts in this and related fields who have increased my knowledge and understanding. These include scholars at the Wellcome Institute for the History of Medicine who have given friendly help and professional advice, lent books and papers, obtained material and advised about how to obtain more, in particular Dr William Bynum, Dr Catherine Crawford and Dr Roy Porter. I also thank Imogen Bloor MRCOG, for discussions about modern gynaecology; Dr Peter Dally for helpful comments; David Doughan for sharing his deep knowledge of nineteenth century and modern feminist literature; Lesley Hall, who seems to have read (and remembered) just about everything in the field; Jo Manton, who discussed the project with me at an early stage; Ornella Moscucci, who lent proofs of her splendid book *The Science of Woman* before it was published; Wendy Savage FRCOG for insights into current problems in gynaecology; Dr Norma Williams, medical gynaecologist and an old friend. I also thank David Brady for help in my search for medical illustrations, Edwin Mullins for producing ideas and books about Victorian painting, Ruth Lumley-Smith for a quotation and the *Church Times* for a photocopy. I also appreciate the many patients who, over the years, have taught me about attitudes and feelings and how doctors deal well or badly with them. My patients have also helped me to develop a personal method of enquiry into situations that I realise I have transposed from them and their problems to the subject of this book.

I am grateful to the staff of the following libraries for their friendly, efficient help in what was often a difficult task of tracking down material, much of it obscure or hard to find: the British Library; the Fawcett Library; the London Library; the library of the Royal Society of Medicine; the Wellcome Library for the History of Medicine; the Women's Health Centre.

I thank my agent, Shân Morley-Jones; Kate Mosse, my publisher and editor at Radius; my secretaries, Anne Lingham and Diana Tomlins; and Emma Dally, my daughter. All made helpful comments and encouraged me with sustained enthusiasm. Last, but not least, I thank my husband, Philip Egerton, for his constant support, encouragement and tolerance. This long list reveals much of the work and effort that goes into creating a book. The author does only part of it and is dependent on the expertise and goodwill of many people.

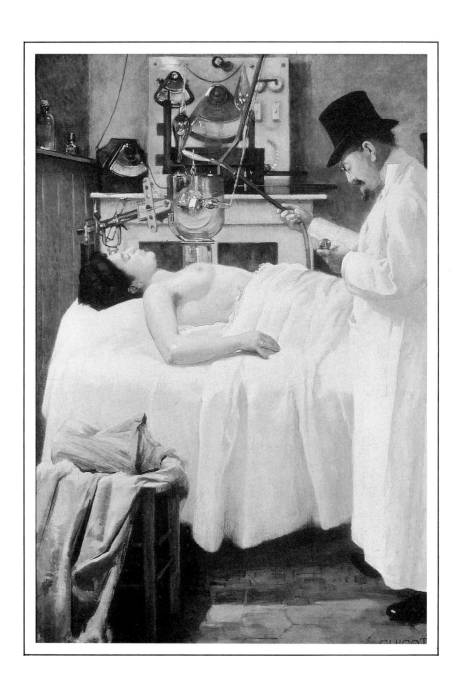

# INTRODUCTION

Many people in the western world, not all of them women, feel angry or worried about gynaecologists. Some believe that the behaviour and motives of certain gynaecologists are unsuited to the modern world and that some of these doctors, even when they are sincere, do not always act in the best interests of their patients. Such anger and criticism have created a new awareness and a need for reassessment but have also led to misinformation and attack. This has been countered by more misinformation and also by the typical reactions of professional groups and organisations when their members feel criticised or threatened – pomposity and pontification, secrecy and vindictiveness.

Doctors and others have diagnosed and treated women's diseases for thousands of years but specialist doctors in the modern sense have existed only since the nineteenth century. They changed the pattern of medical care extensively and the benefit they brought to women was largely unquestioned. Until recently, their activities attracted little criticism from outside. Disagreements in gynaecology, as in medicine generally, were confined largely to its own practitioners and remained within the profession.

Gynaecologists are also obstetricians and so are responsible not only in diseases of women but also in pregnancy and childbirth, where much of the criticism has been concentrated. Since most women visit a gynaecologist at some time during their lives and some visit many times, it is important to try to understand the present disputes and to assess the situation on both sides.

Much of the written history of gynaecology has been produced by gynaecologists, with themselves as heroes. It portrays the subject as a steady advance in knowledge and in humanitarian skill in the relief of human suffering. The beginning of gynaecology is often dated from what has generally, if inaccurately, been labelled the first major gynaecological operation, in 1809. This progress is said to have led to steady improvement in the health and welfare of women. Some of these writers even regard it as an example of the liberation of women – believing that women's liberation consists of advance from the domination of nature to domination by doctors.

There is another side to the story, newer, but just as often misconceived. This is that gynaecology developed at a time of increasing enslavement of women and that it was an instrument of that enslavement. Many people now question the motives behind the acquisition of gynaecologists' knowledge and skill.

Gynaecology is usually described as a branch of medicine or medical science, but it has also played an important part in the history of women. The subject and practice of gynaecology, like the subject and practice of medical history, developed during the second half of the nineteenth century, the very period of maximum prejudice against women, when attitudes towards them were at their most bizarre, in a curious mixture of contempt and idealisation. The intellectual inferiority of women was taken for granted and vigorously and jealously promoted. Most medical history, like general history, was written by men from a male point of view. Today it is still organised in many libraries under categories that suggest a male world dominating human progress, some of it for the benefit of women. Sources which reveal the underside of this progress exist but are often difficult to find. Women and their experiences were scarcely mentioned, even in books about midwifery and gynaecology. Women's history was largely ignored. Women's experience of gynaecology was never regarded as important. Women were essentially and exclusively patients.

So, are we looking at progress towards better health for women or, as some would have us believe, at empire-building on the part of a group of surgeons and the ruthless exploitation of women by men?


During the nineteenth century there emerged a new kind of surgeon who sought greater anatomical accuracy, physiological understanding and technical exactitude than his predecessors. Many of these surgeons had served in the armed forces and had learned their skills in the traditional manner, on the battlefield. When they returned to civilian life, they increased these skills, often by practising on women. Some of them became the first gynaecologists, some remained as general surgeons. Most did both.

The early operations on women patients, through which

gynaecology developed as a body of knowledge and a specialty within surgery were often described by the surgical pioneers themselves as 'experiments'. In view of later developments, this was an unfortunate word to choose, particularly when it referred to patients who were slaves. Were these operations done through chance circumstances? Were they motivated by a desire to relieve suffering, in the accepted language of the time, or were doctors demonstrating their power and a desire to increase control over women? How did women react and how did they feel about it? How far have things changed today? In so far as nineteenth-century surgeons exploited women, does modern gynaecology also exploit them (as many allege) and if so in what ways?

Hostile views refer to 'the gynaecologist's exotic catalog of tortures . . . performed . . . on black female slaves . . . kept for the sole purpose of surgical experimentation'* and to 'Sexual surgery . . . man's means of restraining women . . . by ruthlessly cutting up women's bodies.' Black female slaves were 'garnered' into the backyard 'to provide guinea pigs' for 'monomaniacal' surgeons.

The standard medical view is that gynaecology developed through the brave work of a few pioneers who showed '*almost with a magic wand*' that what had before been incurable and the source of lifelong suffering, could now, thanks to the new wonders of surgery, be cured.

There are arguments for both points of view but the truth may lie elsewhere.

The same kind of discrepancy can be seen in the history of ovariotomy – the misnomer for removal of the ovaries. The operation became common later in the century but gradually fell into disrepute. The disapproving attitude towards it has remained. A typical modern account tells us that doctors removed hundreds of ovaries and were so pleased with themselves that they even handed them round at meetings.

I felt there was something strange in this story so I followed it up. After all, it is normal for doctors to pass round pathological specimens at scientific meetings, a practice not particularly associated with self-satisfaction. At a scientific meeting in 1876, the distinguished early gynaecologist, Spencer Wells, showed his colleagues an ovary with a tumour which he had removed at post-mortem from Harriet Martineau, the writer. He was not gloating but merely making a point which was that had she had an operation instead of being treated with mesmerism, she would probably have been spared much suffering.

* B. Ehrenreich & D. English: *For Her Own Good*, p. 125.

One of the references the author made to the *British Medical Journal* regarding 'removing normal ovaries' was actually a description of the removal of an ovary that had been destroyed by an acute *abscess*. Lawson Tait, another brilliant, if somewhat flamboyant, surgeon, claimed to have uncovered much infection of the pelvis, often with severe sepsis, among the women of Birmingham. The infection often damaged the ovaries irrevocably and made them a source of spreading infection so that they needed to be removed if the patient was to be restored to health. The same situation might arise today in infections which have been inadequately treated. Tait's colleagues in London were sceptical and there were rumours that he had exaggerated. There was also rivalry between London doctors and doctors in the provinces, as well as hostility towards the uncouth, self-promoting and clever Lawson Tait. In 1887, to prove his point, Tait arranged for fifty-eight specimens of septic ovaries to be transported (no mean feat in those days) from Birmingham to London, where he displayed them at a meeting of the Pathological Society of London, chaired by Sir James Paget, a distinguished surgeon.

Another hostile criticism of gynaecologists concerns the use of leeches. 'The common medical practice of bleeding by means of leeches also took on some very peculiar forms in the hands of gynaecologists . . . In some cases leeches were even applied to the cervix despite the danger of their occasional loss in the uterus. (So far as we know, no doctor even considered perpetrating similar medical insults to the male organs).'

Some feminists write as if unpleasant, even sadistic, treatments were given only to women and always with sinister motives. This is not the case. Surgical operations, procedures such as blistering and painful mechanical restraints to curb masturbation were applied widely to men. For instance, the famous German surgeon, Johann Friedrich Dieffenbach, who died in 1847, suggested an operation, and performed it on several occasions, of cutting out half the tongue to cure stuttering, a condition commoner in men than in women.

Many accounts of medical treatment during this period record that leeches were often applied to any part of the body that was swollen or infected, regardless of the sex of the patient and there are many accounts of leeches applied near the male genitals. Leeches were commonly applied to an operation site before and after an operation in order to reduce swelling and inflammation. This surgical custom reached its height in the 1830s and '40s: In 1832, St Bartholomew's Hospital in London bought 97,000 leeches and the Manchester Royal Infirmary spent 4.4 per cent of its total budget on 'that most singular and valuable reptile'. Leeches became so much in demand that the supply ran out and they had to be imported from Turkey.* Some doctors were especially keen on using them, for example the French surgeon Dupuytren, in the first decades of the nineteenth century, seems to have applied six to eight leeches or as many as thirty, where there was infection. He was a pioneer in operations for strangulated hernia, a condition that has nothing to do with gynaecology and which is commoner in men than in women. When patients did badly, Dupuytren used to apply sixty to eighty leeches to the lower abdomen and genitalia and about the anal canal. It may or may not be relevant that when Dupuytren himself was threatened by a fatal illness, he said he would rather die by the hand of God than by that of the surgeons. He refused to have an operation and died twelve days later.

Leeches also appear in the medical history of Louis XIV of France. In 1686, at the age of forty-eight, Louis developed a fistula-in-ano. His physicians treated him with the usual emetics, purges and prescriptions, which included leeches and must have been as unpleasant as leeches on a woman's cervix. None of this was of any avail and in the end the king underwent a dramatic and famous operation, which greatly enhanced the reputation of surgery and equally greatly annoyed the physicians.†

These discrepancies between modern critical accounts and medical histories arose partly because of the way in which the writing of medical history developed and partly in what those who wrote it wanted it to show. Until a few years ago histories of medicine tended

---

* O. & S. Wangensteen, *The Rise of Surgery*, p. 250 gives references.
† This operation was recommended by the king's physician, Guy Fagon, who arranged for Dr Félix to perform it. But Dr Félix needed to practise his technique, so arrangements were made for him to acquire knowledge and deftness in a Paris hospital. People suffering from fistula-in-ano were collected and sent to the hospital for surgery. Tradition has it that some of them did not survive the operation and that the bodies were disposed of at night and the deaths attributed to poisoning. This continued for two months. In November, Félix said he was ready to operate on the king. He operated one afternoon and it was successful. That evening the king was well enough to receive a fairly large assembly of his court. He rewarded Félix handsomely. This incident greatly enhanced the reputation of surgery, which had tended to be despised. The physicians were furious. One might add that it has always been a tradition in medicine, and still is, though not so crudely, to experiment on poor or obscure patients and to use them for the benefit of rich or important patients. A recent case in Britain in which poor Turks were tricked and bribed into donating their kidneys for rich patients shows that the tradition is still alive.

to be 'whiggish' – telling the story of continual new discoveries by dedicated men and of the intellectual conquest of individual diseases for the benefit of humankind. This was the kind of picture that drew many young people (including myself) into medicine until perhaps the 1970s, when the motives of doctors began to seem less altruistic and the original ideals of the National Health Service began to fade. Much of this earlier type of medical history was written by eminent medical specialists, often recently retired, who wrote of the slow unfolding of knowledge in their specialty up to the state of near perfection (acknowledging a few problems still to solve) in which they themselves worked. There is some truth in this approach because scientific knowledge does advance with time and has done so for hundreds of years, even though many social and moral conditions always go with apparent discoveries, and morals and standards of behaviour do not 'advance' but remain unchanged or merely wax and wane. Rather like the 'Kings and Battles' approach to general history, the 'whiggish' way of looking at medical history leaves out an enormous amount, including, for instance, the general state of health and disease among a people (often unaffected by doctors and of little or no interest to them), the actual part played by doctors and how their patients felt about their symptoms and treatment. It also omits the mistakes of 'science' and fashion, and the enormous influence that power politics has had both within the profession and outside, particularly since medicine has been organised, with 'official' institutions such as the Royal Colleges, the British Medical Association, the General Medical Council and so on. Also, most traditional histories of medicine ignore the contributions that women have made, even outstanding contributions. Many histories mention no women except for monarchs, writers and perhaps an occasional patient.

Ideas such as these were built into Britain's National Health Service and had much influence. It was widely believed that once the 'backlog' of disease was dealt with through the treatment of those who had hitherto been unable to afford treatment, disease and the need for treatment would decline, and with it the cost of the National Health Service. This was seen as bringing practice into line with what was known. Both doctors and lay people believed that the major diseases, chiefly infections, were now conquered and that it was only a question of time before the remaining important diseases, for example cancer and congenital abnormalities, were also conquered through similar discoveries. Since popular beliefs about health and disease are often the official medical beliefs of a former generation, many people still think in terms of 'finding the cause' of cancer. Doctors and scientists

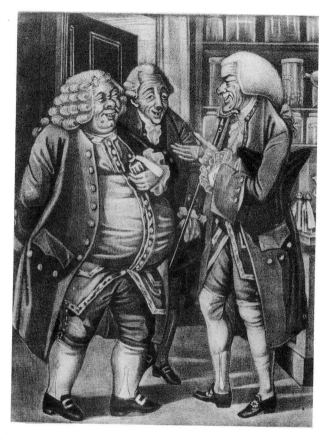

SCENE IN APOTHECARY'S SHOP

no longer think in those terms because in our time this relic of the nineteenth century has become a misleading and expensive fallacy.

In earlier times doctors had been scorned and ridiculed, as we can still see in contemporary cartoons. In the mid-twentieth century they were widely represented as dedicated to science and humanity, though many clearly were not so dedicated. It is true of some individual doctors, but it would be difficult to show that the profession as a whole has ever acted primarily in the interests of its patients or that the institutions that govern the medical profession are concerned with anyone except themselves and their members. As disillusion developed about various health services in different countries, including the National Health Service in England and private medicine in the United States of America, scepticism also grew about the claims, functions and practices of doctors. Social and economic historians, and also

'Marxist' and feminist historians, began to turn their attention to medical history and some became downright hostile. During the last two decades historians have asked questions that were not asked before and these sometimes reveal medicine and its history in a new light, bringing not only a different kind of understanding, but also a realisation of how much more work there is to do.

The new medical history has opened up many possibilities, but some of it tends to suffer because it is written by those who are basically hostile to doctors or by those who lack firsthand experience of disease and of treating patients. Georg Groddeck, a prominent disciple of Freud and famous for his discovery of the 'Id', rose in exasperation at a meeting of psychoanalysts, most of them lay analysts, who were earnestly discussing the 'anal stage' of child development. Groddeck asked ferociously, 'How many of you have even *seen* an anus?' Some of the earnest descriptions and discussions of movements and events in the history of medicine give me the same feeling. Sometimes, when I read not only the hagiography of self-satisfied doctors or the sober accounts of traditional, serious historians, I feel like asking, 'Have you any idea how these women patients felt or what they experienced?' When I read the accounts, often very good in their way, written by 'feminist' and 'new social' historians of nineteenth-century medical practice, I want to ask, 'Do you *really* think that medicine and doctors exist *only* in order to exploit their patients and gain power over them?'

But this new generation of social and feminist historians has started to reveal many aspects of history from a different point of view. This has extended to medical history but so far in only limited ways. Much of what has been written is excellent and thought-provoking, but some of it is conspiratorial and confines itself to the theme of 'how men exploited women'. Too much of it is inaccurate through lack of medical knowledge. For instance, feminist writers often confuse surgical operations which are dubious or exploitive with those which are life-saving, and write as though there was no distinction between the two, sometimes even assuming that both were simply the result of the sadistic desire of men to control women.

Strong views have been expressed that women were oppressed by the rising medical profession and that doctors played, and still play, an important part in the control of women and their relegation to a role confined to homemaking and reproduction. The nineteenth century was an age of social mobility and considerable anxiety. Some of the anxiety was discharged into keeping women in their 'place'. The result was increasing strain and unhappiness among many women, especially as the century wore on. In America there was evidence that the majority of middle-class women were regarded as ill. Britain was not so different.

Probably there has never been a golden age for women, though many people like to think there was and often place it during the Renaissance or just prior to the Industrial Revolution. All through history the position of the majority of women has been inferior to that of men. But the Enlightenment was not enlightened in its attitudes towards women and in many ways added still further to their problems. Its foremost philosopher, Jean-Jacques Rousseau, stated the general male viewpoint when he wrote

> The whole education of women ought to be relative to men, to please them, to be useful to them, to make themselves loved and honoured by them, to educate them when young, to care for them when grown, to counsel them, to console them, and to make life sweet and agreeable to them – these are the duties of women at all times and what they should be taught from their infancy.

For Alexander Pope, poet of the Enlightenment, 'Most women have no characters at all', and Napoleon Bonaparte, at that time dominating Europe, said that in his opinion 'Nature intended women to be our slaves . . . they are our property; . . . Women are nothing but machines for producing children.'

Nineteenth-century sexual repression was not fully developed until about the middle of the century. But the idea that woman's place is in the home was not invented by the Victorians and the qualities that were demanded of the Victorian woman were not peculiar to that time. Nurturance, intuitive morality, passivity and affection were traditional 'feminine' characteristics. The genteel lady of fashion was becoming the ideal of Anglo-American femininity, and her qualities were gradually assumed to be unalterably rooted in biology. Doctors gave strong support to this belief. By the middle of the century the revolution was complete, though the ideas behind it continued to develop to the point of absurdity later in the century. This was the period which Olive Schreiner* claimed that modern civilisation had robbed woman of her 'ancient domain of productive and social labour'.

The historian Alice Clark studied this problem extensively and became convinced that industrialism impoverished women's lives and

---

* O. Schreiner: *Women and Labour.*

damaged both their moral qualities and their capacity as mothers.*
Even those who have disagreed with this† agreed that it was true in the
professions, particularly the healing professions, which had long been
the sphere of women.

During the late eighteenth and nineteenth centuries the medical
profession became organised as a profession along traditional
masculine lines. This was particularly damaging to women healers and
tended to undermine or exclude traditional 'female' characteristics
from 'official' medicine.

There are many ways in which medicine and its practitioners can
become corrupted and fail to serve its clients. Not least is the tendency
to uphold the established order and to find 'scientific' reasons for
doing so. This tendency is virtually inherent in all regulatory
organisations and, as these increased in numbers and power, it was to
become an important trend during the nineteenth century. As the
profession became more organised and knowledgable, weakness,
bigotry, greed, power-seeking, hypocrisy and corruption in doctors
were increasingly focused on women.

The medical profession developed in a way that was particularly
harmful to women. It usurped their traditional function of the care of
the sick. It changed this function to suit itself, with far-reaching
consequences, both for better and for worse. It used this unique
position much less to improve the health of women than to enhance its
own power. It used, and often grabbed at, women as patients in order
to consolidate and support itself. While doing this it neglected the
health of the poor and the disease-producing conditions in the towns.

Further, some doctors perverted scientific knowledge to their
own ends and added the weight of their 'expertise' to the perversions
of others. Later in the century they reinforced and contributed to the
nineteenth-century idea that the 'normal' state of women was to be
sick or diseased. This was used to oppose women's education and
entry into the medical profession with all the rationalisations it could
muster. As a result, traditional 'feminine' virtues and traits were
widely lost from medical practice. The emphasis was much more on
discovery and control, power and acquisition. Medicine developed
differently from the way in which it might otherwise have done.

Male doctors took great pains to support the belief in 'a woman's
place' and many used their considerable power and influence to ensure

---

* A. Clark: *Working Life of Women in the Seventeenth Century.*
† For example, I. Pinchbeck: *Women Workers and the Industrial Revolution, 1750–1820.*

it. Some of the things they wrote and said, allegedly with the backing of 'science', look remarkable today.

So why *did* men struggle so hard to keep women in their place? And do they still? Why did they distort science to justify their beliefs? Were there others with different views? Did women submit readily and if so, why? How *did* they feel? What were their expectations? What really happened? This book is an exploration of these questions.

# I

# PIONEER DOCTOR

In her remote farmhouse in Kentucky, Mrs Jane Todd Crawford, in peril of her life, could be saved only by an operation which no one had ever survived and which, with few exceptions, had been performed only on the dead. Ephraim McDowell, her surgeon, could visit her only by riding sixty miles across a country without roads.

The year was 1809, still pioneer days in America. The population was scattered, communications were poor and doctors were scarce and ill-trained, if trained at all. The country was still recovering from the Revolutionary War more than thirty years before: Europe was devastated by the Napoleonic wars. Wars give valuable education to surgeons and the need for surgery had greatly increased since the invention of gunpowder in the mid-fourteenth century. Common advice to would-be surgeons was to go to war. At this point, surgery concerned largely the outside of the body and speed was its first essential. All surgeons measured amputation time in seconds. Lisfranc of Paris could amputate the thigh of a corpse in ten seconds. Dominique-Jean Larrey, Napoleon's brilliant army surgeon, recalled the amputations he did during the Battle of Borodino on the route to Moscow in 1812, 'I performed in the first twenty-four hours, about two hundred'.*

Abdominal surgery did not exist in any way that would be recognisable today. Few surgeons even contemplated operating internally: it was far too dangerous. By the beginning of the nineteenth century much was known about surgical technique, especially in the great medical centres such as Edinburgh and Paris. Surgeons studied anatomy intensively and practised operating on corpses. They knew

---

* This averages one every seven minutes. He said that about seventy-five per cent recovered.

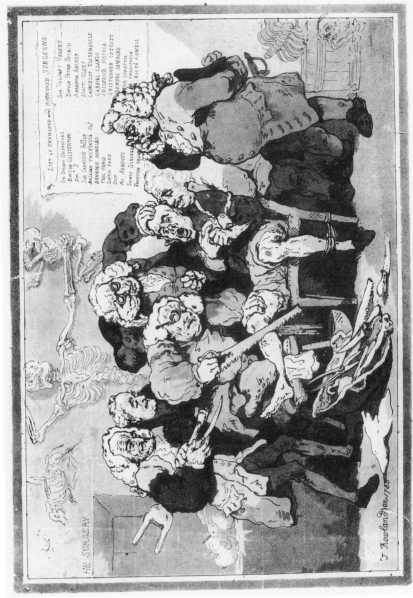

AMPUTATION

what procedures were needed to relieve longterm pain and suffering in certain conditions, though few dared to carry them out. Without anaesthetics, knowledge of germs or efficient methods of stopping bleeding, surgery was hazardous and nearly always complicated by shock, serious bleeding or infection. To do a big operation on a living person required a pioneer spirit, courage and an independence of mind in both doctor and patient that was more likely to be found in the backwoods than in a large medical centre. Even if a surgeon in a teaching centre possessed these qualities, he was likely to be inhibited by opinion and surveillance from those around him, and also by a hospital rule that no serious operation was to be undertaken without the sanction of the honorary medical staff after a general consultation. Even if such a rule had not actually been formulated, it was likely to exist unspoken. This was not surprising, since surgery had a high mortality-rate, sometimes a hundred per cent. Life was not easy for the surgeon-pioneer.

A surgical operation is an ordeal today but in those days it was immeasurably worse, excruciating for the patient and distressing for those who watched and often also for those who performed it. Few enjoyed their work, even when they were deeply involved in it. When he was young, James Simpson, who later became one of the greatest of surgeons and who introduced anaesthesia for childbirth, was so upset when, as a medical student, he saw his first operation that he rushed out of the building and tried to enrol as a law student. Yet he must already have been accustomed to pain and the sight of others enduring it in a way that no young student is today. It is difficult for us to envisage the suffering of our forbears. Pain and disability existed on a scale far beyond our experience. Until the late nineteenth century, in every household at any one time, there was likely to be at least one person in severe pain, even if this was only from toothache, from which, in that era without preventive dentistry, people were liable to suffer frequently until the last tooth had been pulled (without an anaesthetic, of course).

Until the middle of the nineteenth century, there were no anaesthetics and no antenatal care. Childbirth was often excessively painful, lengthy and obstructed. It was impossible to repair its longterm complications or to put right an internal catastrophe. Since there was no knowledge of germs, an operation wound nearly always became infected. The agent of infection was often the doctor, who was likely also to be working with infectious patients or in the post-mortem room. A serious fracture or infection in a limb was likely to be treated by immediate amputation, done with varied skill and probably in only a few seconds to minimise the shock of such a procedure on a conscious person. There was virtually no means of easing trouble in one of the great cavities of the body – abdomen, chest or cranium – because it was too dangerous to open them. A catastrophe in one of them proceeded inexorably to its natural conclusion, which was usually death. A woman with a complicated pregnancy or a serious gynaecological disorder was likely to have a very tough time indeed, with a high risk of losing not only her baby but also her life. In the American Civil War almost all abdominal and head wounds proved fatal.

Did people in the past feel pain less? This seems unlikely but they were certainly more used to it, made less fuss about it and regarded it as inevitable.

Pain is one of the medical mysteries of this period. There was so much of it, with so little relief. It was all around and of great concern to many, but no one seems to have applied his mind to the problem: no one seems to have realised that a general and relatively simple solution might be available. Yet anaesthetics had already been discovered. Instead of being used in the way that now seems obvious and which might have been equally obvious then, it was to be another forty to fifty years before they were used in surgery. Why?

Joseph Priestley had discovered nitrous oxide or 'laughing gas' in 1770. In 1800 Humphry Davy published a large monograph on the subject. He had tested it on both animals and humans and had himself breathed it several times a day for several months. He described its exhilarating, hysterical, laughter-producing effects and even suggested that it might be used to control pain in surgery. In 1818 Faraday made a similar discovery with ether. So why the delay? Anaesthesia, like many new scientific concepts, was an idea before its time. When that time came, in the middle of the nineteenth century, it was used widely and rapidly. Few scientific discoveries have been so readily accepted.

Some historians and others have suggested that the delay occurred because the patients didn't need any relief from their pain and that a change took place in the middle of the century, when sensitivity to pain increased. Silas Weir Mitchell, the famous nineteenth-century doctor, associated this apparent change with the disappearance of official torture and the rack at the end of the eighteenth century. 'Civilised man has of will ceased to torture, but in our process of being civilised we have won, I suspect, intensified capacity to suffer. The savage does not feel pain as we do: nor as we examine the descending scale of life do animals seem to have the acuteness of pain-sense at which we have arrived.'* Women, like 'savages' were regarded as being lower in the evolutionary scale than men, so presumably it was thought that they also felt pain less acutely. Most of Weir Mitchell's patients were women.

It seems more likely that if sensitivity to pain increased, as it appeared to, it was the *result* of anaesthesia and the realisation that pain was not inevitable. Before the time of anaesthesia, pain seemed to be inevitable and both surgeons and patients agreed about it. Samuel Johnson saw physical pain as part of 'the pain of being a man', but, although he suffered from many physical diseases, including bronchitis, asthma, dropsy, and later stroke, he regarded the mental pain of his fits of depression as infinitely worse and vouched he would rather have a limb amputated if it would heal his stricken understanding.

Others were terrified of pain. Lady Holland described how she 'prayed for death . . . a spasm terrifies me, and every moment of the fragile tenure of my bliss strikes a panic through my frame'.† An old patient of Sir James Simpson recalled the pain of an amputation in pre-anaesthetic days.

> Of the agony it occasioned I will say nothing. Suffering so great as I underwent cannot be expressed in words, and thus fortunately cannot be recorded. The particular pangs are now forgotten; but the black whirlwind of emotion, the horror of great darkness, and the sense of desertion by God and man, bordering close to despair, which swept through my mind and overwhelmed my heart, I can never forget, however gladly I would do so.§

Things had not changed since Defoe wrote in his *Journal of the Plague Year*, about victims 'unable to contain themselves, [who] vented their pain by incessant roarings, and such loud and lamentable cries were to be heard as we walked along the streets . . .'

The relief of pain has always been a preoccupation of doctors. Hippocrates in *Epidemics* recognised that pain is a personal experience, coloured by many things – 'How must one value pain? Look at fear, patience, timidity.' Eighteenth-century surgeons were strongly aware of pain and tried to ease it with wine, medicine and comfort. There are many indications that pain was the great preoccupation and patients wanted relief from it above all else. Surgeons regarded pain as inevitable but tried to avoid as much as possible by working fast, often

* Silas Weir Mitchell: 'Civilization and Pain', *JAMA*, 18, 1892, p. 108.
† Ilchester (ed.): *Lady Holland's Journal.*
§ V. Robinson: *Victory over Pain: A History of Anaesthesia.*

doing the operation in seconds. They did few major operations and dealt mostly with leg ulcers, infections and accidents. Despite the pain, there is evidence that some people were keen to have operations and other treatment. It was coming to be realised that for most conditions surgeons were more effective than physicians. John Brown, when working as an assistant surgeon in Chatham in 1830, wrote to his father about the long queues of waiting patients.* He said that there were twenty-five surgeons in the town which, although it was a naval base with a dockyard, was small. He said that all these surgeons were 'well-employed' and in fact 'the people have as ravenous an appetite for and can as little do without medicine as without bacon or beer'. He was working for a surgeon-apothecary and was referring here to the drugs side of the practice, but he also describes the considerable amount of minor surgery that they did, particularly for leg ulcers, infections and accidents.

Many patients seem to have been remarkably compliant, perhaps knowing and dreading the fate that awaited them if they did not submit to operation. Some may have been unusually docile. Some certainly begged for more. One of these was Mrs Driver, whose breast was removed by Richard Kay because of cancer.† A new cancer had appeared under the old wound. This was a common complication and was dangerous because it meant that the growth had not been arrested. She returned to the surgeon, 'being determined to undergo a second amputation'. Kay examined her and found growths around 'six or seven inches square'. He notes, 'I took off the Skin ... I dissected from her ... five hundred different distinct Schirrous Knots or young Cancers.'

It is not surprising that the patient was 'sick and very poorly after the Operation'. But next day Kay notes, 'I left Mrs Driver pretty easy'. But if she really had five hundred new cancers, her 'ease', and indeed her life, cannot have lasted long.

A special study of pain§ has suggested that pain and the inability to function was the starting-point of the notion of ill-health. Submission to surgery was, in the authors' view, not the result of ignorance or docility but came 'out of a rational calculus of pain'.

There was resistance to the idea of relieving pain. This was largely moral and religious and reached its peak later in the century over the question of the relief of pain in childbirth. There was a sense of inevitability that moralists found comforting. The idea of the ubiquity

* *Letters of John Brown.*
† Brockband & Kenworthy, eds.: *Diary of Richard Kay*, (1716–51), p. 142–3.
§ R. & O. Porter: *In Sickness and in Health.*

of sickness, death and woe had been prevalent for many centuries and was reinforced by Christian ideas of original sin. 'Put all the miseries that man is subject to together,' wrote John Donne *'sicknesse* is more than all . . .' Moreover, people were accustomed to witnessing other people's pain and suffering as well as experiencing their own. For instance, crowds flocked to public executions and clearly regarded this as a normal thing to do. 'A very great press of people,' wrote Pepys of the execution of Sir Henry Vane in 1662, 'the Scaffold was so crowded that we could not see it done.' There was also a great deal of open and public interest in other people's illnesses, which were freely discussed and described.

These were some of the reasons why, in the early days of 'scientific' medicine, medical advances, and particularly advances in surgery, were likely to come from unusual individuals working under difficult conditions. A comparable situation today is found in doctors and medical students working in places in the Third World that lack medical resources and specialists. Desperate situations lead to desperate remedies and these doctors often do things and perform operations which they have never done before and would certainly not undertake under normal western conditions. As a result they gain greatly in experience and sometimes make original observations and discoveries. They may or may not save the patients who would otherwise certainly have died.

The practice of surgery, especially gynaecological surgery, was ready for huge advances, although it was still crude and distressing. 'Scientific' medicine had been greatly encouraged during the eighteenth century, when the spirit of the Enlightenment promoted inductive thinking and the rejection of, or at least a change in, superstition. But the progress of scientific medicine was hampered by the inability to solve certain basic problems. Today, most medical advances are made by specialised teams working in big centres. Early in the nineteenth century, 'research' was not organised in this way and virtually everything that was discovered came, as some still does, from simple observation or individual action.

The subject of women's diseases was not a separate specialty. It was part of general surgery or else was dealt with by physicians. The few gynaecological procedures and operations that were performed were done by surgeons who were also involved in such matters as sewing up wounds, setting bones and amputating limbs.

The major operations that led to gynaecology becoming a specialty in its own right were also those from which modern surgery developed. Before this, surgery was largely external, so much so that the early surgeons were also the skin specialists. Few, if any, dared to open an abdomen, chest or skull, even though they knew a good deal about them and what needed to be done when trouble arose in them. Even half a century later it was just as hazardous. They also knew that if surgery was to advance, these forbidden cavities would have to be explored and conquered and that the conditions most available to exploration were gynaecological.

Many of the early surgical pioneers came from the American South between the Revolutionary and the Civil wars. The South was less populated and less regulated than the North, yet was in touch with the rest of the world. There were also slaves there. Many of the early operations, or 'experiments' were carried out on slaves whose gynaecological condition had made them unsuitable for work on the plantations and whose owners therefore lent them willingly to the surgeons to be 'repaired'.

Apart from the doctors' desire to explore and to learn new skills and slave owners' realism, materialism and greed, what feelings and motives lay behind these early operations which were so important in the development of surgery? Firstly, many slave patients were keen to cooperate and were delighted when the operations succeeded. The need for some of their operations can be traced back to the appalling conditions in which many slaves had to live and give birth. These conditions sometimes led to longterm complications so horrible that they could be remedied, if at all, only by these heroic new gynaecological operations. Secondly, the existence of slaves may have meant that some doctors operated on them more freely than they would on whites. Also, the harsh conditions under which most people, even free people, lived, may have helped to create a climate of opinion even among prosperous whites which influenced them towards submitting themselves to surgery. Certainly some of the early gynaecological patients were not poor and some of the early experiments were done on women who came from distinguished families in the South. Jane Todd Crawford was a cousin of Mrs Abraham Lincoln, though in 1809 that was in the future. Early in that year, at Hodgenville, only thirty-five miles from the Crawford farm, Abraham Lincoln himself had been born in a log cabin similar to the Crawfords'.

In 1809 Jane Todd Crawford, forty-seven years old and the mother of four living children, was apparently pregnant and her child overdue.

Her belly was swollen. One day in December she began to have pains but labour did not start. Two doctors saw her but it is unlikely that they gave her an internal examination and in fact quite likely that they did not examine her physically at all. Traditionally, doctors listened to the patient, who was then helped to enlarge on the description of symptoms. The doctors would then look at the tongue and skin, and perhaps the urine and faeces, and then pass judgment, often referring back to authority. In Jane Crawford's case they decided that there were complications and that the delivery would be too difficult for them to manage. They sent for Ephraim McDowell who lived sixty miles away in Danville and was well known as the best surgeon in the area. He rode sixty miles to see her as had, presumably, the person who bore the message from her doctors asking him to come. With such communications, consulting a specialist was often a formidable task.

In the United States in the early nineteenth century there were few formally trained physicians and few schools of medicine. The general public, so soon after the Revolutionary War, was hostile to 'professionalism' and 'foreign elitism' and the system of training doctors in America was even more rudimentary than it was in Britain. In America, anyone who wished could practise the art of healing. There was, however, an increasing number of doctors who had been formally trained. They asserted, often incorrectly, that they were more skilled than lay practitioners, and they tended to treat the middle classes. But there was no real medical science at the time. Their methods consisted largely of bleeding, purging, poisoning with mercury and, later, easing pain and distress with opium. The nineteenth-century philosopher, physician and author Oliver Wendell Holmes, once remarked that if all the medicines used by 'regular' doctors in the United States were thrown into the ocean it would be so much better for mankind and so much worse for the fishes, an opinion shared by some people today. But there were already a number of skilled surgeons and, despite their crude methods and lack of knowledge about certain essentials, they knew that there were many conditions which physicians could neither cure nor improve but which surgeons, at least in theory, knew how to alleviate.


Ephraim McDowell's ancestors came from Argyle in Scotland and emigrated to Northern Ireland during Cromwell's protectorate. An ancestor, another Ephraim, fought with the Covenantors and then emigrated to Pennsylvania. Ephraim was born in 1772 in Rockbridge county, Virginia, the sixth son in a family of eleven. When he was quite small the family moved to Danville, Kentucky. He received only rudimentary education, perhaps because the Revolutionary War broke out when he was three years old. At the age of nineteen he was apprenticed to Dr Alexander Humphreys at Staunton, Virginia. We know little about McDowell's apprenticeship, apart from a confused story concerning a brush with the law over the corpse of a black person that was being used for dissection.

Apprenticeship of this sort was the usual means of becoming a doctor, particularly a surgeon. It had begun in England soon after the Norman Conquest as a form of technical training. It spread from London, and became the basis of the system in America. Its nature and history are well documented because it was illegal to practise a trade or craft (including that of surgeon-apothecary) without a certificate of apprenticeship. Apprentices usually started at the age of fourteen.* The system had advantages and disadvantages. For example, there was no control over any doctor who wished to take apprentices and choice was largely selection by parents. What the apprentice actually did varied according to the wishes of the master. As with apprenticeships in other trades, the young doctor usually lived in the house of his master for several years, followed him as he did his work, was taught how to do it himself, and increasingly assisted with it. Sometimes he was vital to the running of the practice. Sometimes his 'training' included moral training. Sometimes, at least in a big city such as London or Edinburgh, he would then attend private lectures in medical subjects and perhaps 'walk the wards' of the local teaching hospital. Sometimes he set up in business on the strength only of his apprenticeship.

The distinguished nineteenth-century surgeon Sir James Paget was an apprentice from 1830. He thought the system was dull and lengthy but that through it he had, by being left to himself for much of the time, acquired an unusual disposition for scientific pursuits. A few years later†, an apprentice wrote that 'the period of apprenticeship is passed in menial servitude instead of obtaining professional knowledge'. In *Middlemarch*, George Eliot referred to it as 'that initiation in makeshift'. When John Keats was apprenticed to Thomas Hammond, a surgeon-apothecary of good repute in Edmonton, he was expected to sweep the surgery, light the fire and help the groom.§

In 1793, aged twenty-one, McDowell crossed the Atlantic. In

* J. Lane: 'The Role of Apprenticeship in Eighteenth-Century Medical Education in England', in W.F. Bynum & R. Porter: *William Hunter and the Eighteenth-Century Medical World*; I.S.L. Loudon: *Medical Care and the General Practitioner*.
† *British Medical Journal*, 3 July, 1847.
§ Newman: p. 24. See also Robert Gittings: *John Keats*, 1968.

Edinburgh, perhaps the most advanced medical centre in the world, he registered for medical classes and remained there for two years, the standard length of time for a medical student to study. He probably did not take a degree but he heard discussions and learned many things that he could never have learned in America, or elsewhere in Britain. These included dreaming into the future and discussing techniques that might be used for operating on ovaries and other diseased women's organs. There were many discussions about the possibility of doing various operations that were clearly needed but which were dangerous.

The teacher who most impressed him and influenced his ideas was John Bell, whom many idolised.*

John Bell, a native of Edinburgh, was the leading British anatomist of the period. Despite the difficulty in obtaining corpses for dissection at that time, he had managed to become a gifted and accomplished surgeon. Then, as now, dissection of the dead was regarded as the basis of surgery. Since the time of Henry VIII in the sixteenth century the only bodies legally available for dissection were those of criminals who had been hanged. Using the bodies of executed criminals in this way was regarded as a form of *post-mortem* punishment. Even these were difficult to obtain, partly because of resistance by criminals' relatives and partly because of corruption among those who dealt with them. There was bodysnatching long before Ephraim McDowell arrived in Edinburgh. In 1711 the Edinburgh College of Surgeons recorded that 'of late there has been a violation of sepulchres in the Grey Friars Churchyard'. Ten years later Edinburgh apprentices had a clause put into their contracts that they were not to violate graves. Meanwhile, the Barber-Surgeons Company in London, who controlled the surgeons, was fining its members for conducting dissections in their own homes and was bribing execution-ers and their assistants to let it have bodies. The hangman even received a Christmas box from the Company each year while the friends of executed criminals did everything they could to stop the bodies from going to the anatomists. The disinterred body of the hanged highwayman Dick Turpin was found in a surgeon's garden. The great William Harvey had even dissected his own father and sister.

The shortage of bodies affected the training of doctors, as it has at several periods since. For example, the establishment of the 'welfare state' in Britain after World War II led to a shortage of bodies for

---

* Gross: *Lives*, (n.1), p. 209–10.

dissection and they had to be imported for the purpose. As a student, Bell had complained, 'In Dr Monro's class, unless there be a fortunate succession of bloody murders, not three subjects were dissected a year'. Nevertheless, at the age of twenty-three Bell was appointed a fellow of the Royal College of Surgeons of Edinburgh and surgeon to the Edinburgh Royal Infirmary. For ten years he taught anatomy and surgery at the Extra-mural School in Surgeon's Square and it was there that he taught Ephraim McDowell. A few years later his younger brother Charles began to publish his famous textbook but at the time when McDowell was a student in Edinburgh textbooks were scarce and the theory of surgery was usually learned in a single course of lectures, mostly given in the evening and paid for by students's fees. McDowell learned run-of-the-mill surgery, tumour removal, treatment of wounds, amputation and something of the new blood-vessel surgery.

In the eighteenth and early nineteenth century, medical education was private. There was no public or state provision of instruction. The surgeons who ran the schools had to find their own corpses. During the eighteenth century there was growing interest in anatomy and increasing demand from the public for good doctoring. The combination increased the black market in corpses. Anatomists bought them from graverobbers and then sold them, dismembered, to students, at a profit. Every buried corpse was at risk. Charles Bell is known to have received bodies from bodysnatchers.*

By the late eighteenth century, London's underworld had realised that money could be made from graverobbing and the crime became professional. There was also hypocrisy among the authorities. When graverobbers were caught, they were usually given light sentences. This was because the government needed surgeons for its armies. A surgeon or student caught with a stolen corpse would be fined five pounds.†

There was immense public opposition to graverobbing. It affected many people's strongest feelings. People cared deeply about the remains of their loved ones, as they still do. Public hostility was directed more against the bodysnatchers than against the surgeons. The medical profession had long been demanding reform. It was not until the late 1820s that officialdom began to take an interest. A select committee was appointed and recommended change several months before the famous Burke and Hare 'bodysnatcher' murders came to light. In 1832 the Anatomy Act was passed and is still the basis of British law in this sphere. It allowed the use of bodies of paupers who

---

* For more on this subject see R. Richardson: *Death, Dissection and the Destitute*.
† More on this subject can be found in Harvey Graham: *Surgeons All*.

were too poor to pay for their funerals. What had long been a feared and hated punishment for murder became a punishment for poverty.

One of the skills that was most needed and that some surgeons were eager to practise was that of opening the abdomen, repairing damage or abnormality there, and closing it without the patient dying of shock, haemorrhage or, some days later, infection. The abdomen seemed more accessible than the other cavitities of the body, the chest and skull, but it was strictly forbidden to operate on it in any medical centre. In Edinburgh, students were solemnly warned that the abdomen was forbidden territory. Throughout medical history, as elsewhere, taboos and prohibitions have been strongest when they were soon to be broken. There had been some experiments, mostly with Caesarian section, but the mortality-rate had been close to one hundred per cent. These operations were especially dangerous when the surgeon had to cut through the peritoneum, as he would mostly have to do. The peritoneum is the large sheet of membrane that lies in folds inside the abdomen and covers most of the internal organs, enabling them to slide freely over and across each other. The peritoneum still engages the respect of surgeons today, and the way it is handled is still controversial. In the early nineteenth century it was a formidable obstacle.

Nevertheless, there was already speculation about operating on ovarian cysts. One of the subjects Bell was in the habit of discussing with his students and colleagues was the possibility and apparent impossibility of removing large cysts that were disabling the patients. He realised that the future of surgery lay with this operation and that the first successful abdominal operation was likely to be for removal of a large ovarian cyst, but he did not dare to do it himself.

The use of words in this subject can be confusing. A cyst is usually a lump or mass containing fluid. 'Ovarian cyst' is a term that is still used today, even when the lump is solid. McDowell used the long-established term 'ovarian dropsy'. 'Dropsy' is an old medical term for accumulation of fluid, used most commonly for generalised 'oedema' or swelling of the tissues, particularly in certain forms of heart failure. The term 'ovarian cyst' was first used by Isaac Baker Brown in 1850.

The ovaries produce the female ova or eggs and correspond to the male testes, which produce spermatazoa. Although ovulation was not discovered until 1831, and even then was not properly understood, much was already known about ovarian cysts and, in theory, how they might be dealt with. The testes descend from the abdomen during foetal life along the inguinal canal in the groin and into the scrotum. The ovaries remain inside the abdomen and sometimes develop cysts or collections of fluid or other tissue. Few of these are cancerous or dangerous in themselves but they tend to increase in size and are unaffected by purely medical (ie non-surgical) treatment by diet, drugs, manipulation, or any other traditional methods. Even tapping the cyst and withdrawing the fluid through a hollow needle was seldom satisfactory. The fluid nearly always collected again and the procedure had to be repeated, often many times, and at some risk, for sometimes the patient died.

Some years earlier the famous eighteenth-century surgeon John Hunter, also an Edinburgh man, had written, with the typical attitude of his age and many others, that he could see no reason why a woman should not suffer spaying safely, as did other animals. But his brother William said of ovarian dropsy that 'the patient will have the best chance of living under it who does the least to get rid of it'. He was, however, the first to suggest that large cysts should in theory be removed.

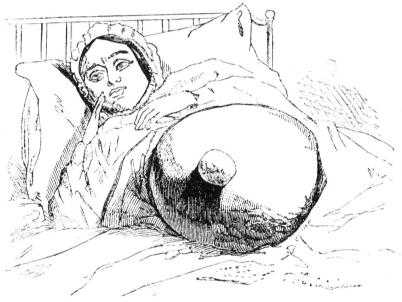

A FORTY-THREE YEAR OLD WOMAN, NOT PREGNANT, BUT WITH A LARGE OVARIAN CYST

Some of the cysts reached an enormous size and big ones were debilitating. Some were so large that the sufferer could hardly move at all. Some of them weighed more than the patient herself. Old textbooks contain amazing drawings of women anchored to their beds by these huge tumours. They grew in otherwise healthy women and often ruined their lives by continuing to collect fluid and growing to a huge size. One cyst on record weighed 149 pounds. Another, repeatedly tapped, produced over 6000 gallons of fluid. Some of these cysts were doubtless malignant, infiltrating surrounding tissues and spreading their own tissues to other parts of the body: many were certainly benign in that they did not function in this way but these could grow to an enormous size and be very disabling. In the distant past there had been a few cases of surgical removal of the ovaries, mostly under rather odd circumstances and of doubtful authenticity. One that is often repeated is that of the sow-gelder in seventeenth-century Holland who was said to have cut out both his daughter's ovaries in order to keep her in at night. We do not know whether or not this story is true.

Ephraim McDowell returned to Kentucky with increased knowledge and skills. His ability in diagnosis was far superior to that of the two physicians who had sent for him. He examined Mrs Crawford for her 'difficult labour' and found that she wasn't even pregnant. He wrote later in the *Eclectic Repertory and Analytical Review*, for October 1816, 'The abdomen was considerably enlarged, and had the appearance of a pregnancy', but the huge swelling was due to an enormously enlarged ovary. He could move the tumour easily from one side to the other, which suggested that it was not malignant but he knew that there was no way he could help her except by trying to remove it. Left alone, it was likely to ruin her life or even kill her.

One can only guess his thoughts. In Edinburgh he had learned so much about this condition and had heard so many discussions about how to relieve it. He had also been taught that it was too dangerous to attempt. But here was the desperate situation that might lead to the desperate remedy. In his own words, 'I gave to the unhappy woman information of her dangerous situation. She appeared willing to undergo an experiment.'

It was probably lucky for her that no hospital was available, but McDowell was not prepared to operate in her house. He told her he would do the operation only if she came to visit him in Danville. The journey appeared to him to be 'almost impracticable by any, even the most favourable, conveyance'. There wasn't even a road. He didn't think she would be able to get there.

He must have been surprised when, a few days later, Mrs Crawford arrived at his house. She had left her youngest son Tommy, six years old, with relatives and had ridden all the way on horseback, cross-country, having forded several rivers on the way, and supporting her large tumour on the horn of her saddle. She must have wanted the operation very much, and indeed have been a redoubtable and courageous woman, prepared to gamble a miserable and probably shortened life for one that was longer and healthier, at the risk of losing both. She would have known that she would have to endure severe pain and must have decided that it was worth it.

McDowell operated in his own house, aided by his assistant and nephew, James McDowell MD. He normally did his operations on Sundays because he was then not so busy with his other patients, but this was Christmas Day. They laid Jane Crawford on a table: a famous mural of the occasion depicts a homely room with a chest of drawers, an open fire, surgical instruments on a wooden pedestal table and a bed behind curtains in the wall. In addition to the McDowells, two other men are in attendance and a black woman stands in the doorway.

Mrs Crawford's operation lasted for twenty-five minutes. She recited the Psalms throughout. McDowell wrote later that her tumour was 'so large that we could not take it away entire . . . We took out fifteen pounds of a dirty gelatinous substance after which we cut through the Fallopian tube and extracted the sack, which weighed seven pounds and one half . . . .' Some years later he described the 'cherry bounce' that he gave the patients on whom he operated. It contained both opium, in the form of laudanum, a preparation of opium and alcohol, still sometimes prescribed, and extra alcohol. He did not say so, but it seems likely that he gave such a concoction to Mrs Crawford.

When the operation was over the doctors applied dressings, put her to bed, and prescribed the usual antiphlogistic regimen of soothing and cooling substances applied to and round the wound.

Mrs Crawford made an uninterrupted recovery. On the fifth day after the operation, McDowell found her on her feet and making her bed. He gave her 'particular caution for the future'. In twenty-five days, she rode home 'in good health which she continued to enjoy'. She lived for over thirty years more.

Ephraim McDowell had done what would today be called a salpingo-oöphorectomy, removing both ovaries and Fallopian tubes. Like his contemporaries, he referred to the operation as 'Extirpation of the Ovaries'. Later in the century it became known as 'ovariotomy' and became one of the famous and classical operations that were to play an important part in surgeons's – and in women's – lives, in ways undreamed of by Ephraim McDowell.

McDowell had to endure harsh criticism. One story is of doubtful authenticity but demonstrates something of the mood of the time. It is said that while McDowell was operating on Mrs Crawford the house was surrounded by a hostile crowd of doctors and others who were ready to lynch him if Jane Crawford died.

McDowell didn't record the case for seven years and then, at the insistence of his friends, in 1816 he wrote it up. This delay was not as unusual at that time as it would be today, when 'writing up' and publishing papers are regarded as all-important and doctors' careers depend upon them. McDowell was then criticised for lack of detail and some people refused to believe that he had done the operation at all.

In Britain James Johnson, editor of the *Medico-Chirurgical Review*, was sceptical and said so angrily in print in 1825. After a major operation today a patient is usually out of bed and active after only a few hours, but this would have seemed almost unbelievable to medical experts of the day. They would have found it incredible that an abdomen could be opened without inevitable subsequent infection, including peritonitis and 'hospital fever'. Doubtless circumstances favoured Mrs Crawford's recovery. Her operation took place in a private house in a small country town, far from the dangerous infections that lurk in hospitals even to this day. Having avoided the very real dangers of an operation under these circumstances, she escaped the almost universal danger of serious infection and so her convalescence was not interrupted by illness and debilitation.

Part of Dr Johnson's criticism and disbelief came from his idea that McDowell had not visited his patient until the fifth day after the operation, but this was probably a misunderstanding due to the way in which McDowell had described the case. He mentioned visiting her only on the fifth day, but since the patient was in his own house and it was an experimental operation, it seems unlikely that this was his first sight of her after the operation.

A few years later Dr James Johnson apologised publicly to McDowell for his disbelief. He acknowledged his error and asked 'pardon of God and of Dr. MacDowel [sic] of Danville' for his mistrust.

Three years later McDowell replied to his critics in a second article.*
As with many good doctors, writing for publication clearly had low

* Ephraim McDowell: 'Three Cases of Extirpation of Diseased Ovaria,' *Eclet. Repert.*, p. 242.

priority for him, though his accounts are vivid. He said, among other things, 'I think my description of the mode of operating, and of the anatomy of the parts concerned, clear enough to enable any good anatomist, possessing the judgment requisite for a surgeon, to operate with safety. I hope no operator of any other description may even attempt it. It is my ardent wish that this operation may remain to the mechanical surgeon forever incomprehensible.' He seemed to regard a good surgeon as a special kind of anatomist, which was the way in which he had been trained.

A famous French surgeon, Auguste Nélaton, in an interview on 10 October 1868, told his colleague F-J. Delstanche that McDowell first tried ovariotomy as an experiment on slaves at the behest of their owners and that ovariotomy was therefore the result of avarice.* No one has been able to verify this story. Nélaton or Delstanche may simply have got it wrong, perhaps in confusion about the black corpse that McDowell seems to have dissected.

McDowell died at the age of fifty-eight, ironically of an abdominal catastrophe. By that time he had done thirteen more ovariotomies: one of his ovariotomy patients was the wife of a general. Only one patient died. This was a far better record than that of most early ovariotomists. Another patient on whom he also operated had, like Mrs Crawford, travelled far to see him. Nineteen-year-old James Polk travelled to Danville, Kentucky, from his home in Columbia, Tennessee, hoping to be relieved by the skill of McDowell. McDowell performed a successful lithotomy for bladder stone, one of the operations in which he was skilled. Some years later Polk became president of the United States. So much for the myth that the early surgeons operated only on women and slaves.

The story of Ephraim McDowell and his daring operation is dramatic but its significance has often been overlooked. McDowell was not the first surgeon to do the operation and little was known about his part in the history of ovariotomy until Samuel Gross lionised him in his *Lives of Great American Doctors*. Since then he has been given all the razzmatazz of the 'reconstructive' history that is particularly common in the New World.

* Félix-J. Delstanche: 'Visite à M. le docteur Nélaton,' *J. de Méd., Chir., et Pharmacol.*, Brussels, 48, 1869, p. 318-322, quoted in Wangensteen, *The Rise of Surgery*, p. 643.

Nevertheless, he was a pioneer. His operation was successful. By risking her life, he gave Jane Todd Crawford a new life forty years before anaesthetics became available. He also inaugurated a whole new phase of medical history by showing the path that surgery was to take. One might even say that he heralded the early divorce of gynaecology from surgery. For reasons one can only guess, gynaecology became a specialty in its own right much earlier than other specialties such as orthopaedics and ear, nose and throat. Thus he inaugurated the new treatment of women.

McDowell was a pioneer before his time. Much more influential in the development of gynaecology and even more famous was another American, J. Marion Sims. He first organised gynaecology as a medical specialty. Known widely as the 'father of gynaecology', he devoted his life to developing treatments and institutions for women's diseases.

# II

# EXPERIMENTS ON WOMEN

Views of the famous nineteenth-century American surgeon J. Marion Sims vary from adulation to hatred. Sims is God-like; Sims is the Devil. He pioneered bravely in the cause of women; he experimented on female slaves. He kept slaves in a barn in order to experiment on them; at his own expense he built a new floor on to his hospital to accommodate those patients who could not pay but were in dire need of his services. He operated on at least one slave, Anarcha, more than thirty times without an anaesthetic; he cured her. He invented new operations and procedures which were to benefit and teach all future gynaecological surgeons; he invented procedures for torturing women. He was a woman-hater and disliked all women ardently and gynaecology in particular. He cared for his patients so much that he paid for all their needs, board and lodging as well as treatments, from his own pocket, sometimes for several years. For doing this, he ran into financial difficulty and was criticised by his colleagues and family.

Sims is widely known as the 'father of gynaecology'. Certainly he made the subject a respectable part of the medical profession. His prowess has often been described, yet a book used in many university courses in America states, 'It should not be imagined that poor women were spared the gynaecologist's exotic catalog of tortures simply because they couldn't pay. The pioneer work in gynaecological surgery had been performed by Marion Sims on black female slaves he kept for the sole purpose of surgical experimentation.'* This view is supported by Mary Daly, who writes, 'Sexual surgery became The Man's means of restraining women. J. Marion Sims, known for his hatred and abhorrence of female organs, remedied his problems (becoming very rich in the process) by ruthlessly cutting up women's bodies.'†

* Ehrenreich & English: *For Her Own Good* p. 124–5.
† Mary Daly: *Gyn/ecology*, 1978, p. 225.

The only evidence I could find of this 'hatred and abhorrence of female organs' was Sims's admission, in his autobiography,* that in his early days as a doctor he disliked gynaecology. Most doctors probably did and certainly still do. Many medical students of both sexes tend to find gynaecology the most difficult of all medical subjects to adapt to. There are many reasons why it imposes a strain. This can be partly due to the unaccustomed exposure of female organs, the contact with women so exposed, the sexual connotations and their suppression in the mind, and last but not least, the characteristic smell, which many find unpleasant or disturbing. One might even suspect the motives and fantasies of a student who felt comfortable with gynaecology from the start. However, those who attack Sims for his initial dislike have not usually themselves been exposed to the reality of the subject. Thus the attack continues, 'He began his life's work "humbly", performing dangerous sexual surgery on black female slaves housed in a small building in his yard'. Another frequently quoted book tells us that Sims '. . . garnered diseased black women into his backyard – to provide guinea pigs . . .'.† Sims himself describes it differently, stating simply, 'I went to work to put another storey on my hospital'.

We are also told that Sims:

> rapidly moved up the professional ladder . . . where he charged enormous fees to the rich, Sims used the 'knowledge' gained through the pain and mutilation inflicted on poor patients . . . There were plenty of victims . . . Sims did not differ essentially from his gynaecological colleagues in intent, attitude, or method. He simply was more monomaniacal and ambitious than most men . . . he was an object of adulation . . . the students recognized him as 'one of the immortals' . . . Such men are 'Immortal' in the sense that they pass on death and fear, their only true offspring.§

Such views are found on both sides of the Atlantic. The respectable and interesting work *The Midwife Challenge* by Sheila Kitzinger, published in 1988, states, 'One notable example of a physician who achieved god status as early as the nineteenth century was J. Marion Sims . . . He profited by the system of slavery in his surgical experiments in vaginal repair surgery. This man . . . was able legally to take possession of black women's bodies and to perform surgery on them at his will. He actually bought some of the subjects of

* J. Marion Sims: *The Story of my Life.*
† Barker-Benfield: *Horrors of the Half-Known Life*, p. 103.
§ Ehrenreich & English: *op.cit.*

his experiments. One woman . . . endured thirty sessions of surgery without anaesthesia before Sims was satisfied with the job he had done. Sims became a hero for generations of obstetrician-gynaecologists who followed him, many dreaming of achieving world-wide fame.'

In contrast to these accounts a standard American account of the very same events states, 'It remained for James Marion Sims (1813–83) . . . to change the whole situation "almost with a magic wand" '.*
Another highly regarded history tells us, 'To Marion Sims of America must always belong the credit of first demonstrating that these . . . could be cured.'†

Which of these accounts is true? Suffice it here to point out that, at the end of a long period of research, Sims's work certainly advanced medical knowledge, showed how suffering could be relieved, and led to increased medical power. At the same time, providing ammunition for later critics, Sims refers continually in his autobiography to 'my experiments'.

Surprising as it may seem, these descriptions all relate to the treatment of one gynaecological condition, fistula, which was not uncommon in the days of dangerous childbirth and ignorant obstetrics though it is rare in the western world today. A fistula is an abnormal passage or connection between two organs or between one organ and the outside of the body. The types of fistula that concerned Sims were vesico-vaginal fistula, connecting the vagina and bladder, and recto-vaginal fistula, between the vagina and the rectum. Some patients, including his first successful case, the slave Anarcha, suffered from both.

Fistula is usually caused by difficult or mismanaged childbirth in which the head of the child becomes wedged against the soft tissues and cannot be moved onwards by the mother's exertions in labour. If it rests too long on the soft tissues, the blood supply to those tissues is cut off, gangrene develops, and the tissues that have been deprived of oxygen die. After a few days the dead tissue sloughs off, leaving a hole. The condition is particularly likely to occur in women who have suffered from rickets, since this disease deforms and flattens the pelvis, making the passage of the baby's head difficult or impossible. Rickets is a disease caused by lack of vitamin D, a substance that is found in certain foods and is also synthesised by the body when it is exposed to sunlight. Thus rickets is particularly likely to develop in people who

* Edwin Jameson: *Gynaecology and Obstetrics.*
† J.M. Munro Kerr & M. H. Phillips: *Historical Review of British Obstetrics and Gynaecology*, 1954.

are poorly fed and deprived of sunlight. Black people are particularly vulnerable to it because dark skins absorb light less easily than do white.

A fistula can develop wherever the baby's head presses for too long against the soft tissues of the vagina, whatever the cause. It leads to continual and permanent incontinence. It had long been known to be incurable. A few surgeons had tried to close the hole, or to fill it with some kind of pessary, but the results were poor. Some surgeons acknowledged as well as recognised the tragedy. One nineteenth-century textbook described it as:

> . . . one of the most distressing and intolerable accidents to which females are subject . . . the result is inexpressible distress to the patient. The escape of faeces or urine is attended with so marked and irrepressible an odour, that the patient is placed *hors de société*. Obliged to confine herself to her own room, she finds herself an object of disgust to her dearest friends and even to her attendants. She lives the life of a recluse, without the comforts of it, or even the consolation of it being voluntary. It is scarcely possible to conceive an object more loudly calling for our pity and strenuous exertion, to mitigate, if not remove, the evils of her melancholy condition.'*

An even more graphic account came from a renowned Berlin surgeon, Johann Friedrich Dieffenbach (1792–1847):

> A vesico-vaginal fistula is the greatest misfortune that can happen to a woman, and the more so, because she is condemned to live with it, without the hope to die from it; to submit to all the sequelae of its tortures till she succumbs either to another disease or to old age. There is not a more pitiable condition than that of a woman suffering from a vesico-vaginal fistula. The urine constantly flowing . . . and heated, . . . producing the most intolerable stench. The skin . . . becomes inflamed and covered by a pustulous eruption. An insupportable itching and burning sensation tortures the patient, so much so, that she scratches the skin to bleeding. Many tear the encrusted hair out . . ., calling on death to relieve them from their suffering. The comfort of a clean bed, that grave for all sorrows and afflictions, is not their lot, for it will soon be drenched with urine. Many of the wealthier classes are, therefore, condemned forever to the straw. The air of the room of the unfortunate woman nauseates the visitor, and drives him off. The husband has an aversion from his own wife; a tender mother is exiled from the circle of her own children. She sits, solitary and alone in the cold, on a perforated

* Fleetwood Churchill: 1840, p. 381.

chair. This is not fiction, but naked truth; and the cure for such an evil is the prize for which we all labor.*

This was the life faced by the women who were victims of this horrible condition. Nearly all of them were young, some very young. Anarcha was only seventeen when it happened to her.

Vesico-vaginal fistula had been known for thousands of years. A large one was found in the mummified body of a Nubian woman named Henhenit who was buried near Thebes in about the year 2050 BC. She was about twenty-two years old and had an abnormal pelvis which would have impeded delivery of a baby's head. Before the nineteenth century little was written about the subject, probably because no one knew what to do about it. It was well known that it occurred, but being incurable and horrible, formidable to contemplate and impossible to treat, it was usually ignored. One early twentieth-century surgeon-writer, Howard Kelly, was unable to find any reference to it before the sixteenth century. During the seventeenth century, a Swiss, Johann Fatio had twice operated successfully and in the eighteenth century there were several attempts. Smellie, the famous man-midwife recorded that he was called to two cases in one day.†

Apart from occasional cases due to cancer rather than childbirth, a modern gynaecologist might work for a lifetime without seeing a case. During the first half of the nineteenth century it was quite common and a recognised problem. As the subject of surgery prepared to advance into a new era, James V. Ricci, the distinguished gynaecologist and historian in his field says the profession made 'a determined pain-staking and almost desperate effort to effect a cure'. This took fifty years of experimentation. The misery caused by the condition, its permanence, and the fact that it was not fatal in itself, doubtless meant that there was no shortage of human 'guinea pigs' for these experiments. When people are desperate and their lives made intolerable, they will endure almost anything that offers even remote hope.

All the early operations were done before anaesthetics were discovered, but the women who submitted to them seem to have been undeterred. I have found no record of any who said that the pain of surgery was worse than that of childbirth and several which said it was bad but not as bad as the labours they had experienced. Of course, the condition had usually been caused by a labour that was complicated,

---

* Quoted from M. Schuppert's *A Treatise on Vesico-Vaginal Fistula*, New Orleans, 1966, p. 7.
† Described in Ricci's *One Hundred Years of Gynaecology*, 1800–1900, p. 524.

protracted and obstructed, but there were similar reports from those who endured other operations and whose labours had been easier. On the other hand these reports come mostly from the surgeons themselves who might be thought to have a vested interest in the women's satisfaction.

Some surgeons tried to make the hole smaller and experimented with various sutures, often practising on corpses. Others, such as Desault, tried to fill it with pessaries, some of them fanciful and weird. Among those who operated there was an occasional success, for example William Cumin, surgeon at the Royal Infirmary, Edinburgh, tried an unusual method, by which, Ricci claimed, he cured a fistula which developed in a woman eight days after the birth of her baby. The description of what the unfortunate woman had to endure is appalling. The surgeon tells us:

> The instrument which I employed consisted of an oval steel spring covered with leather, and made so as to clasp around the pelvis and fasten over the sacrum with shape to pass under the thighs, and prevent it from shifting upwards. In the centre, which rested on the symphysis pubis, a piece of metal was screwed on so as to admit between it and the spring, a curved stalk which could be slipped up or down and fixed with a screw when properly adjusted. At the lower extremity of this stalk was an aperture through which a catheter was passed, and introduced into the bladder – then secured in its place by means of narrow tape.

It is impossible to believe that this cumbersome contraption was in any way a cure. Even if it worked, it must have caused enormous discomfort and secondary problems, including infection. Cumin does not say how long he followed up the case.

Other surgeons invented complicated instruments, which sometimes took hours to fix or which caused the death of the patient. Others devised suitable apparatus which would minimise the inconvenience of the constant dribble, for example 'elastic gum bottles'. These were placed in the vagina with pieces of sponge large enough to cover the area of the fistulous opening. At intervals the patient would press the sponge with her fingers and allow the urine to pass into the 'bottle'. Every two hours the patient was catheterised and at night the vaginal urinal was removed. Still others took wax casts of the vagina and made rubber bags of the shape to catch the urine.* One surgeon even published a book of over 400 pages on the treatment of fistula.†

* Colombat d'Isère describes the various methods in his *Diseases of Woman*, American edition, 1850, p. 247.
† A.J. Jobert de Lamballe.

Until Sims did his work, the treatment of fistula was very much a hit-and-miss affair. There were at least six different basic methods of treatment in vogue, a sure sign that no one really knew what to do. Some of the techniques used were not really even feasible, for example obliteration of the vulva and closure of the vagina. Others were more successful, but only occasionally. Eighteen years before Sims, an M. Gosset of London had combined the three essentials for successful operation: the position of the patient, the use of the vaginal speculum and non-irritant wire sutures.\* Little notice had been taken because he had operated on only one case and did not recognise the importance of what he had done. There were a few attempts to operate in America where surgeons tended to be more adventurous than in Europe, but none was notably successful. Sims credited Hayward of Boston with the first repair but it was Sims himself who showed the way, overcame the difficulties in a manner both logical and imaginative, blazed a trail for the whole of future surgery and became, for better or worse, the father figure of gynaecology.

We know a good deal about Sims because he wrote his *The Story of my Life* twenty years before his death and his life is well documented in his later years. He was a native of South Carolina, as any Southerner would know from his name, Marion being a typical South Carolina name in a state where both a county and a lake are so called. As a young man he was not particularly interested in medicine and did not wish to be a doctor. His father wanted him to be a lawyer but this attracted him even less. He describes his father's reaction when he spoke to him. 'Well, I suppose that I cannot control you; but [medicine] is a profession for which I have the utmost contempt. There is no science in it. There is no honour to be achieved in it; no reputation to be made, and to think that MY son should be going round from house to house . . . with a box of pills in one hand and a squirt in the other . . . is a thought that I never supposed I should have to contemplate.'

Nevertheless, the young Sims was apprenticed to Dr Churchill Jones, an eminent local surgeon. In 1833 he entered the Medical College at Charleston, South Carolina, and later studied at Jefferson Medical College in Philadelphia. He wrote later that when he graduated, he felt 'absolutely incompetent to assume the duties of a practitioner'.

---

\* *Lancet*, 1834, 1, p. 346.

His first two patients died and he became disheartened, feeling that he was not made to be a doctor and that he had chosen the wrong profession. When he recovered his interest, he moved to Montgomery, Alabama, and became known as an able surgeon. He tells us unequivocally, 'I was very successful as a surgeon'.* He tells the story of a young woman who came to consult him because she had a hideous hare-lip and was so ugly that she felt obliged to wear a veil, even at home with her family. She begged him to operate and he was reluctant. The year was 1844, before the new advances that surgery needed had occurred. However, she persuaded him – perhaps he was not hard to persuade for, on his own admission, he was quick to use the knife – and in doing so was aware of his extraordinary talent and skill. Proudly he tells us '. . . in the course of a month she was entirely cured . . . she was a very presentable person indeed, and really a pretty woman.' It must have been enormously satisfying for him and the way he describes it suggests that it increased his courage for further experiment.

In 1845 he was called to a girl of seventeen who had been in labour for three days. This was the slave Anarcha. Sims could see the baby's head and that it was pressing against the soft tissues. He knew at the time that there was danger that these damaged tissues might die, but there was nothing he could now do to prevent it. He delivered the baby easily with forceps but three days later there was extensive sloughing, the wall of the vagina broke down and Anarcha lost control of her bladder and rectum. A month later, he saw another case of vesico-vaginal fistula, equally incurable. A few weeks later he was consulted about another. Then yet another. All were incontinent, excoriated, miserable, and begging him to help. Sims was so upset he could not help them that he became seriously interested in the problem, although admitting that, 'If there was anything I hated, it was investigating the organs of the female pelvis.' This is probably the remark that has caused some writers to assume that he was a woman-hater. But it is a common feeling among doctors of both sexes. Gynaecology tends to be messy and smelly. To practise it with interest and pleasure requires training, a certain orientation and also specific equipment. Probably most doctors of both sexes have always had to overcome an initial distaste and reluctance to become involved in it.

Soon after this Sims was called to Mrs Merrill, a middle-aged woman who had fallen from a horse. He found her uterus retroverted, that is, pointing backwards instead of forwards. He had been taught in

---

* Marion Sims: op. cit., p. 210.

medical school that patients with this condition should be examined in the 'knee-elbow position', kneeling on a table and leaning forward onto their elbows. The idea was that the doctor could then manipulate the uterus, replace it in its normal position and relieve the pain.

This is what seems to have happened according to Sims, who described it in some detail. There is some irony in the fact that, although he seems to have relieved Mrs Merrill, the whole procedure would be, by our standards, a waste of time. No one now believes in traumatic retroversion of the uterus. The fifth edition of Tindall's *Jeffcoate's Principles of Gynaecology*, 1987, states categorically, 'Formerly it was suggested that a sudden and violent physical movement could displace the uterus backwards for it to become gripped by the uterosacral ligaments. This is said to produce severe pain in the lower abdomen or back associated with collapse. This syndrome, which in the past was described in young (and wealthy!) nulliparae, is no longer acceptable.' Another well-known textbook, Philipp, Barnes and Newton, *Obstetrics and Gynaecology*, 1986, does not even mention the condition.

However, Sims believed in what he did, he relieved the patient's distress and while performing the manoeuvre he made an important discovery. He realised that in this position the vagina blew up with air and this enabled him to see the whole area and gain an excellent view of any fistula. Suddenly he realised that he could operate on a fistula in a way that might cure it. He became deeply interested in working out how to do it. With enormous enthusiasm he devoted himself to the problem of 'relieving the loveliest of all God's creations of one of the most loathsome maladies that can possibly befall poor human nature . . . Full of sympathy and enthusiasm, thus all at once I found myself running headlong after the very class of sufferers that I had all my professional life most studiously avoided.'*

Sims collected patients on whom to operate and soon had seven young black women, all of them slaves and apparently all longing to be free of their affliction and prepared to suffer for it. He obtained permission from their owners, who all seem to have cooperated. This is not surprising considering that he was offering to keep and treat the patients at his own expense until he had cured them. A slave with a fistula was unlikely to be of much use to her owner. Anarcha had been destined to work in her owner's house after the birth of her baby, but her fistula made that impossible.

He wrote, 'I went to work to put another storey on my hospital

* Marion Sims: op. cit.: Ricci, op.cit., (p. 127) quotes from the Sims Anniversary Discourse given before the New York Academy of Medicine, 1858.

. . . I was very enthusiastic and expected to cure them, every one, in six months. I never dreamed of failure, and could see how accurately and how nicely the operation could be performed.' But he was disappointed. His first attempts were unsuccessful, and he used to lie awake at night wondering how he might improve his techniques. Later he wrote, 'My repeated failures brought about a degree of anguish that I cannot now depict even if it were desirable. All my spare time was given to developing a single idea, the seemingly visionary one of curing this sad affliction.' He refused to operate further until he had solved it, although the patients begged him to 'try only one more time'. He realised he needed to stitch higher up than he could reach. 'This puzzled me sorely. I had been three weeks without performing a single operation. [The patients] were clamourous, and at last the idea occurred to me about three o'clock in the morning. I had been lying awake for an hour, wondering how to tie the suture, when all at once an idea occurred to me to run a shot, a perforated shot, on the suture, and, when it was drawn tight, to compress it with a pair of forceps, which would make the knot perfectly secure. I was so elated with the idea, and so enthusiastic as I lay in bed, that I could not help waking up my kind and sympathetic wife and telling her of the simple and beautiful method I had discovered of tying the suture.'

He tried it on 'Lucy' and it was a 'complete failure'. In conquering the fearful problem of fistula, Sims showed not only great surgical skill but remarkable resourcefulness and ingenuity. He rationalised and combined what was already known. He invented his special speculum, special catheter, wide denudation and a novel way of introducing silver wire – with silk thread. Typically, he searched long and hard to find the right thread for suturing, consulting many people including jewellers and others used to working in silver. He always devoted much attention to detail, for example, exactly how to insert the sutures (he used silk attached to specially made silver wire) and where and how to space them etc.

Soon afterwards he invented a silver suture and operated yet again on Anarcha. It was her thirtieth operation in four years. This time it worked. He then successfully operated on 'Lucy and Betsey'. He wrote, 'My efforts had been blessed with success, and . . . I had made, perhaps, one of the most important discoveries of the age for the relief of suffering humanity.'


Recently Sims has been widely criticised for exploiting slaves and has even been accused of exploiting them in a sadistic manner, but the evidence does not bear this out, especially when he is seen against the background of his time. He lived in an area of slavery at a time when few questioned its morality. Ideas about the need for total obedience from slaves and the absolute authority of the master encouraged random violence and mindless brutality in families that held slaves and in those who lived among them, but there is no evidence of this in the young Marion Sims. Like most doctors before and since, he does not seem to have questioned the social and moral climate of his day but concentrated on relieving suffering wherever he found it. Probably he found so many cases of fistula because the conditions in which many women lived and gave birth were so appalling.

A vivid account of these conditions has come down to us from the English actress Fanny Kemble. She married a planter who owned many slaves in Georgia and South Carolina. During the time when she lived on his plantations she kept a journal.* The condition of the slaves and the way they were treated upset her greatly. Although she writes emotively, her journals, kept over many years, reveal her as an experienced observer. She was particularly disturbed by the childbirth practices among the slaves. One day she interviewed nine black women who had, between them, borne fifty-five children, twenty-seven of whom were dead. They had also had twelve miscarriages between them. Fanny saw the infirmary where they gave birth.

> ... these poor wretches lay prostrate on the earth, without bedstead, bed, mattress, or pillow, with no covering but the clothes they had on and some filthy rags of blanket in which they endeavoured to wrap themselves as they lay literally strewing the floor, so that there was hardly room to pass between them ... Here lay women expecting every hour the terror and agonies of childbirth, others who had just brought their doomed offspring into the world, others who were groaning under the anguish and bitter disappointment of miscarriages – here lay some burning with fever, others chilled with cold and aching with rheumatism, upon the hard, cold ground, the draughts and damp of the atmosphere increasing their sufferings, and dirt, noise, stench, and every aggravation of which sickness is capable combined in their condition. There had been among them one or two cases of prolonged and terribly hard labor; and the method adopted by the ignorant old Negress, who was the sole matron, midwife, nurse, physician, surgeon, and servant of the infirmary, to assist them in their extremity, was to tie a cloth tight round the throats of the agonized women, and by drawing it till she almost suffocated them she produced the violent and

* Frances Kemble: *Journal of a Residence on a Georgian Plantation in 1838–1839*, 1863, reprint ed., 1961, with an introduction, John A. Scott, Athens, Georgia, 1984.

spasmodic struggles, which she assured me she thought materially assisted the progress of the labor.

In 1852 Sims published his 'On the Treatment of Vesico-Vaginal Fistula'. It became a classic. The following year he sold his practice because of ill-health and moved to New York.

He soon began to feel the need for a 'great hospital to be devoted to the treatment of the diseases peculiar to women', where he could continue his work. Whether this need was to help the women in need or whether it was to help the growing ego of Dr Sims is debatable. It seems likely that both were true since Sims was a proud and self-promoting man as well as being a pioneering doctor. He managed to obtain the goodwill of a number of eminent physicians and also of Henri Stuard, a man of great social and financial prestige. Sims gave a lecture, formed a committee, mostly of ladies, and rented 83 Madison Avenue. Here he encountered opposition, particularly from the medical profession. Ricci claims that prominent doctors said a hospital for women wasn't needed because there was little to be done and the field was too limited. Anyone, they thought, could apply silver nitrate through a cylindrical speculum to an ulcerated cervix, an astringent solution for a discharge and a pessary for a prolapse. That was all there was to gynaecology and it didn't need a special hospital. However, Sims got his way, money was found and the hospital opened in 1855. It was the first women's hospital in the world.

By chance the first patient Sims admitted to the new hospital suffered from vesico-vaginal fistula. She was Mary Smith, an immigrant who had recently arrived from western Ireland, 'a pitiable, ill-smelling, repulsive creature with extensively excoriated vulva, the result of constant escape of urine.' A huge encrusted mass filled her vagina. Sims thought it was a calculus or stone. With much effort on the part of the doctor and much suffering for the patient, he removed the mass. It turned out to be a wooden float from a fishnet with which her doctor in Ireland had tried to plug the hole. Most of the base of the bladder and part of the urethra (the tube connecting the bladder with the outside of the body, through which urine passes), were destroyed. The case seemed hopeless but again Sims set to work and the patient endured many operations. In the end Mary Smith's organs were re-made and her bladder function was partly restored. She became an orderly in the hospital and worked there for many years. Meanwhile the hospital flourished and soon Sims had to appoint an assistant. Later other surgeons were appointed through the governing committee.

When the American Civil War began, Sims, a Southerner working in the North, was unhappy. He moved to Europe in 1861 and became prosperous and famous. In 1862 he returned to New York but left again for France where he built up a lucrative practice and became physician to the Princess Eugénie. In Paris the famous surgeon Nélaton asked him to attend an operation on a French countess who suffered from a vesico-vaginal fistula. Like Sims's earlier operations, it created medical history. Anaesthetics were now in use. Under chloroform, the patient stopped breathing. When Nélaton saw what had happened he uttered a cry that became famous: '*Head down!*' As a boy he had noticed that mice over-anaesthetised with chloroform and apparently dead, could be revived by swinging them round by their tails – centrifugal force drove blood to their heads and revived them. So he ordered the countess to be suspended upside down while he applied artificial respiration. She survived.

In Europe, Sims wrote and published a good deal, particularly his 'Clinical Notes on Uterine Surgery', which were translated into German. He also organised the Anglo-American Ambulance Service.

In 1872 he returned to practise in New York and to the hospital he had founded. However, there had been changes there which he did not like. An impulsive man who tended to attack people with whom he disagreed, he soon quarrelled with the hospital committee and with the other doctors. Being rather autocratic in manner, particularly after so much success in Europe, where he had become used to being lionised, Sims caused offence by appointing his newly qualified son as surgeon to the hospital. He had always found it hard to work as one of a group, and the Board of Lady Managers resented his attempts to resume control. There were two main subjects of dispute. One was the Board's objections to his cancer patients, who smelt unpleasant, were deemed unsuitable for the hospital and therefore were banned. The committee also objected to the 'great crowd of doctors and students watching operations' and claimed that 'a due regard for the modesty of patients' demanded that the number be limited to fifteen. They made a regulation limiting the number of spectators to this number. Sims regarded the operations as important teaching sessions through which a proper knowledge of gynaecological surgery would be disseminated. In 1874 he threatened in anger to resign and then, somewhat reluctantly, found that he had to do so.

In 1876 he was in the ascendant again and was elected president of the American Medical Gynaecological Society. After he died, in November 1883, the *British Medical Journal* assessed him in an obituary as 'the establisher of that branch of medical science which before his day had been looked upon as a mere accessory to obstetrics'.

The first statistical report on birth trauma as a cause of vaginal fistulae was by a London surgeon of whom we shall learn more later, Isaac Baker Brown. He presented it to the Obstetrical Society of London in 1863* and said:

> With regard to the cause of vesico-vaginal fistula, of the 58 cases admitted into the London Surgical home, 47 were over 24 hours in labour, and 39 were as much as 36 hours or more; 7 were two days; 16 were three days; 3 were four days; 2 were five days; 2, six days and 1 seven days.
>
> In the whole number of cases, instruments were used in 29, exactly one-half, and in 4 only of these was the labour less than twenty-four hours, and with seven exceptions the patients had been in labour for thirty-six hours or more before instruments were used.
>
> Of the 58 cases, in 24 only the injury happened at the first labour; in 7 at the second; in 5 at the third; in 4 at the fourth; in 6 at the fifth; in 2 at the sixth; in 5 at the eighth; in 1 at the ninth; 1 at the thirteenth; 1 at the fifteenth and 2 not mentioned.

These are early examples of medical statistics, a subject then, like surgery, in its infancy. Baker Brown had no hesitation in drawing conclusions from them: 'From the foregoing statistics it is evident that the cause of the lesion is protracted labor, and not the use of instruments or deformity of the pelvis.'

By May 1868 Emmet, who had succeeded Sims as leader in the field of gynaecology, had operated on more than 300 cases of vesico-vaginal fistula and it seemed that the operation was now well understood. In his book *Gynaecology* he paid tribute to the achievements of J. Marion Sims. Emmet was followed by Howard A. Kelly, who reigned from 1901 to 1926 and who wrote a history of the treatment of vesico-vaginal fistula.† Kelly's two-volume *Operative Gynaecology* was as far in advance of Emmet as Emmet was of Sims's book. By then gynaecology was advancing rapidly and had established itself permanently as an important part of medicine.

Much of Sims's work is as relevant today as are the conflicts associated with it. No one now doubts the need for gynaecology. The existence of 'women's hospitals' is still controversial, though for different reasons. The argument now is not that the diseases of women do not warrant

---

* Ricci: op. cit., p. 137.
† 'The History of Vesico-Vaginal Fistula', *Trans. Am. Gynec. Soc.*, 37, 1912, p. 3.

special medical care, but that hospitals devoted only to them lack necessary specialist support in other branches of medicine and also create training difficulties for doctors. The modern treatment of fistula is much the same as the operation that Sims devised. The most recent edition of Jeffcoate's textbook of gynaecology recommends 'dissection and suture', which is precisely what Sims did. Jeffcoate also discusses possible difficulties with suture material, another problem that Sims encountered. In recent years there have again been objections to medical experiments on black women.*

Like Ephraim McDowell, Sims has also received adulation not only from medical historians but also from the profession and public. His statue stands in New York City, by Central Park at Fifth Avenue and 103rd Street, opposite the building of the New York Academy of Medicine. In so far as America has a medical establishment, it is there. Engraved on the statue are the words:

SURGEON PHILANTHROPIST, FOUNDER OF THE WOMEN'S HOSPITAL, STATE OF NEW YORK. HIS BRILLIANT ACHIEVEMENT CARRIED THE NAME OF AMERICAN SURGERY THROUGHOUT THE ENTIRE WORLD.

Sims stands on his plinth and looks down benevolently. Another impressive stone monument to him is in the grounds of the South Carolina state capital, Columbia.

We have looked at some of the more remarkable pioneer surgeons and their just as remarkable patients. In order to understand their achievements more fully, let us take a more detailed look at the state of knowledge at the time, at the prevailing beliefs with which they had to live, and at the obstacles they were likely to meet.

---

* For example, D. Axelsen: *Women as Victims of Medical Experimentation*, Sage: a Scholarly Journal on Black Women, vol. 2, no. 2, Fall, 1985.

# *III*
# *KNOWLEDGE AND BELIEF*

All over Europe the effects of the Enlightenment were becoming apparent. At least for those who read and thought, everything appeared in a new perspective and took on new meaning. In England and America there was a new spirit of enquiry and a new desire to understand and control the world, and especially to conquer nature and the human body. Since the late seventeenth century there had been a growing concern with health, by which the learned *philosophes* who were the foundation of the Enlightenment had come to measure improvement.* The slogan *sapere aude*, 'Dare to Know', which Kant called the motto of the Enlightenment, also meant 'Dare to Experiment', even if this meant at your peril.

Belief in progress, the idea that human history moves more or less continuously towards a desirable future, had begun to grow in the seventeenth century and was to develop still further in the eighteenth and nineteenth. The Enlightenment brought the idea that advances in knowledge led to social betterment, and there was optimism about this, inspired by the visible advances in science and material provision. Belief in progress provided a working faith for many, which was to become stronger during the course of the century. A belief in the steady, cumulative and inevitable expansion of human awareness and power – material, intellectual and spiritual – became one of the basic beliefs of the Victorians. The use of knowledge as power over the environment to improve man's condition was central to Victorian thought. With it went the use of professional science for the improvement of mankind that was to become one of the greatest achievements of the Victorian age. It is difficult to appreciate this today because in our time the idea has become tainted. We have

* See Roy Porter: 'Was there a medical enlightenment?' *British Journal for Eighteenth-Century Studies*.

realised that technological advances are not sufficient to ensure moral and social progress, that science is often distorted in order to support authoritarian attitudes or popular prejudice, and that both can be used for destructive purposes that counter their benefits.

The desire to control one's destiny differed greatly in its application to medical treatment from what had gone before, when people had been more fatalistic about disaster and illness and had accepted that the outcome depended on the will of God rather than on the efforts of man.

The Industrial Revolution affected the position of women at least as much as it influenced the medical profession. More and more goods were made in factories so that there was less variety of work to be done at home. Working-class women had to go out to work, mostly in factories or as domestic servants, and middle- and upper-class women were confined to the home, where a decreasing number of activities were becoming increasingly 'domestic'. Poor women were leaving their homes to work long hours while, for the better off, idleness was becoming a status symbol. Women could not be employed if the status of the family was regarded as important, as it was to the middle and upper classes. Increasingly, women had to be seen to remain in the domestic sphere.

In the early nineteenth century, medicine was moving towards a more 'scientific' approach. It was not a simple increase of 'knowledge' or a transition from healing through magic and superstition to healing through science and rationality. Then, as now, medical thinking was not greatly influenced by magic. Rather, new attitudes, ideas and fantasies arose and gradually replaced or overlaid the old ones. Doctors, particularly surgeons, began to play a more active part in changing the lives of their patients. Medical 'knowledge' was changing from the authority of the ancient writers to the authority of experiments that could be observed, measured and repeated.

It is often assumed that medical knowledge and medical practice improve together in the fight against disease, but in fact they seldom do. For a long time the history of medicine was presented as a series of scientific discoveries and 'breakthroughs' leading to treatments which conquered one disease after another. Many people still think of it in this way and are encouraged by the popular press and by some medical historians to do so. The idea is misleading. So is the idea that such 'breakthroughs' are latent and potential, waiting to be discovered. Even more misleading is the belief that the chief interest of the medical profession is in curing patients, preventing disease or helping people to be healthy. These are the aims of some individual doctors, but the profession as a whole has always existed for itself and for the benefit of those who run it. Even the idea of the 'dedicated' doctor is largely a nineteenth century invention. In the eighteenth century the idea that doctors were selflessly committed to their patients scarcely existed. On the whole doctors were regarded, often correctly, as ignorant objects of ridicule, out to benefit only themselves.

Scientific 'discoveries' are not made regularly or inevitably, and sometimes they are invalid. Even if they would clearly benefit humankind, they are often not accepted or put to use as they might be. Tradition and entrenched power militate against advance. New ideas and information may be ignored until a change of attitude or social need, or perhaps another discovery or invention makes them practicable or brings them to notice. For example, for generations after its discovery, electricity was used largely as a conjuring trick or parlour game. The same was true of the chemicals later used as anaesthetics.

Medical 'advance' may also be illusory, perhaps the result of a change in the natural course of a disease. Sometimes a disease disappears before a 'cure' is discovered, or even before the disease is understood, as happened with 'chlorosis', the 'green sickness' of young Victorian girls. Sometimes the known cause of a disease weakens spontaneously, as did the dangerous haemolytic streptococcus, responsible for many deaths from scarlet fever, septicaemia (blood poisoning) and kidney disease. This organism weakened shortly *before* the discovery of the antibiotics which would probably have conquered it. Sometimes the disease turns out to be different from what appeared, as did general paralysis of the insane, once thought to be a disease of stress afflicting ambitious and successful men – until it was shown to be due to syphilis. Only in recent years has much thought been given to the social background of disease and the way in which this influences not only the way the disease is viewed, treated and researched but also the disease itself.

It is difficult, often impossible, to separate knowledge from belief since belief determines the knowledge that is sought or recognised. Even if a valid discovery is made, for example, the importance of asepsis in surgery, people take time to recognise, understand and accept it, especially when it means relinquishing former beliefs. Some prominent surgeons refused to accept the ideas of antisepsis when it was becoming fundamental to the progress and practice of surgery, yet they continued to do good and successful work without undue complications. Another example is micro-organisms. For years before

Pasteur's discoveries concerning germs (mostly in the 1850s), laboratory workers looking down microscopes had seen small organisms in fluids taken from patients with infectious diseases and had suggested that these should be investigated as possible causes of the disease. But the traditional view was that infection was carried in the atmosphere and so powerful doctors rejected the idea that these small creatures in body tissues might be connected with disease. In the case of cholera, a committee of the Royal College of Physicians actually studied the evidence concerning these microscopic objects and concluded that the findings were valueless because they were not in accordance with prevailing beliefs about miasma, the foul air that they believed was responsible for the epidemics of cholera.

Yet scientific knowledge *does* make progress, sometimes in a spectacular way. Many doctors like to feel that they, and medicine, are part of that scientific knowledge and also that doctors are the heroes of progress, solving problems (though not always posing them), making discoveries, bringing relief to suffering humanity.

Medical ideas and theory have great influence on human behaviour. Ideas that catch the spirit of the time are often used to support the established order. Two such beliefs have had a particularly strong influence in Europe and America and have affected the development of surgery, including gynaecology. One of these is the old and enduring medical belief that loss of sperm weakens the male body and, if excessive, causes severe physical damage. In the ancient world and in many cultures since, the fear was associated with emphasis on sexual moderation but it became involved also in the anti-masturbation panics of the eighteenth and nineteenth centuries.

The other medical belief prevalent in the West through most of its history has been in the extreme wantonness of women and the evil effects of this. This fantasy was epitomised in the *Malleus Maleficorum*, the famous witchhunting manual of the fifteenth century. Such medical theories have dominated whole civilisations and the private lives of many who lived in them.

During the nineteenth century, an important body of doctrine developed round the 'energy concept' which greatly influenced medical views on the physiology of women. Energy was supposed to be transferable from system to system and transmutable from form to form. The quantity was held to be constant. This was just what the medical profession wanted to hear in order to reinforce traditional views about women. The gynaecologists were particularly eager to provide 'scientific' evidence to support it in relation to the female body. Men were thought to be different; they had to be careful not to let sex drain energy away from 'higher functions'. But, because reproduction was the sole purpose of woman's existence, even in permanent spinsters and celibates, doctors agreed that women ought to concentrate their physical energy internally, toward the womb. They should never partake of activities that might use up that energy. At puberty and during menstruation they should cease from all activity. Menstruation was seen as a drain on energy which would not then be available for physical or intellectual activity. Such a theory, if adhered to, would make it impossible for women to receive higher education or compete in any way with men in occupations hitherto confined to them. The idea was taken up by many influential people, including Henry Maudsley, the powerful psychiatrist, who announced: 'When Nature spends in one direction, she must economise in another direction.'* The whole theory is expounded concisely in Patrick Geddes's book *The Evolution of Sex*, published in 1889, which was widely read by everyone interested in social theories.

The theory used by the doctors was that each human body contained a set quantity of energy that was directed from one organ or function to another according to demand. Thus one organ or function could be developed only at the expense of others. This was thought to be particularly true of the sexual organs, which fitted in with the idea that reproductivity was central to woman's biological life. Thus reproductive organs were in almost total command of women and energy used anywhere else was dangerous to them. Naturally, any form of 'domesticity', activity that ministered to the needs of men, was part of the domestic sphere and so was not only permissible but required.

In matters concerning women, background beliefs determining 'scientific' research and knowledge have been even more pronounced. At a time when much was known about general physiology, the physiology of women was largely an unknown field, fed by fantasy and fear with little time or research expended on it.

The great intellectual movements of the early modern period – the Renaissance, the French Revolution and the Enlightenment – did not replace 'superstitious' with 'scientific' medicine, but it is probably more useful to think of the change as one of attitude and imagination leading to a rationale of sickness and health which had the practical effect of facilitating many 'discoveries' and 'advances'.

During the nineteenth century, medicine became more and more

* H. Maudsley: 'Sex in Mind and Education', *Fortnightly Review*, p. 470.

'scientific' in the sense that increasingly it incorporated measurement, systematic and repeatable observation, and experiment. These came to predominate over the old ways of respecting authority and concentrating chiefly on symptoms as described by patients. But medicine is different from the 'pure' sciences in that it aims for more than knowledge and understanding. It aims to improve the circumstances and functioning of the human body, to interfere with nature, to restore to health and cure or prevent disease.

The theory and practice of medicine requires action which depends on beliefs about the possible 'cause' of the condition. Thus, if a divine or magical cause is believed, the treatment will correspond. If the cause is seen as a fault in the mechanism of the body, the treatment will aim to correct the fault. If it is seen as a fault of diet, metabolism or spiritual qualities, then the treatment will aim to correct them. During the nineteenth century most people, including doctors, believed that virtually all ill-health in women was caused by the reproductive organs and they treated women patients accordingly. During the twentieth century many came to believe that most illness was rooted in the unconscious mind; they treated it accordingly. This is a kind of 'rationality', but the rationality is based on a particular kind of premise, belief or fantasy, an internally consistent system that cannot be proved or disproved.

Today, many patients complain that the doctor does not listen to them, and young doctors are exhorted to do this, so it may seem paradoxical that the enormous advances of modern medicine began when doctors ceased to rely on what the patient said and used their own senses to detect what was happening in the patient's body. This attitude ignores many facets of disease, including the personal and the social. It tends to reduce the human being to a machine. It encourages specialisation and narrowing of interests and also accounts for the fact that, on the whole, doctors in the eighteenth century seem to have been better psychiatrists than doctors have been since. Now, in the late twentieth century, these omissions are bringing medicine into some disrepute and doctors are again encouraged to listen to their patients. But despite its limitations, the method of objective examination and measurement transformed the conditions and expectations of human life. It did this even for women, despite the fact that their interests and problems, compared with those of men, have been largely ignored or exploited.

Then, as now, there was much variation in what was known and believed, which often differed according to place, person and doctor.

The new 'scientific' medicine existed alongside much older concepts. What was known in one place did not mean that it was generally known. What *could* have been generally known was often confined, as it is today, to certain areas, groups or hospitals. This is why medical students in a teaching hospital in the early 1950s were taught: 'Have your stomach out in the green belt and you put your foot in it.'*

Knowledge, fashion and popular theories in other sciences tend to become metaphors, or 'models', in medicine. Whatever is fashionable is liable to be used to 'explain' medical processes, particularly those that cannot be studied directly, which includes most of the workings of the mind. So-called 'science' in medicine is often derived from bits of other sciences, which may be used and distorted to fit or support current medical fantasies. Typical examples of such metaphor can be found in the theories of Freud. Mental processes cannot be studied directly and attempts to understand them must be through metaphor. Without saying so, and perhaps even without realising it, Freud adopted for use as metaphor the framework of recent discoveries in geology. As a result, his less discerning followers have always tended to think in terms of 'layers' to be uncovered, 'deep' problems, and 'digging down' through those layers to find the problem, and then 'digging it out'. Exactly what is meant by these terms is seldom clear and, like all metaphors, liable to be misleading.

The idea of conservation of energy, incorporated into the medical practice of the day, was used to support its attitude towards women. Linked with these ideas were those of Darwin, which seemed to many people to demonstrate the superiority of the white Anglo-Saxon male and to support the idea of 'inferior' races and groups, including women. This distortion was strongly supported by the medical profession and was used by many doctors in their attempts to keep women at home and prevent them from being educated.

Thus serious study or activity other than domestic or frivolous, believed to drain women's energy from the all-important reproductive sphere, was regarded as a dangerous state of affairs. Adolescent girls, it was held, could be damaged for life by studying, and this was detrimental to the race. The theory applied only to the middle and upper classes. Working class women, thought to be less developed and more primitive, were expected to work hard all their lives. Thus was science corrupted in the service of belief.

Many doctors seized these ideas eagerly. It was just what they wanted to hear.

---

* 'Green belt' meant 'outside a recognised centre of medical teaching and excellence'.

The attitudes of the Enlightenment also changed attitudes towards health and disease. Disease came to be seen as bad for the national interest, as a natural phenomenon under changed yet natural conditions, as a process to be studied objectively at the bedside, in the dissecting room, and in the laboratory. But the influence of the Enlightenment was not all 'scientific' and it could be sentimental. Rousseau and others saw health as part of man's natural state, which civilisation had spoiled. He believed that mothers should breastfeed their babies, children should wear clothes that did not restrict movements, and so on. It was widely believed to be bad to expose the mind, especially the female mind, to novels. Many people, particularly in the middle class, believed that vice led to disease and that some disease, for example alcoholism and venereal disease, were shameful because they were part of an immoral life.

The idea that health was good in itself gained influence. As society became more secular and less inclined to believe in the next world, health appeared to be increasingly desirable, both as a personal aim and as an ideal for society. Ideas arose of trying to prevent disease as well as cure it, for example in variolation and, later, vaccination against smallpox. Epidemics and new diseases had traditionally been regarded as the punishment of God but the strength of this idea lessened under the new influences.* Edwin Chadwick, the great English public-health reformer, was not the first to urge that illness should be prevented in order to save the public expense. An eighteenth-century pronouncement insisted, 'Every Able Industrious Labourer, that is capable to have children, who so Untimely Dies, may be accounted Two Hundred Pounds loss to the Kingdom.' Chadwick was the first who put this idea into extensive practice. He was not a doctor and it is typical of the situation and of the medical profession that he was not. Nevertheless some doctors were interested in the health of the nation. In 1848 the great pathologist Virchow claimed that epidemics had a place in *cultural* history.

Folk medicine was still ubiquitous, as it still is today. However, a search through the *Gentleman's Magazine* from its foundation in 1731 to beyond the close of the eighteenth century revealed no indication of magical healing, even for cancer, even though the magazine was the leading miscellaneous magazine of its age and was read by gentlemen and scholars.† Hundreds, perhaps thousands of entries covered medical matters and there were also remedies and

* See Charles Rosenberg: *The Cholera Years*.
† Roy Porter: 'Medicine and the Decline of Magic'. Society for the Social History of Medicine, Bulletin 41, December 1987.

contributions from readers. A collection of family recipe books also revealed no evidence of magic though this continued to exist alongside 'scientific' medicine, as it still does. The historian Roy Porter suggests that this was because social changes brought new remedies for anxiety, such as new drugs from the New World. Healing was traditionally the preserve of women. Tacitus had noted that among the Germanic peoples few men dared intrude on the mysteries of physick, the monopoly of women and 'They take their injuries to their mothers and wives who do not fear to examine and treat their wounds.'* This had remained true down the centuries. Illness was common in the pre-industrial world and later. Doctors were scarce, expensive and ignorant. Healing was largely women's work, a tradition brought to America from Europe. In Mallory's 'Morte d'Arthur', when surgeons failed to cure a wounded knight, he was treated by a highborn lady with a reputation for skill in medicine. Every woman was expected to understand the treatment of minor ailments and to prepare her own drugs. There were handbooks on the subject, and even private coaching in 'the knowledge of herbs'. *The Compleat Serving-Maid* in 1700 stated that all housekeepers should 'have a competent know-ledge in Physick and Chyrurgery, that they may be able to help their maimed, Sick and indigent Neighbours; for commonly, all good and Charitable Ladies make this a part of their Housekeepers business.'

On the whole the lay practitioners were safer and more effective than the 'real' doctors. They preferred mild herbal remedies, dietary changes and personal care. Often they knew more than the doctors, but even when they did not, they were likely to do less harm and in the past many people on both sides of the Atlantic, including many men, had preferred them to 'qualified' doctors, to whom the 'wise women' were often superior. Sir Ralph Verney advised his wife to 'give the child no phisick but such as midwives and old women, with the doctors approbation, doe prescribe; for assure yourself they by experience know better than any phisition how to treat such infants.'† It was said that the philosopher Thomas Hobbes took little physick and preferred 'an experienced old woman' to the 'most learned and inexperienced physician'.§ In frontier America there were many lay practitioners, not only women but also ex-slaves, Indians and patent medicine salesmen. Folk medicine was a mixture of commonsensical remedies, based on the accumulated experience of nursing and midwifery, combined with inherited lore about the

* Quoted in A. Castiglione: *A History of Medicine.*
† *Verney Memoirs*, 2, p. 270.
§ *DNB.*

healing properties of plants and minerals. It also included certain types of ritual healing, in which prayers, charms or spells accompanied the medicine. Much of it reflected the curative power of the medieval church.

Ideas that may seem magical to a modern person were still prevalent. There was belief in mysterious potions and formulas. In 1725, at Godalming, a day's ride from London, Mary Toft 'gave birth' to a litter of rabbits. Prominent doctors made fools of themselves by believing this. The king was seriously interested and instituted an inquiry into it. Such ideas were to persist even into our own time.

All these ideas co-existed without difficulty. Yet by the beginning of the nineteenth century, developments in society, new knowledge and to some extent the efforts of the medical profession had resulted in some improvement in health. Infant mortality, always an indicator of the health and well-being of a community, was falling. It was lower in the United States than in Britain, probably largely because of the absence of crowded, unhealthy towns with their open drains and epidemics. Even so, most parents lost at least one or two of their children. During the next century, the number of births a woman was likely to experience fell by half and the infant mortality-rate fell by more than half. Gradually during the twentieth century these figures fell by as much again. People came to have confidence in the survival of their children and no longer felt the need to produce them in such large numbers.

Despite changes in attitude, medical and surgical knowledge that was reliable and could be tested was still scanty in the early nineteenth century. As we have seen, surgery was still primitive and largely confined to the outer parts of the body because without anaesthetics it was impossible or dangerous to do internal operations. Amputations were extremely common (about a quarter of all operations in some London hospitals) and were done for many reasons, including despair. For example, a limb with a severe infection or fracture was likely to be amputated because otherwise it would almost certainly kill the patient.

Even this was an advance. In earlier times people had been more fatalistic. They regarded a misfortune as an act of God and waited to see what God would do, often praying. A story has come down to us of a small boy in 1322, before the days when surgeons were likely to be consulted even for serious damage to the human body. Seven-year-old Robert and other small boys were playing with 'certain pieces of timber in the lane':

One piece fell on Robert and broke his right leg. In course of time Johanna his mother arrived and rolled the timber off him and carried him to the shop, where he lingered until the Friday before the Feast of St Margaret, when he died at the hour of prime, of the broken leg and of no other felony; nor do the jurors suspect anyone of the death, but only the accident and the fracture.*

As we have seen, surgeons learnt many of their skills by operating rapidly under conditions of emergency or desperation, often on the battlefield. They also, however, spent much time in slow and detailed study of the human body. Anatomy was the basis of surgery and had come to be taught through dissection of human bodies, following a long period when it was taught through the authoritative books of the ancients. For centuries post-mortem examinations, designed to discover the cause of death, had been either illegal or concerned only with unusual features or legal questions. Anatomy became a science in its own right only in the mid-eighteenth century.† Its practical aim was to correlate the course of the disease and its symptoms with the changes noted after death. This has been a valuable medical technique ever since. Surgeons had developed it more than physicians probably because surgical conditions were usually more obvious, visible or palpable. Advance was made when Auenbrugger taught, in 1761, that changes in sound that could be heard when percussing the chest gave information about changes inside, but this knowledge was not used. In 1819 René Laënnec introduced the stethoscope, which encouraged doctors to use new methods. Twenty years after the publication of Laënnec's book, there was no mention of the physical examination of patients in examinations for would-be licentiates of the Royal College of Physicians (the LRCP examination). It was another thirty years before the stethoscope was widely used, nearly a century after the knowledge was available.

Gradually, all this led to the abandonment of old classifications of disease and the establishment of others more specific, for example typhoid fever, gastric ulcer, multiple sclerosis and diphtheria. Hospitals began to house groups of patients with the same disease instead of just the indigent poor. The patients became 'material' for study and charitable treatment. Hospitals developed statistical methods and, for example, showed that bleeding a patient early in the course of a pneumonia did not improve the chances of recovery.

* From the *Calendar of Coroner's Rolls* quoted in *The Faber Book of Reportage*, 1987, p. 39.
† Particularly after the publication of G.B. Morgagni's *De Sedibus et Causis Morborum* in 1761.

In England, bills of mortality, stating the numbers of deaths from various causes, had begun in the sixteenth century. Their purpose was largely to chart the progress of epidemics. They were used in the seventeenth century as a basis for vital statistics. Mercantilism, with its advocacy of national industries in the interest of a positive balance of trade, led to calculations of the economic advantages of health and the loss incurred to the national economy through sickness and untimely death. In 1714 it was suggested that parliament make provisions for the improvement of medicine so that the population 'may, once in Sixty or Seventy Years, be Reprieved from destruction and consequently, the Number of the people in the Kingdom, in that time, may be doubled, and many Millions of the Sick may be recovered from their Beds and Couches, in half the time that they usually are now.'*

Diagnosis in surgery was usually easy since most conditions treated by surgeons could be clearly seen. Thus the process of diagnosis formed a much smaller part of the teaching of surgery than it does today.

At the turn of the century medical standards were low. Physicians were only just emerging from studies which encouraged them to discuss the authority and traditions rather than study their patients. Interest in experimental science had declined since the important discoveries from Harvey to Newton: it had probably never been great. But the spirit of excitement in enquiry was beginning to revive, much of it inspired by the development of chemistry and the technology of metals. Many 'scientists' and most members of the Royal Society were doctors because this was the only way they could make a living. There was a gradual shift in interest from general culture and philosophy to 'useful knowledge'. The idea grew that the business of a physician was to heal and not to study and speculate, and that this could be learned only from studying the various forms of sickness.

Stimulus for this came from fighting quackery, which had increased greatly. The physicians objected to the intrusion of people who had avoided the long and expensive training. Available knowledge of medicine was so small that it was a question not of skill or standards of practice but of professional privilege. Outcry against quackery led to the Apothecaries Act of 1815, but the physicians played little or no part in this. They were busy arguing and quarrelling amongst themselves and they were obstructive for some years, while they considered only their own restrictive interests. As a result, when the act was finally passed, much of the power in the

---

* John Bellers: *An Essay Towards the Improvement of Physick.*

profession and responsibility for medical education was given to the apothecaries.

Gradually the revival of science influenced medicine and was applied to it. Laennec's stethoscope was an example of a more scientific approach to clinical medicine. His book on auscultation (1819) encouraged others to correlate what was found by auscultation of the living heart and lungs with what was found at post-mortem. This led to the development of clinical medicine and of physical examination in the diagnosis of disease.

Thus the great change in the first half of the nineteenth century was a shift of emphasis from symptoms to physical signs. It included search for methods by which the newly described changes in organs could be detected and measured in life by examination of the patient. The practice of medicine became increasingly concerned with structural changes and their detection.

It seems astonishing to a modern mind to find how little doctors examined their patients. Physical examination was ignored when it could easily have been done, when it would seem to have been essential to do it and when much knowledge had accumulated about what might be detected. Yet it was not done, or done only in the traditional manner of looking at the skin and tongue and at the fluids of the body in line with traditional theories. The physician took the history, ie listened to the patient's story, then looked at face, tongue, pulse, urine and faeces, but he seldom, if ever, examined a patient. Even Queen Caroline herself was too modest to tell doctors she had an umbilical hernia and when it strangulated (ie when the blood supply was cut off, an acute emergency in 1737), they didn't examine her until the king told them to, although this required no more than a view of the abdomen. Instead, they simply watched her die. Occasionally doctors examined a lump, for example in the case of Edward Gibbon. In 1793 he was sufficiently concerned about his tumour to consult his doctor, and 'after viewing and palping, he . . . examined it again today with Mr Cline, a surgeon'. At Guy's Hospital in 1824 there was no record of the examination of any woman patient. In the previous year there was no record of any physical examination at all. Yet doctors knew quite a lot about women's diseases, especially the kind that were visible at post-mortem, but the way they treated their patients was often determined by their sensibilities and prejudices, through belief rather than knowledge.

If they wished, doctors could find some guidance from their most learned colleagues, though this was not yet widely available to English speakers. During the years 1761–5 the French surgeon Jean Astruc had published a monumental series of volumes about the diseases of women and these had been translated into English. Though greatly different and containing miscellaneous papers and lacking an index, much in these volumes reads more like a modern textbook than anything published in English for the next seventy years or more. In general there was a wide difference between attitudes to gynaecology in France and in Britain and the United States. The French mostly believed that uterine diseases were local in origin with general symptoms depending on and resulting from local pathological changes and they believed in examining directly by hand and speculum. The British and American view was that there was usually a feminine constitutional derangement, often 'nervous', with local manifestations in the pelvis. Gradually the two views coalesced, but not before Anglo-American gynaecology had become dominated and hampered by ideas about the nature, inferiority and the essential modesty of women. Nowhere is this seen more clearly than in attitudes towards vaginal examination.

In medicine today an essential procedure in most serious disease is the physical examination and this was beginning to be customary. Once this is accepted it becomes clear that in gynaecological disorder a vaginal examination is essential. Inspection, palpation and percussion were all known to the ancients, for example Hippocrates, Soranus and Aetius, as essential to the examination of any patient. Soranus showed that rectal examination was important in the diagnosis of pelvic inflammations. The lithotomy position, with the patient on his or her back with legs raised, bent and supported is as old as gynaecology. Soranus and Aetius both used the knee-elbow position in diagnosis, with the patient kneeling with knees and elbows touching. The first known picture of a vaginal examination is in a text by a military surgeon of the Dutch army published in 1789.* It shows the surgeon's index finger touching the cervical os (the mouth of the womb), but this kind of examination was by no means routine and seems to have been uncommon in the English-speaking world. A picture that has been widely reproduced in recent books shows a young woman fully dressed, leaning against what appears to be a desk and staring into space with arms akimbo. The doctor, a handsome young man in a frock coat, is on one knee before her and holds both his arms high under the lady's skirts. Like her, he is staring into space, in the opposite

---

\* Lorenz Heister: *Institutiones Chirurgicae*, 1739.

direction from the lady. The picture comes from a book published in Paris in 1822.* One modern book which reproduces it calls it 'Conventional method of diagnosing pregnancy', while another calls it 'Gynaecological Exam'. It is significant that the original picture is *French*. A search through early British textbooks on diseases of women revealed no comparable illustration. It is typical that a British book which went into many editions from the year 1835 and was highly regarded as being up to date and accurate, did not stress the importance of gynaecological examination until the edition of 1850.

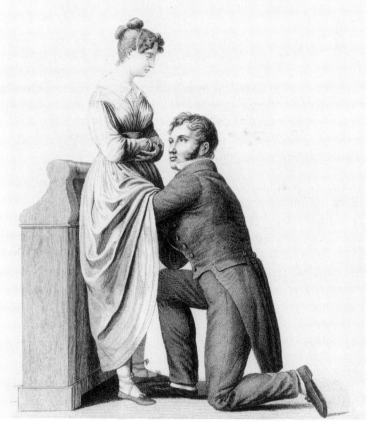

THE MUCH-USED MAYGRIER PICTURE OF AN EARLY NINETEENTH-CENTURY VAGINAL EXAMINATION

In the 1844 edition the author warns:

> To make an examination with the finger or speculum, unless it be plainly necessary, is a flagrant breach of delicacy; and, in the case of

* J-P. Maygrier: *Nouvelles Démonstrations d'Accouchements*, Paris, 1822.

young unmarried women, it is almost a crime . . . But . . . if the disease
be such as cannot be satisfactorily made out or treated without it, then
its use is not only justifiable, but to reject it would be a blameable
neglect of the means without our power for the relief of disease.*

After this concession to modesty he goes on to give a detailed
description of vaginal examination, including the use of the speculum,
which had been widely used in France since the young Récamier
introduced it at the beginning of the century.

Some years earlier the British surgeon Charles Mansfield Clarke
had attributed failure in treatment to failure to examine.

> From the general disinclination of practitioners to make an examin-
> ation, arises in part their want of success in the treatment of these
> complaints . . . It is notorious that many practitioners prescribe for
> complaints of these organs from a mere history of the symptoms given
> by the patient. It is quite impossible in many complaints to depend upon
> these descriptions; and daily experience demonstrates the futility, and
> in some cases, the injury, arising from medicines prescribed upon such
> vague information.†

But these pragmatic comments were soon lost in the linking of
shame with common sense. In spite of increasing knowledge, this sense
of shame increased and reached unprecedented heights in the writings
of some doctors. In America the influential Charles Meigs, a professor
in Philadelphia, firmly took embarrassment into account in his advice,
even when it led to failure to diagnose and treat. He even believed that
modesty was a good reason for not trying to further knowledge in the
field. It is, he says:

> . . . perhaps best, on the whole, that this great degree of modesty should
> exist even to the extent of putting a bar to researches, without which no
> very clear and understandable notions can be obtained of the sexual
> disorders. I confess I am proud to say, that in this country generally,
> certainly in many parts of it, there are women who prefer to suffer the
> extremity of danger and pain rather than waive those scruples of
> delicacy which prevent their maladies from being fully explored. I say it
> is an evidence of the dominian of a fine morality in our society . . .§

Meigs is fully aware of the significance of what he is saying
because he goes on to point out that diseases are, in consequence,

* Fleetwood Churchill: *Outlines of the Principle Diseases of Females.*
† Charles Mansfield Clarke: *Observations on Those Diseases of Females*, 1821.
§ Charles D. Meigs: *Females and their Diseases*, p. 19.

'mismanaged and incurable'. A substantial part of Meigs's book is taken up with what he calls 'Embarrassments in the Practice', much of which consists of complaints about growing laxity and immodesty. He complains about newspaper advertisements for 'utero-abdominal supports':

> When I was young a young woman had no legs even, but only feet, and possibly ANKLES; forsooth, they have UTERO-abdominal supporters, not in fact only, but in the very newspapers. They are, surely, not fit for newspaper advertisements.*

The French could never understand why British and American surgeons did not do vaginal examinations, but even in France the use of the speculum was believed to be a 'serious sacrifice of delicacy', only to be made when it was essential to diagnosis. It was little used in Germany where one distinguished gynaecologist, Meissner, gave the ingenious excuse that it could not be used so freely as in France because German women had a much 'longer and stronger vagina'.

In the 1830s doctors examined the chest more frequently than they had done earlier. However, in 1835 a patient who was under Dr Bright himself had acute rheumatism but the only part of him that was examined was his tongue.† By 1853 the stethoscope was widely used. Nevertheless, the diagnosis of disease by physical examination was the great medical advance of the nineteenth century.

The changes in attitudes that occurred in medicine are epitomised in Claude Bernard's great work *Introduction to Experimental Medicine*, published in 1865. Its ideas are still valid today. They contrast with what the staff at St George's Hospital wrote about John Hunter's lectures in 1788:

> If they had . . . contained principles and rules founded upon judgment and experience, with a regard to the authority of others as well as their own, they would have been highly useful; if, on the contrary, they have leaned to physiology and experiment, with a contempt for all other opinions but their own, they would have been pernicious.

* Meigs: op. cit., p. 24.
† Newman: p. 90

# IV

# PROFESSIONAL ORGANISATION AND ANXIETY

During the nineteenth century the medical profession organised and consolidated itself in a way that greatly affected women patients and their treatment by surgeons. Much of what happened was the result of strife and quarrelling among prominent doctors.

The eighteenth century was a period of comparative peace and prosperity for doctors, but many people held them in low esteem. The cartoons of Gillray and Rowlandson depicted greedy, ignorant and opinionated charlatans leering over their patients and grabbing their fees. This was followed early in the nineteenth century by the image of the pompous humbug in a frockcoat. In a *Punch* cartoon a patient wails, 'Oh, doctor, I'm afraid I'm pretty well at death's door!' 'Don't you worry, dear sir,' replies the doctor, 'we'll pull you through!'*

Later in the century doctors still knew little and were ineffective in curing illness but their popularity increased enormously. This had little to do with their scientific knowledge or practical capabilities but was more concerned with the confidence they managed to inspire, partly due to the mystery in which they shrouded much of what they did. The public, or at least the middle classes, came to believe in them. Their social status rose. People respected and encouraged them, and they organised themselves into a profession enjoying high status and considerable autonomy. Their overall ignorance could be concealed in the one branch of medicine in which activity achieved visible results, however dubious. This was surgery.

The medical profession and its development is probably best understood if it is assumed that doctors are no better or worse than

* Quoted in Vaughan, 1959.

other people and act in their own interests and in accordance with their personal fantasies and satisfactions, although these are not always apparent. Doctors, probably even more than most other people, like to seem to act from motives of which society approves. Success and status may depend on seeming to be 'dedicated', even if this is but a thin disguise. This can be achieved in a number of ways. Firstly, many doctors enjoy solving puzzles and like to earn their livings by so doing and they often benefit patients more than doctors whose aim is to do good. Much interesting or amusing puzzle-solving can be disguised as technology, as dedication to patients or as promoting or maintaining high professional standards, especially if the puzzle-solver also likes his patients or at least knows how to behave towards them. Some of these doctors are the scientists and clever specialists who can do and achieve what is beyond the scope of others. Sometimes they help patients, sometimes they treat them only as experimental, or experiential, material – it is not always possible to tell the difference. Secondly, some doctors are able to feel with and for others as well as for themselves. They have empathy; they can identify with those in trouble and feel satisfied if they can relieve their pain. These are the real doctors, the dedicated doctors. They are good doctors as long as they do not use their feelings for their patients in place of necessary treatment and do not develop a strong desire to control. Thirdly, some doctors, like some other people, are obsessed with acquiring status, power or money. If they are clever, such people may have considerable influence. These are the dangerous doctors, especially when their semblance of helping patients appears genuine.

In 1770 the Reformist physician John Gregory wrote that after a physician has been in practice for a while, 'he becomes haughty, rapacious, careless, and often somewhat brutal in his manners. Conscious of the ascendant he has acquired, he acts a despotic part.'* He also wrote that doctors had acquired 'an affectation of knowledge, inscrutable to all . . . an air of perfect confidence in their own skill and abilities; and a demeanour solemn, contemptuous, and highly expressive of self-sufficiency.'

The desired power may be no more than power over the patient and the satisfaction of using it: it may be more institutional. Power struggles between the three branches of the medical profession – physicians, surgeons and apothecaries – have existed in Britain for as long as there have been doctors and healers. So has the desire and the drive to stay on top and keep out other groups, often supported by

* John Gregory: *Lectures on the Duties and Qualifications of a Physician*, 2nd edn., London, 1772, p. 25. The first edition appeared in 1770.

rationalisation about the need to be exclusive and restrictive and by pious utterances about the interests of the patient. The physicians were the oldest and most respected and privileged of the groups. They used their heads and not their hands. In the words of one act of parliament, they were 'profound, sad, discreet, groundedly learned and deeply studied in Physic'* and their learning was chiefly in classics. One president of the Royal College of Physicians was also the professor of Greek at Cambridge and until the nineteenth century the examinations for membership of the College were conducted in Latin and Greek. The emphasis was on classics rather than on medicine. In 1842 the *Lancet* wrote, 'the information of the medical profession, generally, on matters of natural science is very little greater than that of the people at large. This is an extremely humiliating fact.' In 1847 the *Lancet* wrote, 'Scanty physiology and pathology, decked out in respectable Latin, will stand higher than mere professional excellence'. That important journal was not too scientific itself, for in 1842–3 it published a series of articles on 'the law of seven', showing that seven was the magic number in medicine, and invoking the moon.

Surgeons worked with their hands and only on the outside of the body, which included diseases of the skin (later handed over to physicians). They were mostly trained through apprenticeship and of them the *Lancet* said:

> The Royal Colleges have discovered the most extraordinary ground for creating professional distinction that ever entered the mind of man. With them, the chief qualification for eminence in the healing art is ignorance of one or other half of it. A physician need not know much of physic; an entire ignorance of surgery will be sufficient to give him a respectable standing; a surgeon need not possess any real knowledge of surgery, but . . . if he does not know gout from measles – that will render him 'pure' and make him eligible to receive the highest appointments . . .

In 1979 the historian Youngson described the surgeons as 'uncontaminated with the slightest knowledge of medicine'. During the second half of the nineteenth century, the education they received during apprenticeship was augmented by instruction in medical schools and teaching hospitals and by 'walking the wards'.

Surgeons were despised despite the fact that a few had been honoured with knighthoods. The contempt for them may have been partly because of a widespread revulsion at the realities of surgery

---

* 'Physic' meant natural sciences as well as medicine.

before the days of anaesthetics and partly because many of those who could bring themselves to operate under the conditions that then prevailed were coarse and uncouth. They were, however, powerful and organised and during the first half of the nineteenth century they seem to have been more effective as a body than the quarrelsome physicians. Their status rose after the introduction of anaesthesia, for they could now be seen to be doing something useful even when most patients still died.

Physicians largely confined their attentions to the rich. They lost ground during the eighteenth century when they failed to see the importance of the rising middle class. The apothecaries were originally retail druggists. Then, in 1703, in the case of a Mr Rose, the House of Lords decided that an apothecary might 'not only compound and dispense, but also direct and order' remedies for the treatment of disease. He was given freedom to visit and prescribe, but he was not allowed to charge a fee for his visits or his opinions. He could charge only for the drugs that he dispensed.

Inevitably, this led to over-prescribing. Since these prescribing apothecaries foreshadowed the general practitioners, it seems likely that it also contributed to the tradition of expecting a bottle of medicine at every visit and, eventually, to the modern situation, much promoted by pharmaceutical advertising, of 'a pill for every ill'. It also led to the apothecary being regarded as a tradesman in an era when trade was regarded as debased. In grander houses, until recent times, the doctor entered by the tradesman's entrance. Thackeray's elder Pendennis saw retirement as an opportunity to discard his trade of apothecary and become a gentleman.

Despite these social distinctions, the House of Lords ruling greatly increased the importance and scope of the apothecaries. They saw the importance of the new middle class who needed a different kind of medical attention from those who attended the rich and the great. The apothecaries became the general practitioners and this is shown clearly in contemporary fiction. George Eliot's Dr Lydgate set up in practice in 1829 and Trollope's Dr Thorne in 1833. Apothecaries were supposed to hold diplomas from both the Society of Apothecaries and the College of Surgeons to perform all the duties of a general practitioner. In theory they were not even supposed to bleed a patient without a licence from the Surgeons' Company, but in practice there was no need for them to hold any qualifications at all.

In 1804 the Lincolnshire Benevolent Medical Society enquired into the state of medical practice in the county and discovered that for every qualified doctor there were nine 'pretenders'. The Society began to exert pressure to restrain unqualified practitioners. Trying to exclude 'quacks' was always popular in the medical profession and still is. Although there has never been public demand for their suppression, their existence has always been threatening to 'regular' doctors, especially those whose chief interest is gaining and exerting power, for these are the keenest to protect their privileges.

So the standard of most doctors was low and their training was poor. In America the situation was different but no better. Medical practice there broadly followed British trends but it was less structured, spread more thinly over the country, as was the population, and was practised in a fiercely independent atmosphere. At the beginning of the nineteenth century, there were few formally trained doctors in the United States. The general public, with a new sense of national liberation after a bitter war, was hostile to professionalism. In America anyone who wished could practise as a healer and many unofficial practitioners were more skilful than trained doctors. In New Jersey, medical practice was mainly in the hands of women as late as 1818.

As she must have known, old wives' widsom, advice or 'physick' could not ease Mrs Crawford's life with her huge ovarian cyst. It was a condition that no herbs or drugs could touch. Through her courage and determination she was able to take advantage of a trend in medical practice on both sides of the Atlantic which was not always helpful to the sick and was certainly harmful to women who wished to obtain and practise healing skills. This was the trend toward professionalisation, which coincided with the retreat of middle-class women into domesticity.

The restrictive practices of Anglo-American medicine can be traced back to the demands by London associations of physicians, surgeons and apothecaries, whose charters were very similar to those of other companies seeking exclusive privileges for themselves. The charters were granted by a Tudor government whose desire was to control the practice of medicine, to check witchcraft. It was enacted* that 'none should exercise the Faculty of Physick or Surgery within the city of London or within Seven Miles of the same, unless first he were examined, approved and admitted by the Bishop of London, or the Dean of St. Paul's . . .' This was a move against 'quacks', 'that common Artificers, as Smiths, Weavers, and Women, boldly and accustomably took upon them great Cures and Things of great Difficulty, in the which they partly used Sorceries and Witchcraft, and

---

* Statute 3, Henry VIII.

partly applied such Medicines unto the Diseased as were very noyous, and nothing meet therefore.'

By 1830, thirteen American states had passed medical licensing laws outlawing 'irregular' practice and establishing that only 'regulars' were legal healers. Only then were standards in the American medical schools rising, and even then the profession did little research. The great contribution of American doctors to the advance of medicine at this time was in their practice and their daring. The most skilful of them had, like Ephraim McDowell, been trained abroad.

In the United States, though not in Britian, the spread of licensing for doctors was to be reversed in the 1830s and '40s, when most states repealed their licensing requirements. This was due to pressure from eclectic, homeopathic practitioners, to the public's dissatisfaction with the 'heroic medicine' then practised by licensed physicians, and to the distrust of state regulation. Licensing as prime proof of qualification for the practice of medicine was not reinstituted till the 1870s, but this did not help women. What mattered now was graduation from an approved medical college, admission to hospital practice, and referral from other doctors. Women were excluded from all these things.

So medical education was of poor quality and in some ways deplorable. The aim for physicians was to produce a cultured and highly educated gentleman with, secondarily, some knowledge of medicine. The amount of medical knowledge required was only the art of treatment by drugs and the writing of complicated prescriptions. Few schools demanded attendance for more than two years and in America few provided clinical experience or had any affiliation with hospitals. Elizabeth Blackwell, the first woman doctor in America and Britain, found that midwifery lectures usually provided a professor with more opportunity for dirty jokes than for the dissemination of knowledge.* Many physicians had only one year's training in medicine after their general education was completed. Elizabeth Blackwell's took fourteen months.

During the second quarter of the nineteenth century many medical schools opened in England. They were connected with hospitals rather than with universities and anatomy figured prominently in their syllabuses. At the same time public schools were opening for boys of the middle classes. Medical education in Scotland was different since it had a long tradition of university instruction derived largely from Holland.

* *Pioneer Work*, 1895, p. 257–59.

During the first part of the nineteenth century there was a greatly increased interest in scientific study, and this did much to raise the status of doctors, despite the fact that 'physic' was not 'science'. People tended to be impressed by science and by pseudo-science. The extent of quackery led to a drive to improve medical education. It was thought that there were too many people practising medicine and the healing arts. During the Napoleonic wars, France had responded to the need for more doctors by improving army doctors, but Britain had simply encouraged the semi-qualified. In 1804 a movement started in the Royal College of Physicians to control the situation but there was so much politicking and squabbling that they lost sight of what was happening and lost control of the situation. In 1815 they were so much in disagreement and disarray in the College that the power went to the Society of Apothecaries, who were henceforth entrusted with organ-

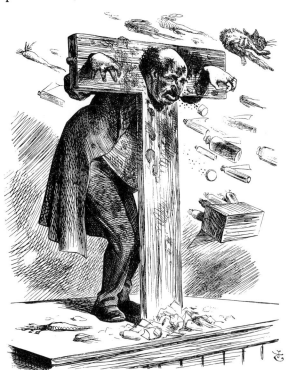

A QUACK IN THE RIGHT PLACE;
Or, What we Should Like to See.

PUNCH PUBLISHED MANY CARTOONS INDICATING HOW SOME PEOPLE FELT
ABOUT DOCTORS

ising the examinations and given responsibilty for most medical education. The Royal College of Physicians went into obscurity.

From the beginning there seem to have been ambiguous and ambivalent attitudes towards fees. In theory, the physicians did not charge fees; in practice they were skilled at collecting them. Many treated the servants for free and the family of the house for fees. Later in the century it became the custom for the doctor to charge lower fees for servants than for the gentry. In 1840 an inaugural lecture at St George's Hospital began with the words, 'You are about to begin your medical studies. The sole objects of such studies are two: first to get a name; secondly to get money.'*

There were also genuine attempts to improve standards of practice and behaviour. In 1832, the year of the Great Reform Bill, 'more than fifty medical gentlemen' assembled in the board room of the Worcester Royal Infirmary to hear Dr Charles Hastings, a relative of Warren Hastings, deliver an address proposing the inauguration of a medical association 'both friendly and scientific', to be called the Provincial Medical and Surgical Association. This association became the British Medical Association, an organisation that is still flourishing and powerful. It is the nearest thing British doctors have to a trade union and has always represented chiefly, though not exclusively, the particular interests of general practitioners.

During the first half of the nineteenth century, surgeons were pushing forward, ever keener to practise their increasing skills on living patients. The adoption and use of anaesthetics revolutionised their position and gave a huge impetus to their art. In the climate of the time, this encouraged further experimentation on women patients. One might think that women would have been reluctant to undergo operations of doubtful technique and validity, especially when they were not suffering from life-threatening conditions. Some no doubt were reluctant, but many were willing, often raised to be obedient and dutiful in serving the superior male and enhancing his status. As Virginia Woolf was to remark, women have always served as looking-glasses 'possessing the magic and delicious power of reflecting the figure of man at twice its natural size'. In any case it had been apparent for some time that if the patient could face the treatment and did not die of shock, haemorrhage or infection, surgeons were much better able to help their patients than were most other doctors. This was true in spite of the primitiveness of their instruments. For instance, the clinical thermometer had been invented but it took twenty minutes

---

* Quoted in Atlay's life of Acland.

to register and was the size of a small umbrella. Nevertheless, improvements were on the way and all that the Medical Act of 1858 really did was to consolidate them. The act also founded the General Medical Council for Medical Education and Registration, later known simply as the General Medical Council or GMC. It was in charge of medical education and discipline. It was in theory free from direct political control but had no powers of compulsion.

The act probably turned out as well as it did because the GMC had so little power and did almost nothing. The improvement had already taken place, and it is doubtful whether the GMC ever became an asset to standards, education or behaviour in the medical profession. By 1862, only four years after its inception, it was already being attacked, as it still is today, for pomposity, verbosity, ineptitude and irrelevance.

By the second half of the nineteenth century there was a professional upper middle class alongside the business class. It consisted not only of the doctors but of the other professions as well. Throughout the century the old professions, medicine and law, restructured themselves to emphasise expertise, expanded in numbers, and achieved enhanced status. New professions such as the engineers joined them. The population was increasing and the professions were growing at an even faster rate. Between 1841 and 1881 the nation's population rose by sixty per cent, whereas the seventeen main professional occupations increased their numbers by 150 per cent, thereby constituting a substantial proportion of the middle class.*

One of the characteristics of these professional men was the comparative freedom they had achieved from the struggle for income. Once established, professional men could generally rely on a steady income. They were, however, greatly concerned with their status and one of the features of the growth of the professions in England was that they tended to ape the aristocracy and aspired to full social acceptance.

An occupational group does not gain a professional monopoly by proclaiming itself to be expert. It needs to convince others of its technical skill and superiority. It also needs authority in law to select its own members, regulate their practice and exclude others as it wishes. For this it needs to convince some elite segment of society of the special value in its work. Thus the rising medical profession needed the patronage of the ruling class. In Britain, top doctors began to socialise with the aristocracy. In America, the doctors eventually

* See W.J. Reader: *Professional Men*, 1966.

received support from rich people such as the Carnegies and Rockefellers.

In the United States, new, tough laws concerning the licensing of doctors established the doctors' monopoly in state after state. The midwives, their last opponents, were driven out. Publicly, the attack was launched in the name of science and reform. Women had almost no place in the system except as subordinates. Training for doctors' helpers became essential with the new technology. Nurses had become necessary and the Nightingale idea that they should be parallel with doctors rather than subservient was dropped. The doctor diagnosed, prescribed, perhaps operated, and moved on. He needed an obedient and skilled helper.

One of the most marked features of the organisation of the doctors into a profession was the exclusion of women and the insistence that they would participate only in subservient tasks. Professionalism in medicine, as in other professions, was institutionalised as a male upper-class monopoly. Because there were now so many doctors, more patients were needed. Inevitably, most of these were women. New symptoms began to develop. New groups in the population, such as younger women, began to demand treatment. New diseases were described and both old and new symptoms were labelled with new diagnoses. The middle class at least became more conscious of symptoms and less tolerant of them.* The idea continued to grow that women were more sensitive, sick and vulnerable than men and were in special need of the fatherly doctor to look after them. One English doctor expressed it thus: 'Men are less inclined to resort to physic for every passing ailment; they have less time and opportunity for doing so; from greater vigour of constitution and a more nourishing diet they are less seriously affected; their nervous system is less excitable and their moral sensibility less acute.'† Of course, traditionally women have always tended to do what is expected of them. Doctors became increasingly dependent on women for their living and worked hard to increase both the use of drugs and the demand for them. After some years of this, Bernard Shaw caught the spirit of it when he wrote *The Doctor's Dilemma* in 1906 and made Sir Ralph Bloomfield Bonington say '. . . the world would be healthier if every chemist's shop in England were demolished. Look at the papers! full of scandalous advertisements of patent medicines! a huge commercial system of quackery and poison. Well, whose fault is it?

* Edward Shorter: *A History of Women's Bodies*, p. 109.
† Charles Cowan: 'Report of Private Medical Practice for 1840', *J. of the [royal] Stat. Soc. of London*, 1842, 5, Ser. A General, p. 84, quoted by Shorter.

Ours, I say, ours. We set the example. We spread the superstition. We taught the people to believe in bottles of doctor's stuff; and now they buy it at the stores instead of consulting a medical man.'

Shaw knew how important the sale of drugs was to a doctor's livelihood and in the preface he says that doctors 'must believe, on the whole, what their patients believe, just as they must wear the sort of hats their patients wear ... When the patient has a prejudice the doctor must either keep it in countenance or lose his patient.' Thus in essence 'medical practice is governed not by science but by supply and demand; and however scientific a treatment may be, it cannot hold its place in the market if there is no demand for it.'

Doctors concentrated their attention almost exclusively on individual patients and not on the enormous problems of public health that faced the nation. Although much more could have been done for the health of the nation, it was the study and treatment of disease that attracted the medical profession. Most doctors have always found diagnosis and treatment more interesting than prevention and this is still the case. To keep their patients and acquire more, they had to be seen to be doing something, so active treatment became the vogue. Once its main dangers had been overcome through anaesthetics, asepsis and efficient haemostasis, and even before those achievements, surgery seemed to be the most likely source of new treatments, and women were becoming ready for it.

Meanwhile the status of doctors rose and became much higher than it was before or has been since, though their knowledge was of little practical use in the treatment of disease. Few people today would describe doctors, as Robert Louis Stevenson did in 1887, as 'the flower of our civilisation', but many people still think of the history of medicine as the story of finding 'wonder cures' for one disease after another (plague, syphilis, diphtheria, tuberculosis, pneumonia, AIDS) on the path to the conquest of *all* disease.

Anxiety, both public and private, played an important part in the development of the medical profession, including gynaecology, and emerged as part of the growing insistence on respectability, which can itself be seen as arising from anxiety. Some of this anxiety was a legacy from the eighteenth century and some developed during the nineteenth century; some was contained in attitudes towards doctors and women, while some was inherent in the minds of individuals.

Life in eighteenth-century London was uncertain and insecure. This was described by Dr Johnson, who loved London.

> Here malice, rapine, accident, conspire,
> And now a rabble rages, now a fire;
> Their ambush here relentless ruffians lay,
> And here the fell attorney prowls for prey;
> Here falling houses thunder on your head,
> And here a female atheist talks you dead.

The thinker and reformer Francis Place repeatedly asserted that ruin through idleness and extravagance was the rule rather than the exception in the London of his youth. He described many men with good businesses who became destitute through dissipation and gambling. Debt played an important part in the degradation. Place pointed out that it was not the custom of the time to bring up families respectably and send children out in the world comfortably. London life centred on the tavern, the alehouse and the club, all of them low in morals and culture. This was very different from the background of respectability that was to play so important a part in the development of gynaecology.

There were similar conditions and situations elsewhere in Britain and the United States. The effects of industrialisation, the growth of factories, the strain on families, the fear of revolution, the new spirit of enterprise and discovery were all among the influences that tended to increase anxiety.

There were enormous changes in the early nineteenth century. In 1808 the tax on coffee was reduced. Coffee became the favourite breakfast drink for working men, replacing porter and gin. New coffee houses began to open and drunkenness declined. There was increasing prosperity, though the background of uncertainty remained. There were also serious health problems, particularly epidemics associated with the growth of towns.

There were problems of power and status. Industrialisation brought with it profound changes in the balance of power within society and this led to serious tensions amid inadequate institutions. Class tension became very high. There was also widespread puritan anxiety, associated with establishing and maintaining moral standards.

The relationship between public and private anxiety is complex. 'Public' anxiety can increase or diminish 'private' anxiety or be a focus for it. Modern examples include nuclear weapons, cancer, AIDS, environmental pollution and illegal drugs. In the nineteenth century there was mounting anxiety about many things and the second half has often been labelled 'the age of anxiety'. The many sources of this anxiety included anxiety about 'the mob' and democracy, about social status in a rising middle class, or else about going bankrupt in a world where many new businesses failed and there was little insurance and no welfare state or 'safety net'. There were also anxieties specifically related to medical matters such as catching disease, for example cholera and tuberculosis, and about the dangers of childbirth. A number of doctors wrote about the anxiety of many women as they approached childbirth. As several thousands of women died in Britain each year while giving birth, this was not surprising.

The medical profession as an organised whole displayed much anxiety and, in addition, individual doctors had their own anxieties. There were problems of status and finance, of power and politics. There were also therapeutic problems. There was great ignorance and, however much they postured, doctors had little power over disease and were seldom able to do much to help except provide comfort and moral support. Yet they had to be seen to be doing something. Also, paying conspicuous attention to individual patients diverted attention from other failures, for example in public health, where much more could have been done.

This was all part of the anxieties of the middle classes who were mastering the new environment, forging a place within it and trying to establish boundaries, particularly against the encroachments of the working class and the urban poor. After the end of the Napoleonic wars, many large country houses kept artillery in readiness, lest they be attacked by the mob* and incidents such as Peterloo in 1819 seemed to justify this. Later in the century there was again fear of foreign invasion, in the 1850s from Napoleon III and in the '70s from Prussia. There was also widespread fear of free thought, which was believed to lead to eternal damnation. Many individuals felt anxious almost to the point of despair. For example, in 1848 Thackeray wrote to his mother of 'a society in the last stage of corruption, as ours is. I feel persuaded that there is an awful time coming for all of us.' In an earlier letter in the same year he wrote 'The question of poverty is that of death, disease, winter or that of any other natural phenomenon. I don't know how either is to stop.'

Some of this anxiety was focused on the ideas of the age, both the new and the less new. There was Malthusian anxiety: fear that the

* See W. Houghton: *Ideas and Beliefs of the Victorians.*

population increased geometrically and resources arithmetically. This often went with anxiety that middle-class women were failing to reproduce at a suitable rate and that the country was in danger of being over-run by the lower orders, inferior races or other undesirables. Darwinism increased anxiety because it introduced a new relativism that seemed to attack the old certainties, not only those concerning the origins of humankind but also and most particularly those concerning the purpose of God in creating the world. Faith became for many a sort of desperate hope.

Inevitably, all this anxiety invaded and affected human relations and the feelings people had about each other, particularly men and women. Late in the century Matthew Arnold expressed the feeling of individual dependence succinctly in the last verse of his poem 'Dover Beach'.

> Ah, Love, let us be true
> To one another! for the world, which seems
> To lie before us like a land of dreams,
> So various, so beautiful, so new,
> Hath really neither joy, nor love, nor light,
> Nor certitude, nor peace, nor help for pain;
> And we are here as on a darkling plain
> Swept with confused alarms of struggle and flight
> Where ignorant armies clash by night.

This is the kind of feeling that expressed itself in a desperate need for a home and a wife who was constantly in it, ready to minister to her master's needs. The sharp assertion of the different roles of the sexes was expressed, among many others, by Freud in his letters to his fiancée. Freud was expressing typical sentiments of his time.

Large numbers of Victorian men of the growing middle classes and the emergent professional classes, aspiring to be gentlemen, felt a strong need to possess a personal haven of peace, created by a woman who was always there and whose sole purpose was to maintain and manage that haven and minister to the needs of the man who provided for it, to which he could retire from the cares and anxieties of the world. Because of industrialisation, middle-class women had much less to do than their forbears, and there were many more of them. Retreat into domesticity and running households of rising domestic standards suited many of them and continued, albeit in exaggerated and sometimes absurd form, the traditional relationships, described by one of Tennyson's characters:

Man for the field and woman for the hearth:
Man for the sword and for the needle she:
Man with the head and woman with the heart:
Man to command and woman to obey;
All else confusion.

No one expressed the need for domestic peace more forcibly or more dramatically than John Ruskin, whose own impotence and inability to make his wife happy doubtless contributed to his insistence on the position and place of women. It was, he said, a woman's task to provide a 'temple of the hearth', and 'the place of Peace', sheltered from terror, doubt, division, and all the anxieties rampant in the hostile society of the outer world. Outside it was the role of the husband to 'encounter all peril and trial', and he would often be wounded or subdued, and 'ALWAYS hardened'. Inside, it was the role of the wife to create an oasis of peace and emotional stability – not only to maintain the outward appearance of order and comfort, but to build around every domestic scene 'a strong wall of confidence, which no internal suspicion can undermine, no external enemy break through'. She was the priestess of the Victorian religious cult of hearth and home, and on her shoulders 'fell the burden of stemming the amoral and irreligious drift of modern society.'

The archetypal celebration of Victorian marriage was, of course, Coventry Patmore's long poem 'The Angel in the House'.

Doctors also had much anxiety about their social status. Neutral observers often raised the question 'Is a medical man a gentleman?' The upper and upper middle classes discussed whether the doctor should enter by the front door or by the back. This may have contributed to the intolerance of doctors and their tendency to adopt a committed stance and make pronouncements on many matters in which they were ignorant. In 1862 the *Lancet* thundered: 'The demonstrations achieved by medical science have needed and still need to be pressed upon public men with incessant energy, in order to effect the necessary reforms.'

But science played little part in these struggles. In order to become accepted as experts, doctors did not need to demonstrate their expertise; both they and their authority needed to be accepted not as scientists, but socially. Their authority increased because the public was increasingly separated from knowledge of their work. The power of the doctors as experts was not the power to heal or to demonstrate their knowledge: it was the power to give the appearance of knowing, and therefore to judge. The doctors gained in stature not because of what they could do but because they could name, describe and explain. The tradition of medical secretiveness is only just beginning to break down now as the twentieth century nears its end, and it is still strong. The secretive tradition still causes problems, for example for patients (and doctors) who believe they have been wronged yet are denied access to the papers which might prove or disprove it. That centre of medical professionalism, the General Medical Council, is still aggressively secretive about its proceedings, even those that took place in the nineteenth century.

The establishment of an organised profession brought its own anxieties. This period saw the transformation of a group of medical practitioners into a profession with its accompanying autonomy and high status: the barber-surgeons became university graduates. There were financial problems, concerned with making a living. There were problems of politicking and power struggles within the profession. When women began to demand entry into the profession, they created much anxiety among the men. Elizabeth Blackwell, Britain's first woman doctor, qualified in America in 1848, the year of the Women's Rights Convention at Seneca Falls. This was ten years before the Medical Act of 1858. The anxiety about women was partly due to the prospect of competition, partly because it outraged custom and countered received belief and prejudice, and partly because middle-class women were the best patients. The whole process involved the challenge of crossing boundaries which inevitably provoked a response in the form of rituals, beliefs and taboos in order to clarify, reinforce and maintain the existing social structure.

To a great extent, these anxieties turned against women and doctors reinforced society's attitudes. Few people at the time regarded women as people in their own right, few could see them as anything except appendages to men. These beliefs and prejudices, much more powerful than logic or scientific knowledge, were increasingly strengthened not by exploration and discovery, but by pontification and intellectual processes based on emotion. Ignorance tends to evoke pontification, especially in those who wish to conceal that ignorance from both others and themselves or in whom ignorance of the facts liberates the expression of strongly held beliefs. The tendency to pontificate is strongest in those accustomed to authority and the medical profession was becoming accustomed to this. In authoritarian people and organisations the preservation of apparent omniscience is sometimes deemed to be more important than the truth.

Pontification is related to an uncomfortable mental state which arises when a person possesses knowledge and beliefs which conflict with a decision he has made. Known technically as 'cognitive dissonance', this is well described by Norman Dixon in his excellent book *On the Psychology of Military Incompetence*. Once a decision has been made and an individual is committed to a given course of action, the psychological situation changes decisively. There is less emphasis on objectivity and more partiality and bias in the way the person views and evaluates the alternatives. This is what seems to have happened in many Victorian people, particularly doctors, regarding women and everything to do with them, including sexuality and its manifestations.

Pontification is one of the ways in which people try to resolve this discomfort. By loudly asserting what is consistent with some belief they have adopted or some decision they have made and ignoring the contrary, they can make themselves feel more comfortable.

# V

# SCIENCE

The philosopher-doctor Oliver Wendell Holmes said that 'the truth is that medicine, professedly founded on observation, is as sensitive to outside influences, political, religious, philosophical, imaginative, as is the barometer to changes of atmospheric density.' Nowhere is this displayed more completely than in the history of Victorian science. During this period knowledge and contemporary belief influenced not only the development of medicine but also the position of women in society, and science itself was used to bolster up these beliefs.

Science tends to grow from the established ideas and institutions of its age. During the nineteenth century different professional and educated groups of men united to 'prove' the inferiority of women, thus preventing them from sharing education or occupation with men and from competing with them. The strongest powers of science were invoked to keep women in their 'place' and to prevent them from being educated or becoming doctors.

Scientific support was needed to bolster old beliefs about the inherent inferiority and weaknesses of women and about their moral purity. By the 1860s the power of religious arguments that denigrated women and reinforced their inferiority and traditional role was declining. Increasingly, responsibility for the moral welfare of women was being taken over by doctors. The power of old arguments against the employment of women was also diminishing. The increasing number of unsupported middle-class women was becoming obvious everywhere. In 1848 Charlotte Brontë wrote to William S. Williams, 'It is true enough that the female market is quite overstocked . . . Is there any room for female lawyers, female doctors, female engravers, for more female artists, more authoresses? One can see where the evil lies, but who can point out the remedy?'* The women's rights movement was felt as a potential threat to the social order in England.

* Quoted by Clement Shorter in *The Brontës and their Circle*, 1914.

Experts in many different fields responded to the demand. Never before had powerful men combined so openly in order to use and distort 'scientific knowledge' to a degree that now seems ludicrous. They were desperate to keep women in their 'place'. Some doctors supported this strongly.

By the middle of the century the cult of male superiority was being shaken a little from below, but at the same time the cult of Victorian domesticity for middle-class women was at its height. Many middle-class women were content to stay at home, raising their large families in ultra-domesticity and perhaps, if time permitted, doing good works such as visiting the poor or working for one of the many charities that were springing up. Some women who did not enjoy these activities managed to circumvent them and lead interesting and fulfilling lives. This was easier to achieve for women who were intellectual, political, eccentric by nature or upper class. But some women set their sights on greater independence, notably in education and the vote.

The belief in male superiority relieved anxiety in many men and was shared by many, perhaps nearly all, women. The idea that this belief might be false was so upsetting that it was seldom uttered, even by feminists or those who believed that women should have more opportunities. For those who felt threatened by any hint of women becoming more active or educated, the only means of stifling the incipient demands of women was by massive rationalisation. Rationalisation, the justification of belief, opinion and feeling through 'facts' and intellectual explanation and argument, is a powerful defence against anxiety and often difficult to counter. The peace of mind of many men, including many who were intelligent and successful, depended on it. The rapidly advancing scientific knowledge of the age was clearly the most appropriate vehicle with which to control women's demands, preferably for ever. It seemed that truth and goodness depended on maintaining the *status quo* and protecting it with 'scientific' proof. Subjects most suitable for this included physics, evolution, anthropology and medicine, notably gynaecology and psychiatry. The organised medical profession has always tended to uphold the established order strongly.

One example of the many scientific theories that were used to support the ideas of women's inherent weakness was that of the conservation of energy, described in Chapter three (p. 38). Another rich field for this kind of argument was evolution and anthropology. In 1868 Paul Broca, a distinguished anthropologist and neuroscientist, spoke to the Anthropological Society and said that they must begin to study the 'condition of women in society'. Unchecked female militancy threatened to produce a 'perturbation of races' and to divert the orderly course of evolution. The subordinate position of women had for far too long rested only on assumptions of female inferiority.

These arguments were often extreme, switching from one to the other according to what seemed most plausible in the fight against the liberation of women. Some men who seemed sympathetic to the women's cause, for example Herbert Spencer, were actually the strongest opponents of changes for women. Increasingly, medicine and the medical profession became powerful with an essentially male power that, as it grew, depended increasingly on women for its patients and its 'clinical material', just as the domestic base that supported successful men was also provided by women. Old beliefs and prejudices gained new strength and took on new meaning and medical opinion backed these prejudices and theories and added to them eagerly. The power of the medical profession was increased because many 'scientists' were also doctors. Typical was the attitude of the *Lancet*. It was a medical journal with a strong reforming tradition and it ran a continuous campaign to improve medical standards, yet it opposed the entry of women into the medical profession and, in 1869, revealing the true limits of its broadmindedness and innovativeness, promoted the idea that women who wished to have a profession should become hairdressers, saying, 'Surely this is an employment to which women are perfectly suitable . . .' It justified this by announcing, 'Many women have a great aptitude for routine duties, which men commonly find so irksome.' Victorian men regarded it as part of nature that women should do the chores and liked to think that they were specially adapted for this.

Ideas that women were intellectually inferior, less aggressive and more passive than men, and naturally inclined to domesticity were all supported by 'scientific' observation. Women believed it themselves, as people do believe what is universally acknowledged and seems to be self-evident. Even women of great talent or genius believed it, for example Caroline Norton and Elizabeth Barrett. The latter wrote to Robert Browning in 1845:

> *There is* a natural inferiority of mind in women – of the intellect . . . not by any means of the moral nature – and that the history of Art and of genius testifies to this fact openly . . . I believe women . . . all of us in a mass . . . to have minds of quicker movement, but less power and depth . . . and that we are under your feet, because we can't stand on our own.

The background to the tremendous changes in attitude and

knowledge that occurred during the second part of the nineteenth century was the theory of evolution, which permeated scientific thinking and encouraged scientists in different disciplines to look for the laws governing nature and their speciality. Science was the pursuit of *law* and scientists hoped to find the universal laws of society. There was increasing emphasis on group differences. Race was a burning social question in England and America, and there was much anxiety about idiots, criminals, pathological monstrosities and children, as well as women.

Scientists and medical men seem to have been more anti-feminist than literary men, lawyers and businessmen – or they provided fewer supporters of feminists. Abraham Jacobi, married to Dr Mary Putnam Jacobi, in America and Alfred Russel Wallace in England were among the few scientists who showed any understanding of the women's cause. When Helen Gardiner sought aid from American neurologists in combatting William Hammond's theory about sex differences in the brain, she found none who believed in women's suffrage or equality. Men tended to view women as a group instead of as individuals. Refusal to see them as individuals was a common stance of anti-feminists, not peculiar to science, but the scientific method strongly reinforced it. Science categorises, generalises, seeks for general truths and widely applicable laws and facts. In 1892 Karl Pearson described the process in his *Grammar of Science* as 'orderly classification of facts followed by the recognition of relationship and recurring sequence'. Thus the subject under discussion was usually *woman* rather than women.

The argument that women were inferior was also strengthened by the theory of evolution and by those who disseminated and adumbrated it. The evolutionary arguments used for the purpose of subjugating women were often inconsistent and they also changed with time. They showed three fundamental shifts of emphasis. Firstly, the dynamic view of past evolution became a static view of present and future, as though all evolution had led to the pinnacle of achievement, namely the white, middle-class male of the nineteenth century. Secondly, natural laws which had governed changes in the past and had determined the evolution of women rapidly became social laws for maintaining the *status quo*. Thirdly, the idea of competition between individuals, essential to evolutionary theory, was replaced by the idea of competition between groups or races. In this way women became classed with 'lower' races that were not in a position to compete with men.

The most important influence on the application of theories of evolution to the social order was Herbert Spencer. His influence was vast and his writings widely read. He made Darwinism seem understandable to the middle classes and adapted it, as Darwin did himself, to suit the theories of the time. Spencer believed that Victorian society was the zenith of evolutionary development and believed that the future would prove it. He was prepared to use any evidence in attempts to support his belief and to insist that it always came to the required conclusions.

Spencer's concern about women's rights is revealed in the several chapters he wrote on the subject in various works. In his early works he seemed in favour of improvements for women, but this was deceptive. He believed in 'a diminution of the political and domestic disabilities of women, until there remain only such as differences of constitution entail'. This sounds open-minded but the 'constitutions' of women, physical, mental and moral, became increasingly prominent in his writings. His rationalisations were complicated. He was convinced by the argument stemming from the theory of conservation of energy. He cited examples of species in which the individual is sacrificed to produce the next generation. He insisted that the individual development of women was impossible because of the demands of reproduction. To him celibacy was not a choice because it meant only that the woman was not fulfilling her duty to the race. In other words, no matter what she chose, a woman could not escape her destiny. His ideas were echoed by many others, such as Geddes and Thomson, in their *Evolution of Sex*, published in 1899.

A new and growing science was anthropology, the study of *man*. Anthropologists and those associated with them were among the most enthusiastic in creating and adapting theories which, in their view, demonstrated women's inherent inferiority. Comparative anatomists made detailed studies of the brains of men and women which anthropologists and general writers then used to support their theories. One of their arguments was that men and women had developed at different rates and in different ways and so the higher the degree of civilisation, the greater the difference between the sexes and the more each should be confined to its separate sphere. A society organised its labour according to the characteristics of its men and women. Thus, 'the lower we go among savage tribes, the less of this diversity there would seem to be; so that it appears to be a direct retrogression to assimilate the work of the highly developed woman to that of her mate; and if perfection is to be the aim of our efforts, it will be best advanced by further divergence of male and female characteristics.'*

* *Saturday Review*, 1871.

Many anatomical studies of the brain were published in the 1860s. Adolphe Quételet in Belgium did measurements, known as craniometry, which were widely discussed. Although phrenology had been discredited, this was its lingering, more respectable, form. There were arguments about which angles and lines to use in the measurements. Comparison between the brains and skulls of different animals were extended to comparisons between different humans. These workers also calculated the volume of the brain by filling the cranial cavity with lead shot and deducting that fraction of the volume that in living organisms would be filled by tissue other than brain. The idea was often no more than to 'prove' that women, along with non-Europeans, were inferior. In other words, again, the intention was to emphasise the superiority of the middle-class, white male and to ensure that everyone else served him. Another popular argument was that if women were equal, there would be some societies where they ruled.

It was also suggested* that there was probably a 'natural law' which governed the way the mental structures of the two sexes had evolved, since it was 'universal' throughout the human race, and still more because it was a good and not an evil. Woman excelled in the faculties most useful to her, as man excelled in the faculties most required by him. Evidence supporting this was to be found in anatomical studies.

Thus did the circular argument continue. One 'scientist', a Mr Peacock, in 1863–4 reported the weights of five negro brains and concluded from this that the average weight for negro men was 44.34 ounzes and for women was 43.5 ounzes. Another claimed that the female skull was more 'child-like than the male skull'.† There was much talk of 'savages' and 'deviants', 'throwbacks' and 'degeneration'.

Anthropology as a subject emerged during the nineteenth century and was organised in a way that reflected some of the intellectual preoccupations of the time. It used to be known as 'ethnology' (and in some libraries it is still so classified) and has been traced back to Quakers in their humanitarian defence of blacks threatened with extinction by the 'giant efforts of modern commerce' and by the 'system of colonization hitherto pursued'.§ Gradually 'ethnology' was replaced by anthropology, humanitarian concerns were separated

* Cox in *Distant*, 1875.
† John Cleland: 'Variations in the Human Skull'.
§ G.W. Stocking: *Victorian Anthropology*, and Ronald Rainger: 'Race, Politics, and Science', *Victorian Studies*, 1978.

from intellectual, and the goal of scientific understanding displaced that of 'protecting the defenceless, and promoting the advancement of uncivilized tribes'. But there were difficulties, including the upheaval that took place in the subject at the very time when women were beginning to demand rights and gynaecology was becoming established. Some played an important part in the history of women as patients.

The Ethnological Society had strong religious, humanitarian and environmental traditions and influences. During the second half of the century the Society was losing its appeal. It was then re-invigorated by a group of men of whom the most dynamic and determined was the secretary, James Hunt, an eccentric man who held strong views about race and who made his living teaching stammerers.

In 1862 there was a row about his racist portrayal of blacks from the colony of free slaves in Sierrra Leone who had been the concern of British humanitarians for the previous seventy years. In a publication of the Society, Hunt had portrayed them in a 'bestial' manner. As a result of the row, he resigned from the Ethnological Society. Then in 1863, he started his own organisation, the Anthropological Society of London, which sounded more respectable than it was. Hunt gave various reasons for initiating this break, but it seems to have been largely in order to propagate his racist views. Like most racists, he was also strongly opposed to women's rights.

Hunt followed the distinguished neurologist Paul Broca and defined anthropology in the very broadest terms as 'the science of the whole nature of man'. He contrasted it with ethnology which, he said, was merely 'the history or science of races' and which, hamstrung by biblical dogma, had become mired in arguments over their unity or plurality. Thus there was serious confusion over who meant and stood for what. One can see why Darwinians at this time were on the whole antagonistic to the Anthropological Society.

Hunt began to organise his new society with big ideas and great dynamism. Within two years, he had five hundred members. He embarked on a big publishing programme, including the Society's own *Memoirs*, a series of translations of foreign works, the *Anthropological Review*, which included the Society's *Journal*, and an abortive *Popular Magazine of Anthropology*. The last two of these were Hunt's personal organs. Even a critic of the Society said there was 'nothing like it in any other scientific body in the country'.

Huxley spoke of it as 'a nest of imposters'. The Darwinians made the Ethnological Society the centre for their 'anthropological' interests and at the same time rejected the term 'ethnology'. Hunt had appropriated the name they would have preferred and they rejected Hunt. Hunt rejected Darwinism and made a point of associating this rejection with the Anthropological Society. His point of view is made well in a paper he gave to his society soon after its founding. Rejecting the origin of man as an insoluble problem at present, he proposed 'merely to classify man as he now exists, or has existed since the historical period' on the basis of anatomical and physiological characteristics, especially 'the form of the cranium'. Three times as many physical anthropological articles were published in the *Memoirs* as in the ethnological *Transactions*.

In contrast, the Ethnological Society, apart from its religious associations, was not incompatible with the questions that evolutionists were asking. It seems that the 'ethnologicals' came from intellectual backgrounds, had philanthropic affiliations, and were interested in history, literature, language and culture. They believed in the monogenic theory that all men were descended from common ancestors (they do not seem to have been so sure about women) and so were in some sense 'brothers'.

In contrast, Hunt's polygenetic view was basically unmodifiable over time and clearly designed only to assert the superiority of white males. The 'anthropologicals' insisted that there were several original races of differing superiority. They were avowedly racist, interested in physical description and showed little interest in historical evidence.

The 'anthropologicals' seem to have come from traditional backgrounds but from marginal positions in them. A modern person might see similarities between them and Nazis in Germany or the National Front in Britain. In contrast, the 'ethnologicals' were from dissenting middle-class backgrounds of the sort from which a new intellectual aristocracy was emerging during this period. More of the 'ethnologicals' were educated and more had been to university, more were successful in established professions and more were members of the Athenaeum and the Royal Society. Among the 'ethnologicals' there were three Liberals for every Tory, but the proportions were the reverse among the 'anthropologicals'.

Hunt's address in the first volume of the *Memoirs* might be the archetype of the traditional racist view of blacks. He asserted that they are different, closer to the ape, incapable of civilisation and so on. In 1866 when Governor Eyre's ruthless suppression of rioting in Jamaica aroused anger and protest among liberals and humanitarians, the news was greeted at the Anthropological Society with loud cheers.

The 'ethnologicals' also tended, like virtually everyone else at the time, to believe that a darker skin was inferior, but they were much more liberal and humanitarian. Galton, who succeeded Hunt as secretary of the Ethnological Society, thought of other races as 'our kinsmen' rather than as aliens. Meanwhile the inner clique of the Anthropological Society called themselves the 'Cannibal Club' and used a gavil in the shape of a negro head. The Society also displayed in its window an articulated 'savage skeleton'.

Attempts to amalgamate the two societies led to acrimony. To strengthen his position, Hunt appointed fellows who hadn't paid their subscriptions and others who didn't belong to the Society. Some of them hadn't even been asked.

During 1869, the last year in which the Anthropological Society operated on its own, it devoted much attention and a whole issue of its journal to laying out the 'scientific' evidence for the inferiority of women. But Hunt died in August of that year and in 1870 the two societies joined to form the Anthropological Institute of Great Britain and Ireland. However, there were more rows and power struggles. The 'anthropologicals' went off and formed the London Anthropological Society and published one volume of a journal but soon realised that they could not survive on their own. They petitioned to rejoin the Institute and were allowed to do so only as individuals, not as a body.

The word 'anthropology' had been made somewhat disreputable. When it seemed that the future Liberal MP, Sir John Lubbock, might become president, Huxley warned him that the title 'President of the Anthropological Society' might hinder his efforts to get into parliament, but he took the risk and was elected.

Meanwhile something strange was happening to the women's movement. Many of its leaders had absorbed the old concept that women are 'different' and therefore should be treated differently. This argument can develop in any way required and has always been used not only by ardent suppressors of women but also by humane and liberal-minded people who feel unable to go against the prevalent ethos sufficiently to believe in the basic equality of the sexes as human beings. Even some struggling women came to believe this. Without thinking it through, and probably without the knowledge or information necessary in order to do this, they took the easy option, as many have done to this day, of arguing that the two sexes are 'equal but different', and complementary to each other. This view was endorsed by many of the more advanced men. It has always been a sort of staging post in feminist theory. A typical 'scientific' view was:

The main characteristic difference between the two sexes I should infer to be this – the male has the most energy, the female the most sensitiveness; and this distinction will, I believe, be found to rule the leading operations affected by those of each sex.*

Resistance to all these theories was difficult even for the most determined women. Elizabeth Garrett Anderson and other pioneer women doctors had to fight against these beliefs and prejudices. Some doctors did not approve of the way in which scientific theories were being used and, though they themselves were imbued with the prejudices of the time, they tried to be fair and to help these women even if they did not approve of them. Such a one was the eminent surgeon Sir James Paget. But, as is usual with prominent people, he would not step out of line. Few influential doctors were prepared to protest at the misuse of science.

The women's movement developed as part of the movement for egalitarian justice that had become strong in the eighteenth century. It was now undermined by these 'scientific' concepts. Inevitably, limits allegedly imposed by 'nature' on human nature or human potential would be used by some groups to assert superiority and exercise power over other groups. And so it happened.

We can follow the same thoughts from Mary Wollstonecraft's *Vindication of the Rights of Women*, published in 1792, through J.S. Mill's *Subjection of Women*, published in 1869, to Simone de Beauvoir's *The Second Sex*, 1953, without noting any substantial increase or decrease in the force of the argument.

The impact of nineteenth-century science gave vigorous and persuasive reinforcement to the traditional dogmatic view of sexual character that not only strengthened the opposition to feminism but disengaged the ideals of feminists themselves from their philosophic roots. One example of this was Margaret Fuller herself. In 1855 she propounded the idea of woman's special genius and said that male and female were 'two sides of the great radical dualism'.

Both scientific and feminist thought challenged traditional belief and authority. Both had a missionary element and so at times they coalesced, even in the same individual, against a common orthodoxy.

Thus the tendency to develop ambiguous connotations of the concept of female 'genius' led people astray. Appeals to women's limited 'nature' and peculiar 'genius' threatened the women's movement.

* Harris, 1869.

An example of someone whose thinking was distorted by this new emphasis was Thomas Wentworth Higginson, who was devoted to an idea that could have been enormously helpful to women. This was that 'Great achievements imply great preparations and favourable conditions . . . Give an equal chance, and let genius and industry do the rest.' But Higginson's thought was diverted to other paths when he was influenced by the historian H.T. Buckle.* Buckle asserted that women had a special 'genius' for deductive and intuitive modes of thought and then concluded that new opportunities for women would be opened by the feminine ethos of modern social development. He said that women had powers 'equal but not identical' with those of men and offered them, in return for their education, a vague promise of influence on 'philanthropy, culture, arts, affections, aspirations'.

There were advantages in this approach. In a society basically hostile to the advancement of women and deeply insecure in its sexuality, it must have appeared much less threatening than demands for full equality. Many people were working for improved opportunities for women in much quieter, more modest, ways. For example, there was the Society for Promoting the Employment of Women which had been started by a country reader of the *Englishwoman's Journal*, at the offices of the *Journal*. The aim of the Society, which was, initially, to win a fuller, more interesting life for middle-class women, was soon extended to the working class.

Few saw the dangers inherent in this approach. It would be all too easy to let philanthropy, arts and so on fall by the wayside, as indeed happened. In 1851, John Stuart Mill and Harriet Taylor, writing on 'The Enfranchisement of Women', published in *Dissertations and Discussions*, 1873, commended the Seneca Falls Women's Rights Convention of 1848 for having *failed* to 'entertain the question of the peculiar aptitudes either of men or women, or the limits within which this or that occupation may be supposed to be more adapted to one or the other.' But during the following decades this point of view became increasingly obscured in a trend that was strongly reinforced by Victorian 'science'.

Between 1850 and 1870 the evolutionists Darwin, his cousin Galton, and Huxley, were drawn into the arguments about sexual character and, by analogy, social development. Herbert Spencer, who applied evolutionary ideas to social situations, wrote extensively about

* H.T. Buckle: *The Influence of Women on the Progress of Knowledge.*

woman being a case of arrested development. Huxley believed that
women should have legal and political emancipation but believed that
there was 'natural' inequality between the sexes.* In *The Descent of
Man*, published in 1871, Darwin even had a chapter 'Differences in
Mental Powers of the Two Sexes' in which he wrote:

> It is generally admitted that with women the powers of intuition, of
> rapid perception, and perhaps of imitation, are more strongly marked
> than in man; but some, at least, of these faculties are characteristic of
> the lower races, and therefore of a past and lower state of civilization.

Darwin gave no scientific evidence for this statement. He quotes
only from Mill's *Subjection*, thus reversing its meaning. There is no
suggestion in any of these writings that woman's failure to achieve
great things might be the result of her cultural subjection. Darwin
declared that 'the chief distinction in the intellectual powers of the two
sexes is shown by Man's attaining to a higher eminence, in whatever
he takes up, than woman *can attain*' (my italics). Then he softens it a
little with, 'It is indeed fortunate that *the law of equal transmission of
characters to both sexes* prevails with mammals; otherwise it is
probable that man would have become as superior in mental
endowment to woman, as the peacock is in ornamental plumage to the
peahen.' (Again, my italics.)

In 1869 Galton published his *Hereditary Genius*. The qualities of
genius he described were largely traditional masculine qualities and
his 'geniuses' were mostly men. The women he included were mostly
only those whom he thought demonstrated the hereditary nature of his
heroes' genius. He was also markedly attracted to the more extreme
traditionally masculine professions and activities such as military
commanders, 'Senior Classics of Cambridge', oarsmen and wrestlers.
He also had the self-satisfied idea, in marked contrast to Higginson,
that great potential could never be repressed by circumstances,
however uncongenial to it. If a man is gifted 'with vast intellectual
ability, eagerness to work, and power of working, I cannot compre-
hend how such a man should be repressed.'

Cesare Lombroso echoed this when he wrote, 'if there had been in
women a really great ability . . . it would have shown itself in
overcoming the difficulties opposed to it.'†

---

* See his *Emancipation – Black and White*, Science and Education: Essays, New
York, 1914.
† *Man of Genius*, 1891, London.

Later in the century, Havelock Ellis, along with others, furthered the discussion in the inaugurating volume of the *Contemporary Science Series*, edited by him. Many people joined in this discussion, typically Geddes and Thomson re-analysed Darwin's theories, attacked both schools of feminism and said they both spoke 'as if the known facts of sex did not exist at all'. They insisted that the two sexes were 'complementary and mutually dependent'. Males were 'katabolic', and females were 'anabolic'. They connected women with altruism and sacrifice.


In 1873, just as real progress was starting to be made in women's education and medical training, Dr Edward Clarke published his *Sex in Education*. This short book was to prove a formidable opponent to women's advancement. Women are delicate, he insisted. Education is over-pressure and exhaustion. Education turns women into men. Menstruation is an insuperable barrier to women's education. These were but common rationalisations of old tales, but belief in them was increasing.

The leading psychiatrist, Henry Maudsley, a continual opponent of women's rights and founder of the Maudsley Hospital in London, added his weight to the argument in his 'Sex in Mind and Education', published in the *Fortnightly Review* in April, 1874. The menstrual myth gave him a 'scientific' justification for his anti-feminism. He prophesied a gloomy future for the high-school or college girl. It was true, she might *appear* to enjoy her studies, but could a young girl 'bear without injury an excessive mental drain as well as the natural physical drain which is so great at that time?' Nor was physical harm only to be feared. 'The consequences of an imperfectly developed reproductive system are not sexual only; they are also mental. Intellectually and morally there is a deficiency . . . the individual fails to reach the level of a complete and perfect womanhood.' In some cases 'nervous and even mental disorders declare themselves'. Women could not afford to risk any menstrual disorder, since irregularity or suppression was associated with other diseases. He concluded that women could never hope to equal masculine accomplishments, because their physiology acted as a handicap, body and mind being 'for one quarter of each month during the best years of life . . . more or less sick and unfit for hard work'.

There was widespread anxiety that men would suffer if women were allowed to step out of the home. A typical writer refers to women's 'horrible and vicious attempt to unsex themselves – in the

acquisition of anatomical and physiological knowledge, the gratification of a prurient and morbid curiosity'.*

These men were merely publicising prejudices that were widespread. They were expressing their own anxieties and cloaking these in
'scientific' terms.


Thus were 'science' and belief used to influence women's positions. In
the next chapter we shall look at problems specific to women. It is
particularly important to do this since the arguments about women's
education were so closely tied up with debates on menstruation, a
subject deserving greater analysis than we have so far been able to give
it.


* Walter Rivington: *The Medical Profession*, p. 135–6.

# VI

# DOMINANT ORGANS

The idea prevailed throughout the nineteenth century that the uterus was the central and controlling organ in women, that it was closely connected to the nervous system (which it is not), that it influenced not only the genitalia but also the rest of the body and that any stress or 'shock' could have a profoundly deleterious effect on female functioning. This was the prevailing doctrine on both sides of the Atlantic and as much on the continent of Europe as in the English-speaking world.

Although these ideas can also be found in earlier centuries, they had been background beliefs rather than the basis of aggressive ideas and tactics. In former times women's sexual appetites had been seen as stronger and more difficult to discipline than those of men. Reproduction and birth were regarded as normal and relatively un-complicated. There was little concern about sexual 'abnormalities' such as masturbation or homosexuality. During the nineteenth century all these things became prominent and women came to be seen as frail, with nervous systems that were easily unbalanced. There was universal belief that the uterus and its appendages were under the direct control of the nervous system. This belief was false but since the discovery of hormones was far in the future, the assumption was not unreasonable. It seemed to account for many things, for example, 'This connection between the uterus and the sensorium may account for the greater number of instances of madness which occur in females than in males.'* In 1833 Walter Channing, Professor of Obstetrics at Harvard, wrote a comprehensive article entitled 'The Irritable Uterus'. Another reminded his readers 'The Uterus, it must be remembered, is the *controlling* organ in the female body, being the most excitable of all, and so intimately connected with the ramifications of its numerous

* Charles Mansfield Clarke: *Observations on Diseases*, 1821, p. 62–3.

nerves, with every other part.'* A characteristic of such writing is the unquestioning belief that women are dominated by their generative organs. Typically, one of them writes.

> Accepting, then, these views of the gigantic power and influence of the ovaries . . . that they are the most powerful agents in all the commotions of her system; that on them rest her intellectual standing in society, her physical perfection, . . . all that is great, noble and beautiful, all that is voluptuous, tender and endearing; that her fidelity, her devotedness . . . and all those qualities of mind . . . which inspire respect and love and fit her *as the safest counsellor and friend of man*, spring from the ovaries.†

The italics are mine and reveal the common secret fear behind most such outpourings – the fear middle-class men had of losing control not only over the huge class of servile women but also over their own wives who succoured and protected them from uncongenial tasks.

Emphasis on the ovaries and uterus also produced the idea that *all* or nearly all illness or dysfunction in women stemmed from these organs. Some doctors supported this strongly and were prepared to propound aggressively. For example, one of them insisted that 'The influence of the ovaries over the mind is displayed in woman's artfulness and dissimulation.' Virchow, probably the greatest pathologist of the nineteenth century, wrote 'Woman is a pair of ovaries with a human being attached; whereas man is a human being furnished with a pair of testes.' Others accepted these ideas passively without thought or analysis. Elizabeth Garrett Anderson and other early women doctors had to fight against such beliefs and prejudices, often while also wondering whether or not to believe them.

One factor that militated against honest attempts to understand was the fact that, in the environment of the expanding profession, doctors needed to earn a living. Professionally, it was convenient, often irresistibly convenient, to regard women, especially middle-class women whose husbands could pay fees, as creatures dominated by their reproductive organs. Many of them *were* idle, neurotic and attention-seeking and could easily be persuaded to have extreme treatments and operations and so provide work, fees and the 'clinical material' needed for the perfection and exercise of new medical skills.

A typical statement from a doctor at the top of the medical profession comes from the obstetrician Robert Barnes:

> Any disease occurring in a woman will almost certainly involve some

* F. Hollick: *Diseases of Women.*
† Bliss, 1879.

modifications in the work of her sexual system. On the other hand, the ordinary or disturbed work of her sexual system will influence the course of any disease which may assail her, however independent this disease may seem to be in its origin.*

Once it was believed that women were totally dominated by their sexual organs, it was easy to say that they should devote their entire attention to caring for these – in the widest possible sense which included, invariably the 'duty' of domesticity and keeping husbands happy.

With these ideas accepted without question and assumed to be true in every discussion, it was easy to say that woman was inherently sick and that to be a woman meant that the greatest care had to be taken, even in small matters, all being preferably under medical supervision.

It seems obvious to us that women are incapacited during labour and that this form of incapacity is not shared by men, but we do not regard this as an excuse to disqualify women from anything they might wish to do when they are not in labour. To the Victorians it seemed equally obvious that women were also incapacitated by menstruation, an idea that had very different implications, but seemed to be so true that writer after writer either assumed it to be true or said it was so self-evident that there was no need to prove it. This belief implied that women were inherently sick, patients rather than healthy people. It strengthened the argument that they were inferior. If they were continually sick, they could not be educated with men, as some women were now demanding. Also, the medical profession was growing fast and the idea of 'the curse' as an illness, part of the overall pathological nature of womanhood, helped doctors in their search for more patients and new illnesses.

The idea that women are sick simply because they are women had a long history, but it became prominent only during the nineteenth century. Aristotle had believed it† and St Thomas Aquinas wrote that woman is a 'misbegotten male'.§ Women had long been regarded as close to children and idiots because of their supposed lack of control over feelings and the apparent predominance in them of feeling over reason. These ideas were now exaggerated, strengthened and emphasised, probably partly in response to the development of organised movements for women's suffrage and the founding of

---

* Robert Barnes on 'Diseases of Women' in R. Quain's *A Dictionary of Medicine*, p. 1237.
† *Generation of Animals*, Bk. II, 732a.
§ See 'Articles on the Production of Woman' in his *Summa Theologica*.

institutions of learning for women. In the 1860s women were also beginning to qualify as doctors. They were achieving these things despite many difficulties and the strong opposition. Taboos and prejudices are always stronger when they are about to be broken.

In the mid-nineteenth century the 'aberration' of woman, especially woman as a physical, sexual being, seemed to become more a part of everyday life. Different trends and ideas came together and strengthened each other. The idea that women were subordinate to men and that this was the natural order was as old as civilisation. As men's anxiety increased and Victorian morality took hold, so did insistence on this principle and on the idea of woman's inferiority. This gave new strength to the old idea that woman was dominated by her sexual organs and that this was rather disgusting. The inherent weakness of women was much discussed, as was the idea that they were immature and primitive because of their lack of control over feelings and the predominance of feeling over reason. Thus, in a circular argument, the result of years of conditioning about 'ways of thinking' was used to support the idea that it was true and 'scientific'. It was part of the general attitude to illness, which was sentimental and sexist as well as anxious and scared. Undisputed diseases such as cholera, tuberculosis and ovarian cyst were joined in the doctor's repertoire by menstruation, 'delicacy' and 'nerves', as well as 'chlorosis', 'debility' and 'irritability' or 'displacement' of the uterus.

So, the prevalent idea was that women, or at least middle-class women, were delicate and ailing. Working women, thought to be at a lower stage of evolutionary development, were not so regarded. The middle-class female 'in a decline' was the epitomy of nineteenth-century woman. Meigs, a prominent American gynaecologist, in his textbook for students, refers to patients as 'the dear little ladies', and 'good only for love'. Books written between 1840 and 1900 consistently asserted that a large number of American middle-class women were ill.

More and more conditions were also being regarded as 'diseases' and so were coming under the doctor. Behaviour regarded as socially inappropriate to the passive female role, such as laughing loudly, smoking, talking excitedly and dancing, were regarded as manifestations of organic disorder, often of a gynaecological origin, and even as liable to lead to serious disease such as cancer.* Some said such behaviour was the result of 'self-abuse' or masturbation, an act that excited some Victorians to extremes of pontification and dire warn-

* See S. Edwards: 'Femina Sexualis: Medico-Legal Control in Victoriana'. Bulletin of the Society for the Social History of Medicine. p. 17.

ings about its effects on health and sanity. Dr Savage, a prominent psychiatrist who later became doctor to Virginia Woolf and many others, insisted that the unconventional woman who smoked and declared her intention of doing as she liked, was suffering from 'simple hysterical mania', requiring medical treatment.

Psychiatrists and gynaecologists shared the same outlook and the same way of thinking. The longstanding connection between them was thus expanded. For example, Alexander Hamilton, Professor of Midwifery at Edinburgh, had suggested that female hysteria 'occurs most frequently about the time of the periodical evacuation' between the ages of fifteen and forty-five.* Throughout the nineteenth century such ideas were built upon, often adding a new dimension. For example, following Robert Barnes, John Thorburn, Professor of Obstetric Medicine in the University of Manchester, suggested that menstruation implied 'an increased liability to all forms of explosive nerve disease'.† Thomas Clouston, Physician-Superintendant of the Royal Edinburgh Asylum and the first lecturer on mental disease in the University of Edinburgh was concerned with the connection between reproductive functions and mental health. He wrote:

> The regular normal performance of the reproductive functions is of the highest importance to the mental soundness of the female. Disturbed menstruation is a constant danger to the mental stability of some women; nay the occurrence of normal menstruation is attended by some risk in unstable brains. The actual outbreak of mental disease, or its worst paroxysms, is coincident with the menstrual period in a very large number of women indeed.§

This book was first published in 1883 and had its sixth edition in 1904. Americans shared the same views. In 1866 Isaac Ray wrote, 'With women it is but a step from extreme nervous susceptibility to downright hysteria, and from that to overt insanity.'

Institutions such as the Girls' Public Day School Company and Queen's College, Harley Street, were beginning to make an impression on the life of the nation and were promoting the idea that women could be serious about subjects unconnected with reproduction or domesticity. A few women were now qualified as doctors and an increasing number were struggling for recognition. This showed that women were not necessarily the weak, sick creatures that doctors were describing and doubtless this increased the anxieties of many still

* Alexander Hamilton: *A Treatise on the Management of Female Complaints.*
† John Thorburn: *A Practical Treatise on the Diseases of Women*, London, 1885, p. 157.
§ T.S. Clouston: *Clinical Lectures on Mental Disease*, p. 521.

further. Yet in 1873 the distinguished doctors of the Royal College of Physicians heard, apparently without protest, what must be one of the weirdest series of lectures ever to be delivered to a medical audience. Robert Barnes, Obstetric Physician to several London hospitals, gave the Lumleian lectures. The subject he chose was 'The Convulsive Diseases of Women'. At the time the new specialty of neurology was developing fast and two of its most obvious concerns were epilepsy and 'nervousness'.

Linking women with 'convulsive diseases' could be a clever way of promoting the idea that they were sick and denigrating them at the same time. 'Convulsive disease' is associated with the various forms of epilepsy, which had long been regarded as a shameful disease. People with epilepsy took care to conceal their condition from others, as many still do. People tend to be scared of epileptic fits and to avoid contact with epileptics. Doctors now made much of a disease called 'hystero-epilepsy', a form of epilepsy said to be caused by disorders of the womb. It existed only in their minds but it accorded with the fantasies of the age. There is mention of 'epileptoid' conditions, and sometimes the word 'epilepsy' is used to cover certain forms of hysteria.

In the process of strengthening the connection that was believed to exist between female functions and 'fits', all doctors would have been aware of the fits that occur in eclampsia, a dangerous condition that can develop during pregnancy or labour. During the nineteenth century this frightening illness was much commoner than it is today because good antenatal care virtually eliminates it. Eclampsia was the main reason for the development of antenatal care, but that was not until the twentieth century. A Victorian woman may have had her pregnancy confirmed by a doctor but she was unlikely to see him again until she went into labour. No one was likely to know if she developed a dangerous condition such as eclampsia or placenta praevia until it was too late.

In his lectures Barnes takes pregnancy as a sort of 'model' disease for nearly all other diseases. He discusses particularly convulsions 'because the conditions under which convulsions break out in pregnancy and labour, and the nervous phenomena are so striking and so open to observation that they will best serve as a type which will guide to the more ready understanding of the other varieties of convulsion.' There was no evidence then, or now, that eclampsia, the epilepsy of pregnancy, was related to nerves and he does not dwell on this. He is aiming at the whole condition and, it seems, at every woman. Barnes manages to see 'convulsiveness' in normal physiological phenomena. He says that women are specially liable to convulsions at three periods of life. The first of these is childhood. The second covers the years of menstruation and 'includes, and is continuous with, that of sexual life and reproductive capacity'. Thus, according to Barnes, the female was suffering from convulsions, actually or potentially, from childhood until the menopause. This, too, was part of the beliefs of the day. Many believed that little was left after the menopause. Colombat d'Isère, an expert on diseases of women, patronisingly conceded, 'Old age, always early for a woman, does not always commence as soon as they become absolved of all obligations as regards the species.' Clearly he regarded her function, apart from breeding, as solely to interest and delight men. She still, he writes, 'has left a space, doubtless all too short, in which she may yet interest by the remnants of those charms that serve to recall the memory of those she has lost forever.' He goes on to say that at the menopause the female 'becomes sad, restless, taciturn, she regrets her lost power to please, the enjoyments that are gone forever.'* The idea that women might have lives and interests apart from their sexual and domestic functions does not seem to have occurred to any of the early gynaecologists.

Not content with that, Barnes goes on to describe the third stage of life in which the female is specially liable to convulsions. In his view, it 'runs almost imperceptibly on from the second'. It 'begins with the decay of the reproductive capacity, and is prolonged for an indefinite period.' He then concedes that it is 'seldom prolonged into the age of senility'. Magnanimously, it seems, he allows a senile female to be free of this sickness.

Driving his argument home, Barnes links the 'cramps' of menstrual pain with epileptic fits. He argues that epileptic fits can occur during sexual intercourse and says that irritable women, if they develop albuminuria (protein in the urine) in pregnancy, 'could hardly escape from eclampsia'. Again he is making mental links between the rare and pathological eclampsia and normal pregnancy. He even says that some women have an 'explosive or convulsive cough' in pregnancy.

He goes on to describe labour as 'a series of convulsions' and likens the 'premonitory shudder' before pain in late labour with that of epilepsy. He also compares epilepsy with the second stage of labour, when the foetus is expelled by means of a series of contractions of the uterus. 'The resemblance to epilepsy is . . . so close that the two

* D'Isère, *Traité des Maladies des Femmes.*

conditions can hardly be distinguished.' Then, conclusively, he returns to the subject of the unequivocally abnormal eclampsia. He gave four lectures enlarging on this theme.

To a modern reader Barnes's lectures seem to be bizarre fantasy. Almost nothing in them is relevant to modern practice. This is not simply because the age in which he worked is remote from ours. Eight years before, in 1865, was published one of the classics of medical development, Claude Bernard's *Introduction to Experimental Medicine*, a work that makes sense to modern readers and is still valid for modern doctors.

Barnes was following old traditions of fantasy medicine based on the idea of the frailty of women and on taboo. Colombat related that a certain princess had died after inhaling the scent of a rose; and in 1774 in London a woman was found dead in bed after breathing the odour of 'full-blown lilies that she had placed in a small chamber'. Doctors advised women to refrain from perfuming their apartments with flowers. One might add that this bit of medical nonsense survived till modern times. Even in the middle of the twentieth century, flowers were carefully removed every evening from hospital wards and placed in the corridor for the night. Colombat also advised against tea, spicy foods and waltzing.

The word *taboo* comes from a Polynesian word meaning 'menstruation' and in many different cultures menstruation has given rise to powerful taboos. The Bible tells us, 'And if a woman have an issue, and her issue in her flesh be blood, she shall be put apart seven days'.* Pliny described attitudes in the ancient world when he wrote:

> Contact with it [menstrual blood] turns new wine sour, crops touched by it become barren, grafts die, seed in gardens are dried up, the fruit of trees falls off, the edge of steel and the gleam of ivory are dulled, hives of bees die, even bronze and iron are at once seized by rust, and a horrible smell fills the air; to taste it drives dogs mad and infects their bites with an incurable poison . . . Even that very tiny creature the ant is said to be sensitive to it and throws away grains of corn that taste of it and does not touch them again . . .'†

Few people are anxious to study what is taboo and the medical men of the eighteenth and nineteenth centuries were no exception. They seem to have made few if any attempts to overcome their profound ignorance of a subject about which many of them held beliefs so strong that they were to dictate medical thinking on the subject of women until our own time.

* Leviticus XV, 19.
† Pliny: Natural History. See 'Half the World', p. 86.

Female physiology has never had a high priority in medicine and knowledge of the physiology of reproduction was small. This lack of interest can be seen in the number of original books and articles regarded as important in the history of medicine. Garrison and Morton, a standard work of reference which lists important publications, demonstrates this well. Crammed with references on every subject regarded as important in medicine, it contains few on women's reproductive organs, despite the fact that for centuries these were believed to control and dominate half the adult population. The 1983 edition mentions little more than Fallopius (of the tube), Graaf (of the follicle) and a 1707 account of sterility in women.

Ovulation was discovered in 1831 but its characteristics in the human were not understood until much later. There was no knowledge of the endocrine glands until the end of the century. Menstruation was thought to be similar to the *oestrus* of lower mammals and, at least until the 1950s, popular books on health were advising that the 'safe period' was midway between periods, which is actually the time when pregnancy is most likely to occur. Even when much more was known by scientists, most surgeons were ignorant of physiology. One might expect that those who held high office in important professional organisations might be up to date in their professional knowledge, but this was not the case. For example, in 1891 the president of the American Gynecological Society, T.A. Reamy, did not even know that menstruation can occur only if the ovaries are functioning. He observed with surprise that in his experience of 144 cases of bilateral removal of the ovaries, menstruation had ceased within six months in every case. Even in 1975 the *Columbia Encyclopedia* informs us cautiously that removal of the ovaries *may* result in loss of periods. Many years later surgeons were removing thyroids, adrenals, thymuses and tonsils without any idea of their function.

One of the first experimental demonstrations of the existence of a hormone in the ovary was in 1896 by Emil Knauer, who demonstrated that secondary sexual characteristics developed after ovaries were transplanted into immature and castrated animals. In 1900 the experiment was repeated by Josef von Halben with the same result. Virtually nothing else was discovered in the subject until 1917. There was little impetus or desire to learn more about women. The powerful underlying mystery and source of fear was menstruation and this seldom evoked desire for more knowledge.

Folktales about menstruation were still common, many connected to the moon. Some believed that the foetus was made from menstrual blood. Some toyed with these ideas even while aware of the theories, for example that of John Power who was the first to suggest, in 1831, that ovulation and menstruation might be connected. In the first part of the nineteenth century it was generally believed that the menstrual flow came from an excess of nutrient and that human eggs, like those of rabbits, left the ovary only as a result of sexual intercourse.

In 1845 Adam Raciborski discovered that eggs were ejected spontaneously and in 1861 Eduard Pflüger showed that menstruation did not take place in women whose ovaries had been removed. Slowly menstruation was becoming a subject for scientific study. But it seems that these discoveries stirred up something stronger than logic and observable truth.

In 1840 John Elliotson wrote in the fifth edition of his *Human Physiology*, 'To regard women during menstruation as unclean is certainly very useful.' And he noted, 'In this country, it is firmly believed by many that meat will not take salt if the process is conducted by a menstruating woman.' He does not comment on this.

In 1841 Dr William Acton, a doctor who specialised in sexuality, published his first book, *A Practical Treatise on Diseases of the Urinary and Generative Organs in Both Sexes*. It sold widely and, perhaps more than any other book, expressed the attitude of the Victorian age towards middle-class women. The book was to have three further editions before the author's death in 1875. Sir James Paget, one of the most distinguished of Victorian doctors, wrote of Acton that 'he practised honorably in the most dangerous of specialties'.

Colombat d'Isère held much the same views. He advised removing girls from school when they approached the age of puberty so that a constant watch could be kept over them. He insisted that they should not read 'highly-wrought romances' and should avoid frequent visits to the theatre.

> Those powerful exciting agents, and still more frequently, the violent intimacies formed at boarding school, tear the veil of modesty, and destroy, forever, the seductive innocence which is the most charming ornament of a young girl. Endowed with an organization eminently impressionable, she soon contracts improper habits, and constantly tormented by an amorous melancholy, becomes sad, dreamy, sentimental and languishing. Like a delicate plant, withered by the rays of a burning sun, she fades and dies under the influence of a poisoned breath. The desire for happiness and love, so sweet and attractive in their native truth, are in her converted into a devouring flame, and onanism, that execrable and fatal evil, soon destroys her beauty,

impairs her health and conducts her almost always to a premature grave!*

In the same year as Barnes delivered his lectures, 1873, Edward Clarke of Harvard College published his influential little book, *Sex in Education*. He was by far the most influential of those who believed that menstruation was essentially disabling. He was in an influential position, being a professor of materia medica at Harvard and a fellow of the American Academy of Arts and Sciences. He argued that higher education was already destroying the reproductive functions of American women by overworking them at a critical time in their physiological development. Although women had a right to do anything of which they were physically capable, he insisted that they could not retain their good health if they were educated on the pattern and model of men. This was because at puberty they need all their strength for that and because they were incapacitated by menstruation. Women were now ruining their health by studying. Clarke thought they were already so unhealthy that they would soon be unable to reproduce at all. The population would be depleted within fifty years so that 'the wives who are to be mothers in our republic must be drawn from trans-Atlantic homes'. The author continually reveals his own anxiety.

Many physicians followed Clarke and supported and expanded his views. Some were even more extreme in their condemnation of women's education or in their insistence on the basic sickness of women. In 1877 Lawson Tait, one of Britain's leading surgeons, entered the argument and was strongly in favour of treating women as invalids. Tait was normally pragmatic and commonsensical. He must have known that most young girls experience 'curse pains' during the early years of menstruation, yet he argued in 1877 in his *Diseases of Women* that if there was pain, the girl should be removed from school and that 'for six months, all instruction, especially in music, should cease.' Music, he says, was responsible for 'a great deal of menstrual mischief'. It was 'especially hurtful' because it is 'a strong excitant to the emotions'. He believed that treating girls the same when menstruating as at other times and not making them rest caused 'serious disease in young ladies'. The sufferer from pain should be confined to bed for several days before and after the period. Another gynaecologist insisted that over-stimulation of the female brain caused stunted growth, nervousness, headaches, neuralgia, difficult childbirth, hysteria, inflammation of the brain, and insanity.

* D'Isère, op. cit.

These comments show how, during the late nineteenth century, menstruation came to be regarded more and more as incapacitating. The theories concerning its abnormal nature were reinforced by new scientific discoveries. For example, Raciborski's discovery in 1845 that eggs were ejected spontaneously produced new warnings of dangers to women and injunctions on behaviour that might influence the process of ovulation.

There was an increasing *rapprochement* between gynaecologists and psychiatrists and both were deeply involved in mapping out the dangers that awaited females, many of both kinds of doctor being convinced of the truth of Clarke's theories. These were propagated by Britain's leading psychiatrist, Henry Maudsley, who in 1874 published his *Sex in Mind and Education*. Maudsley used Clarke's theories as a 'scientific' basis for his anti-feminism and supported the theory that menstruation was an absolute bar to higher education.

Maudsley had an influence on British psychiatry which still prevails. He and Clarke were not producing new theories. They were merely publicising the new 'scientific' evidence for prejudices and demonstrating how scientific knowledge reflects rather than determines the moral biases of an era.

Feminists were appalled by what was happening and especially by the likely effects of Clarke's published views that education had already seriously damaged future mothers. But these women were also, inevitably, influenced by these views. It was impossible to escape the Victorian climate of opinion about women and even dedicated feminists found it hard to believe that virtually the whole of society, including the entire medical profession, was wrong about the dangers that awaited women who were active during menstruation or who tried to do things hitherto reserved for men. They tended to think that men were exaggerating rather than inventing the truth and many of them tried to tread carefully so as not to arouse even more opposition and antagonism.* Looking back later in life, M. Carey Thomas, the first president of Bryn Mawr College, reminiscing in 1908, recalled:

> We did not know when we began whether women's health could stand the strain of college education. We were haunted in those days by the clanging chains of that gloomy little specter, Dr Edward H. Clarke's 'Sex in Education'. With trepidation of spirit I made my mother read it, and was much cheered by her remark that, as neither she nor any of the

---

* Marion Harland wrote a tactful reply to Clarke.

women she knew, had ever seen girls or women of the kind described in Dr Clarke's book, we might as well act as if they did not exist.*

In England there was discussion about Clarke's theories. New educationalists and progressive doctors, who were most closely involved in promoting the education of young girls, were deeply disturbed. In 1874, the *Westminster Review* argued that it was nonsense. Britain's first woman doctor, Elizabeth Garrett Anderson, wrote a sharp reply to Maudsley. She questioned whether menstruation was really such an incapacitating affliction as he suggested and said that the idea was 'entirely contradicted by experience'. Emily Davies, struggling to establish Girton College as an institution of higher learning, felt that doctors were being backward and unreasonable. Frances Buss, an experienced educationalist, wrote 'Girton suffers from the determined opposition of medical men. As for me I scarcely expect anything else if a medical opinion is asked in the case of any girl. The smallest ailment always proceeds from brainwork (!!!) never from neglected conditions of health, from too many parties, etc.'† But there was little change in attitudes. It suited society and the doctors to regard middle-class women as patients rather than normal people. Meanwhile the number of doctors was growing. In England and Wales between 1861 and 1891 their numbers increased by fifty-three per cent, from 17,300 to 26,000.§ Dr Mary Putnam Jacobi wrote in 1895, 'I think, finally, it is in the increased attention paid to women, and especially in their new function as lucrative patients, scarcely imagined a hundred years ago, that we find explanation for much of the ill-health among women, freshly discovered today . . .'

Such observations were rare and brave. It is difficult to find texts that in any way criticise the prevailing views. Elizabeth Garrett Anderson argued against the idea that women were invalids.** Mary Livermore, a women's suffrage worker,‡ spoke against 'the monstrous assumption that woman is a natural invalid' and denounced 'the unclean army of "gyneacologists" who seem desirous to convince women that they possess but one set of organs – and these are always diseased.'

Among those who cared for psychiatric patients, a few recognised that the intellectual and vocational limitations of the female role, especially in the middle classes, made women just as mad as the role's

---

* William O'Neill (ed.): *The Woman Movement*, London, 1969.
† Quoted in Bennett, 1990, p. 156.
§ Census finding quoted in Booth's *Life and Labour*, vol. 8.
** *Westminster Review*, 1874.
‡ Quoted in Ehrenreich & English, *Complaints and Disorders*, p. 25.

biology. They lamented the absence of serious and absorbing exercise for 'females of the middle and higher ranks' who, 'have no strong motives to exertion ... no interests that call forth their mental energies.'* Another agreed that feminine vulnerability to insanity was caused by constitutional weakness, but felt it was also due to women's 'imperfect and vicious education'. The pioneering psychiatrist John Conolly also found 'the condition of the female mind' deplorable, even in the highest classes, 'the few accomplishments possessed by them have been taught for display in society, and not for solace in quieter hours'. Since their education provided them with so little of the self-discipline and inner resources psychiatrists deemed essential for the individual's struggle against moral insanity, women were seen as poor mental risks.

Silas Weir Mitchell, the American doctor who invented the 'rest' treatment wrote a number of novels in which sick women were portrayed in a hostile light. Like many others, Mitchell believed that sickness in women developed if they refused to behave as women should and shirked their feminine duties. The idea was widespread that women became sick if they ceased to be submissive and selfless or were aggressive, intellectual, sexual or ambitious. Some literary observers, such as James Fenimore Cooper in *Gleanings in Europe*, and Nathaniel Hawthorne in *Our Old Home*, were appalled at the delicate health of American women. Catherine Beecher took as her chief concern in later life 'the *health of women and children*', which, she wrote in 1866, had become 'a matter of alarming interest to all'. In *Physiology and Calisthenics* she had already written 'there is a delicacy of constitution and an increase of disease, both among mature women and young girls, that is most alarming, and such as was never known in any former period.' In her *Letters to the People on Health* she attempted to back up this view with statistics. She described how she asked all the women she knew to make a list of the ten women they knew best and to rate their health as 'perfectly healthy', 'well', 'delicate', 'sick', 'invalid' and so on. The results suggested to her that most women of her class in America *were* ill. One of her friends wrote to her that among all her women acquaintances in the city of Milwaukee she did 'not know one perfectly healthy woman in the place'. Beecher held the traditional view that they were sick *because they were women*, and that 'female complaints' and nervous disorders were linked with malfunctioning of the female sex organs.

Were there really so many invalids, and, if so, what was the matter with them?

* Rev William Moseley.

There is no doubt that there was much illness, both physical and psychological, in women of all classes on both sides of the Atlantic, though it is impossible to know how much. Epidemics and infections due to insanitary living conditions were commoner in the lower classes in the towns but were by no means confined to them. Fear of the lower orders as contaminating bearers of disease was common in Victorian England. Venereal disease was common, but no one knows how common. Both syphilis and gonorrhoea were rampant in the armed forces and among prostitutes and led to the controversial Contagious Diseases Acts of 1864, 1866 and 1869 which made inspection for disease compulsory for prostitutes. The authorities were worried about the spread and cost of venereal disease in the armed forces. The public reacted variously. There was great fear of it, which led to the coining of the word 'syphilophobia'. There was a widespread form of hypochondria known as syphilis imaginaria. As is usual with what is greatly feared, the subject also provoked levity and a lighthearted attitude, as in this limerick.*

> There was an old party of Fife,
> Who suspected a clap in his wife,
> So he bought an injection
> To cure the infection,
> Which gave him a stricture for life.

Tuberculosis was common but before 1882, when Koch discovered the bacillus responsible for it, it was often difficult to diagnose. Pulmonary tuberculosis, affecting the lungs, was in many ways revered as an ethereal illness becoming to delicate and sensitive females. Among many others, it had already taken the lives of Keats, the three eldest and the three youngest Brontës. Charlotte Brontë, the middle child in the family, probably died of excessive vomiting in pregnancy, a condition known as hyperemesis gravidarum, although her death certificate gave 'Phisis' (sic) as the sole cause of death.† Mrs Gaskell's account of Charlotte's last illness is a classical description of hyperemesis gravidarum and does not suggest that she had tuberculosis. Tuberculosis had also infected Elizabeth Barrett Browning.§

Because of the difficulties of identifying it in many cases, it was often missed or else diagnosed where it did not exist. Sometimes it was difficult to distinguish from other, less specific, disorders which were predominantly middle-class female conditions and were often held to

* Quoted in Ronald Pearsall's *The Worm in the Bud*, London, 1969, p. 228.
† See Winifred Guerin: *Charlotte Brontë: the Evolution of Genius*, Oxford, 1967, p. 566.
§ Peter Dally: *Elizabeth Barrett Browning: A Psychological Study*, Macmillan, 1989.

be caused or controlled by the sexual organs. These disorders were chlorosis, hysteria and, later in the century, neurasthenia. All these were to some extent interchangeable and often overlapped. We see similar patterns today in such conditions as anorexia nervosa, certain forms of anxiety and 'depression', and the many different forms of hysteria, some of them sophisticated and subtle.

Chlorosis was believed to be a form of anaemia and was named because of the greenish tinge it was alleged to give the skin. There is a chapter on the subject in Allbutt's textbook *A System of Medicine*, 1905, giving the accepted medical beliefs of the previous half century. Allbutt says that chlorosis is a 'malady of young women, and primarily of young women at or about the age of puberty . . . consisting in defect of the red corpuscles of the blood, a defect partly of numbers, chiefly of haemoglobin; the plasma being constant or even enriched.' It seems to be distinguished from iron-deficiency anaemia only in the age and sex of the patients (girls between fourteen and twenty-five) and by the fact that they gave vivid descriptions of other symptoms.

To diagnose anaemia accurately it is necessary to measure the number and size of red blood cells (corpuscles) and the amount of haemoglobin (the substance that makes blood red and which carries the oxygen) they carry. The first satisfactory attempt to determine the number of corpuscles in a cubic millimetre of blood had been in 1852 and an instrument for measuring haemoglobin was not invented till 1875.* Before 1870 virtually no blood tests were done, so it was impossible to see the 'blood picture'. After 1870, richer patients often had blood tests but others were still diagnosed without. The diagnosis was often made because of the symptoms, gender and age of the patient. Some women diagnosed themselves and were given home cures. Many adolescents diagnosed themselves: 'I think my blood must be out of order' or 'My friends say I am pale'.

Beliefs varied about the causes of chlorosis. It was often believed to be threefold – environmental, constitutional and moral – with the emphasis on whichever suited a particular doctor's beliefs. Many factors were blamed – living in dark, badly ventilated or poorly lit rooms, poor diet, excessive study, lack of exercise, derangement of the menstrual function, 'impoverished blood', 'disease of the nervous system', 'a morbid condition of the organs of generation', the result of masturbation. Mothers were urged to watch 'unobtrusively' and to leave the girl alone as seldom as possible. Menstruation was always implicated in one way or another. Allbutt advised that in looking for

* Charles Singer: *A Short History of Medicine*, 2nd edn., OUP, 1962.

the cause of chlorosis, 'if epithelial debris be found repeatedly in the urine, masturbation must not be forgotten, and corroborative evidence of the habit . . . detected.'

Those who wrote on the subject of chlorosis, as on so many other topics concerning chiefly women, tended not to distinguish between the sick and the well. The process of diagnosis was complicated by the fact that the pale, enervated girl was the ideal of the time. One researcher in Cambridge* claimed that chlorosis correlated with high fertility, attractiveness and perhaps with the best potential mothers. He asserted that while the 'lips and ears' of a chlorotic girl might be 'pallid', her cheeks were not and her face remained a 'pretty pink and white colour' because her blood vessels were so 'well-filled'. In 1889, Lawson Tait called it 'the anaemia of good-looking girls'. The chlorotic girl was simultaneously 'diseased, fertile and attractive'. It is not surprising that many people today have the idea that chlorosis and its history were no more than fantasy satisfying the prejudices of aging male doctors.

Yet chlorosis was one of the most prominent diseases of the nineteenth century. It was said also to be common in working-class girls, but this may well have been straight iron-deficiency anaemia. As one would expect with a fantasy disease, it simply disappeared. Between 1897 and 1906 at Massachusetts General Hospital, cases declined by ninety per cent.† No one thinks its disappearance was due to medical treatment. The change may have been due to improved nutrition, decline of the prejudice against eating meat, abandonment of corsets and tight-lacing, and an increase in physical activity in young women. The causes may be much deeper.

Hysteria is traditionally a disease or condition of women and the name derives from the Greek word for 'womb', though the condition has long been known to be psychological. Its manifestations change from age to age and from place to place. There is always purposeful over-reaction and often the conversion of unsatisfied desires or internal conflicts into physical symptoms. The patient is seldom consciously aware of what is happening and is deeply resentful if this is pointed out. The symptoms often imitate what the sufferer believes to be 'real'. To give an example, most people who develop hysterical anaesthesia lose the sense of feeling from the tip of the limb in a 'glove-and-stocking' pattern. Loss of sensation in this pattern does not correspond with damage or disease in any nerve and so reveals the diagnosis to the physician. But if a doctor develops hysterical loss of

* Jones, 1897.
† W.M. Fowler: 'Chlorosis – An Obituary', *Annals of Medical History*, 8, 1936, p. 168.

feeling, it is likely to be along the pathway of a particular nerve whose course through the body he learned about in his anatomy classes.

In Victorian times hysteria took the form of 'fits' or paralysis much more frequently than it does today. At that time the diagnosis of various forms of fits and paralysis was not as certain or as sophisticated as today and doctors were more often deceived. The fact that there was often considerable difficulty in distinguishing the symptoms from those of physical disease undoubtedly encouraged the form the attacks took and suggests that many women were eager to be ill and become patients. It may also be that doctors encouraged the development of certain forms of hysteria. For example, Jean-Martin Charcot at the Salpêtrière Hospital in Paris used to give demonstrations of hysterical fits in young women who could apparently produce them to order.*

Hysteria affects men too. For example, it is common under battle conditions. However in women, like chlorosis, it tends to develop characteristics regarded as desirable. Fainting, giggling, displays of emotion and the rapid change from one state of mind to another are still regarded as typically feminine and this was even more true in the nineteenth century. Edward Tilt, writer of textbooks about women, noted in 1881, 'mutability is characteristic of hysteria – *La donna è mobile.*' Against a background of widespread convictions about inherent female invalidism and lack of opportunity for interesting activity, Victorian women may have been more 'hysterical' than women in previous or later generations.

The distinguished psychiatrist E. Kraepelin (1856-1926) believed that seventy per cent of all women were hysterical. There were differences of opinion about the causes. Some, such as Robert Brudenell, saw that social pressures increased the tendency to hysteria in some women. As we have seen earlier in this chapter, most thought it was due to physical disease of the reproductive organs or at least to their inherent derangement.

The other condition that was diagnosed frequently in women towards the end of the nineteenth century and which overlapped with others was 'neurasthenia', meaning nerve weakness. The new science of neurology was becoming organised so it is not surprising that 'nerve weakness' should have become a recognised illness. This was originally an American condition, first described in *American Nervousness* by George Beard in 1868. As long as it remained in America it affected men as well as women. Beard thought it was a functional nervous

---

* It was these demonstrations that started the young Sigmund Freud's interest in hysteria, which led ultimately to the development of psychoanalysis and to a greater understanding of hysteria.

disorder, meaning that it had no organic basis. Nevertheless, Beard's fantasies about the disease were physical and he applied the now traditional concepts about conservation of energy to his ideas about nerves. He believed that the nervous system contained a fixed amount of energy and that any expenditure in one direction left less energy for other activity. He listed more than fifty symptoms of neurasthenia, including paralysis, convulsions, crying fits, tiredness, indigestion, vomiting, loss of appetite, morbid fears, inability to concentrate, sense of hopelessness and temporary blindness. He noted that it was a 'disease of the comfortable classes'. Many of these would seem, by our standards, to be hysterical. Beard, and others after him, tried to make the distinction. The descriptions and their variations are complex and seem related to the idea that symptoms have different meanings according to sex and social class. Neurasthenia was regarded as more masculine and sensible than hysteria. Later Freud equated it with hypochondria.

Beard related neurasthenia to the pressures in society that led to or encouraged the illness. He wrote that it occurred most often in 'civilised intellectual communities' as 'part of the compensation for our progress and refinement'. He described five factors that he believed accounted for its rise: steam power, the telegraph, science, the press and an increase of mental activity in women. Neurasthenic illness was the result of these stresses acting on 'nervous, civilised' people. Weir Mitchell, another famous neurologist, described sufferers as being 'of good position in society . . . just the kind of women one likes to meet with − sensible, not oversensitive or emotional, exhibiting a proper amount of illness . . . and a willingness to perform their share of work quietly and to the best of their ability.' Neurasthenia was often associated with the 'new woman' as well as with the traditional Victorian woman. Dr Margaret Cleaves suffered from it and, in her autobiography, attributed it to unfulfilled desires and ambitions.*

Neurasthenia was definitely more respectable than hysteria or even chlorosis. It was, however, part of the same group of symptoms in different degrees. Virginia Woolf was diagnosed as suffering from neurasthenia and so were Alice James (sister of William and Henry), and Charlotte Perkins Gilman. The latter wrote a novel, *The Yellow Wallpaper*, 1892, which described her 'rest treatment' and the appalling effects it had on her.

Alcott, a noted Boston physician and author of several books on

* Dr Margaret Cleaves: *Autobiography of a Neurasthene*, 1886.

women's health, estimated that one half of American women suffered from the 'real disease' of nervousness. Psychiatrists, neurologists and gynaecologists were all treating different, or sometimes the same, aspects of the same conditions, and all with the prevailing preconceptions about femininity and what women should be like.* In London the Professor of Obstetric Medicine at King's College Hospital had a private nursing home where he treated nervous diseases, about which he wrote a book.† Tuke's famous dictionary, 1892, states in an entry contributed by Robert Barnes.

> The correlation of the sexual functions and nervous phenomena in the female are too common and too striking not to have attracted attention at all times; but it may be confidently affirmed, that it is only within quite recent years that we have had adequate knowledge to enable us to discuss the problems arising out of these relations with scientific precision. Gynaecology, and our knowledge of the anatomy and physiology of the nervous system have advanced . . . so that now we have the clearer and reciprocal light shed by better knowledge.

There was also much straight gynaecological disease. Much of it was due to venereal disease or to the effects of childbirth. The numbers of mothers dying in childbirth did not change significantly until the 1930s. For every death, many were left sick or disabled. Most of these, if they were to be helped at all, needed not 'nerve' treatment but direct gynaecological intervention.

What did women think about it and how did they react? We know, for instance, the difference in feeling about a 'real' and a 'nervous' complaint was already apparent. In 1866 Alice James first became ill with various 'nervous' complaints and later admitted that thereafter she 'longed and longed for some palpable disease, no matter how dreadful a label it might have'. In 1891 she developed the breast cancer that was going to kill her. She expressed pleasure and wrote in her diary that her aspirations had been 'brilliantly fulfilled'. In the next chapter we shall see how women, both real and fictional, saw themselves and how this related to their health and diseases.

---

* See, for example, Andrew T. Scull ed.: *Madhouses, Mad-doctors, and Madmen: The Social History of Psychiatry in the Victorian Era*, Athlone Press, London, 1981.
† W.S. Playfair: *The Systematic Treatment of Nerve Prostration and Hysteria*, Henry Lee, Philadelphia, 1883.

# VII

# WOMEN'S VIEWS ABOUT THEIR LIVES

Before looking in greater detail at the treatment given to women with illnesses – real and imaginary – it seems appropriate to meet a few more patients. We have seen some of the illnesses and complaints from which they suffered and the general attitudes of the doctors towards them, or at least, the attitudes of the doctors who wrote textbooks and tracts. But were so many women sick and did they view themselves as such?

There are difficulties in finding answers to these questions from the women themselves. Evidence is hard to find, particularly for the countless middle-class women who may have been the most affected by the climate of opinion about their allegedly precarious state of health. Even more, we lack evidence from the working class. It was an age when many women kept diaries and journals and wrote large numbers of letters, yet relatively few have survived. All too often the everyday lives of women were regarded as unimportant and the documents thrown away. Even those whose records survive seldom described their intimate feelings about their health, particularly their gynaecological problems, or even referred to these obliquely, with euphemisms. If they recorded such medical events it was likely to be in a letter to a sister or a close friend and was unlikely to survive. If these accounts did survive and the woman was deemed sufficiently interesting and important to have her correspondence and diaries published, editors often omitted the medical details and it would take several lifetimes to track down the omissions. There has long been a feeling among literary and 'arts' people that medical subjects are not interesting, not quite nice, to be despised and certainly not written about or published. Such feelings still exist despite the recent greatly increased interest in medicine and medical history and the recognition of the enormous influence that disease has had on history. Many records of sickness and treatment in the past, even if they were made and have survived, undoubtedly lie buried among papers in many different countries.

The element of chance and luck that are needed for us to possess such material is exemplified in the case of Fanny Burney. Her detailed account of her mastectomy operation in 1811,* which must be one of the most remarkable in the history of medicine, has survived. She wrote it in the middle of the Napoleonic wars in a letter to her sister in England. In 1811 Fanny, then Madame d'Arblay and aged fifty-nine, was living in Paris where she endured a mastectomy for cancer of her right breast. The operation was performed by Napoleon's surgeon, Dominique-Jean Larrey, just before he left for the Russian campaign, during which, at the Battle of Borodino, he amputated 200 limbs in twenty-four hours. The other surgeon was Dubois, surgeon to the Empress. The operation lasted for twenty-five minutes, Fanny was fully conscious throughout and the whole procedure was conducted in silence. A cambric handkerchief was placed over her face but it was so transparent that she could see everything through it. She reported that Larrey's face was ashen grey throughout. Fanny describes her experiences so vividly that a reader can feel with her through the whole gruesome procedure.

She begins by describing the development of the cancer during the previous year, her reactions to it and those of her husband and her woman friend. She mentions pain, which is unusual in the early stages of the condition, but she does not mention a lump, which is usually the first thing to be noticed.

> About August, in the year 1810, I began to be annoyed by a small pain in my breast, which went on augmenting from week to week, yet being rather heavy than acute, without causing me any uneasiness with respect to consequences: Alas, 'what was ignorance?' The most sympathising of Partners, however, was more disturbed: not a start, not a wry face, not a movement that indicated pain was unobserved, & hoped, by care and warmth, to make all succour unnecessary. Thus passed some months, during which Madame de Maisonneuve, my particularly intimate friend, joined M. d'Arblay to press me to consent to an examination. I thought their fears groundless, and could not make so great a conquest over my repugnance.

The growth became worse until 'All hope of escaping this evil being now at end, I could console or employ my Mind in considering

---

* *The Diary of Fanny Burney,* Everyman Edition, 1956.

how to render it less dreadful'. She consulted with surgeons. They diagnosed cancer and advised surgery. Initially Fanny had consulted Monsieur Dubois, but he was too busy with his royal patient to take on the full responsibility for Fanny's operation and, while remaining involved, passed her on to his colleague, Larrey. He also warned her to prepare for great suffering. She wrote:

> M. Dubois had pronounced 'il faut s'attendre a souffrir, Je ne veux pas vous tromper – Vous souffrirez – vous souffrirez *beaucoup*!' – M. Ribe had *charged* me to cry! to withold or restrain myself might have seriously bad consequences, he said. M. Moreau, in echoing this injunction, enquired whether I had cried or screamed at the birth of Alexander [her only child, born in 1794] – Alas, I told him, it had not been possible to do otherwise; Oh, then, he answered, there is no fear! – What terrible inferences were here to be drawn! I desired, therefore, that M. d'A. [her husband] might be kept in ignorance of the day till the operation should be over. To this they all agreed, except M. Larrey, with high approbation: . . . I obtained with difficulty a promise of 4 hours warning, which were essential to me for sundry regulations. From that time I assumed my best spirits *to meet the coming blow*; – & support my too sympathising Partner.

The operation was to be done in her own house. There was nothing unusual about this. It was the custom then and for many years afterwards. If the operation was done in hospital, it was often done on the bed in the ward or else the patient sat in an armchair in the middle of the ward. Since the extreme pain of an operation without an anaesthetic nearly always led to screaming and struggling, one wonders how the other patients felt when they saw it.

But although she was to be in her own house for the operation, Fanny complained that the doctors 'let me make no preparations, refusing to inform me what would be necessary'. When one thinks of the preparations made today even for a home birth, this seems remarkable. Was it an attempt to allay her anxiety? If so, it must have increased it. While waiting for something dreadful to happen, it helps to have something useful to do. Was the doctors' dismissal of her offer an assertion of their own mystique and power? Was it simple thoughtless custom, perhaps derived from their assumption of superiority? Was there some other reason?

When the day arrived, Fanny was given only two hours' warning. 'Dr Moreau instantly entered my room, to see if I were alive.' So little warning would be unheard of in these days when patients are understandably upset when given only a few days' notice. Then Dr Moreau did something which no surgeon would do today: 'He gave me wine and cordial & went to the salon.' Today's patients do not undergo operations in the 'salon' and are not fed just before operations because of the danger of vomiting under anaesthetic.

Fanny rang for her maid and nurse but before she could speak to them, her room 'was entered by seven men in black'. These were the doctors. She became agitated. 'I was now awakened from my stupor – & by a sort of indignation – why so many? & without leave? – But I could not utter a syllable.'

One is reminded here of the lady governors' objections to Sims operating in front of large numbers of spectators and their limiting the number of spectators to fifteen. A hospital operating theatre used for teaching purposes was likely even then to have a tiered gallery for spectators and could accommodate several dozen people but in her own salon when she was to remain awake throughout, seven men must have seemed intrusive. Fanny goes on to describe the preparations for the operation. 'M. Dubois acted as Commander in Chief. Dr Larry [sic] kept out of sight.'

The likely reason that Dr Larrey 'kept out of sight' soon became apparent. He had previously assured her that she would sit in an armchair during the operation but now:

> M. Dubois ordered a Bed stead [sic] into the middle of the room. Astonished, I turned to M. Larry . . . but he hung his head & [sic] would not look at me. Two *old mattresses* M. Dubois then demanded, & an old sheet. I now began to tremble violently, more with distaste and horrour [sic] of [the] preparations even than of the pain. These arranged to his liking, he desired me to mount the Bed stead. I stood suspended, for a moment, whether I should not abruptly escape – I looked at the door, the windows – I felt desperate – but it was only for a moment, my reason then took command, & my fears and feeling struggled vainly against it. I called to my maid – she was crying, & the two nurses stood transfixed at the door. Let those women all go! cried M. Dubois.

Fanny reacted badly when she heard this order, which, she says 'recovered me my voice'. She then had a disagreement with the autocratic doctor. She seems to have felt a need to resist, to impose something of herself on to the situation rather than be totally passive and at the mercy of the surgeons.

> No, I cried, let them stay! 'qu'elles restent!' This occasioned a little dispute that re-animated me – The Maid, however, & one of the nurses ran off – I charged the other to approach, & she obeyed. M. Dubois now tried to issue his commands en militaire, but I resisted all that was resistable.

She was made to remove her dressing gown, though she had

intended to keep it on. She thought of her sisters, of whom she had many, but 'not one, at so dreadful an instant to protect – adjust – guard me'. She regretted that she had refused the aid of several French women friends. She now had to face the operation on her own.

> I mounted, therefore, unbidden, the Bed stead – and M. Dubois placed me upon the mattress, and spread a cambric handkechief upon my face. It was transparent however, & I saw through it that the Bed stead was instantly surrounded by the men & my nurse, I refused to be held; but when, bright through the cambric, I saw the glitter of polished Steel – I closed my Eyes. I would not trust to convulsive fear the sight of the terrible incision. A silence the most profound ensued, which lasted for some minutes, during which, I imagine, they took their orders by signs, and made their examination – Oh what horrible suspension! – I did not breathe – & M. Dubois tried vainly to find any pulse. This pause, at length was broken by Dr Larrey, who, in a voice [of] solemn melancholy, said 'qui me tiendra ce sein?'* – no one answered; at least not verbally.

Here Fanny conveys her sense of utter rejection. The pause, the silence when no one answered 'aroused' her from her 'passively submissive state', for she 'feared they imagined the whole breast infected'.

> . . . feared it too justly, – for again, through the Cambric, I saw the hand of M. Dubois held up, while his forefinger first described a straight line from top to bottom of the breast, secondly a Cross & thirdly a circle: intimating that the whole was to be taken off.

Her response to this was agitation, leading to protest and action. Again, Fanny's urge to be somehow or at least in part in control of herself and her body is evident. She even offered to hold her breast herself to keep it still while the surgeon operated.

> I started up, threw off my veil, &, in answer to the demand 'Qui me tiendra ce sein' cried 'C'est moi, Monsieur!' ['I will, Sir'] & I held my hand under it, and explained the nature of my sufferings, which all sprang from one point, though they darted into every part.

But the surgeons were in no mood to listen to her or to accept her participation. Probably they were disturbed themselves. Before the days of anaesthetics, many surgeons were agitated and upset by the frightful things they felt obliged to do. Fanny's surgeons 'heard attentively' what she was saying, but 'in utter silence'. M. Dubois then 'replaced' her as before, '&, as before spread my veil over my face.'
Fanny realised that her outburst had been in vain.

* 'Who will support this breast for me?'

Immediately again I saw the fatal finger describe the Cross – and the circle – Hopeless, then, desperate, & self-given up, I closed once more my eyes, relinquishing all watching, all resistance, all interference, and sadly resolute to be wholly resigned.

Fanny had already suffered grievously, at least emotionally, yet the operation had not yet even begun. There is a stark contrast between the way she was prepared for the operation and today's smooth 'pre-medication', through which the patient scarcely knows that anything is happening. There is no record that Fanny was even given alcohol or opium to dull the pain.

Her eventual resolution to be 'wholly resigned' was, she recalls thankfully, 'firmly adhered to, in defiance of a terror that surpasses all description, & the most torturing pain' as the operation began.

> . . . when the dreadful steel was plunged into the breast – cutting through veins – arteries – flesh – nerves – I needed no injunctions not to restrain my cries. I began a scream that lasted unintermittingly [sic] during the whole time of the incision – & I almost marvel that it rings not in my Ears still! so excruciating was the agony. When the wound was made, & the instrument was withdrawn, the pain seemed undiminished, for the air that suddenly rushed into those delicate parts felt like a mass of minute but sharp & forked poignards, that were tearing at the edges of the wound, but when I felt again the instrument . . . I thought I must have expired, I attempted no more to open my Eyes – they felt as if hermetically shut, & so firmly closed, that the Eyelids seemed indented to the Cheeks . . .

At this point she thought that the operation was over, but she was wrong. The surgeons still had to remove the bits of the cancer left behind and make sure that none further was left.

> Oh no! presently the terrible cutting was renewed – & worse than ever, to separate the bottom, the foundation of this dreadful gland from the parts to which it adhered – Again all description would be baffled – yet again all was not over . . . and oh Heaven! – I then felt the Knife [rack]ling against the breast bone – scraping it! – This performed, while I lay in utterly speechless torture, I heard the Voice of Mr Larry, – (all others guarded a dead silence) in a tone nearly tragic, desire every one present to pronounce if any thing more remained to be done; The general voice was Yes – but the finger of Mr Dubois – which I literally *felt* elevated over the wound, though I saw nothing, & though he touched nothing, so indescribably sensitive was the spot – pointed to some further requisition – & again began the scraping! – and, after this, Dr. Moreau thought he discerned a peccant attom – and still, & still, M. Dubois demanded attom after attom – My dearest Esther, not for

Weeks, but for Months I could not speak of this terrible business without nearly again going through it! . . .

She seems to have been surprised, not at her own fortitude but at her exhaustion, which perhaps reveals something of what people were accustomed to enduring in the early nineteenth century.

When all was done, & they lifted me up that I might be put to bed, my strength was so totally annihilated, that I was obliged to be carried, & could not even sustain my hands and arms; which hung as if I had been lifeless; while my face, as the Nurse has told me, was utterly colourless. This removal made me open my Eyes – & then I saw my good Dr. Larry, pale nearly as myself, his face streaked with blood, & its expression depicting grief, apprehension, & almost horrour [sic].

Her diary is less explicit. In it Fanny refers simply to 'my then terrible situation; hovering over my head was the stiletto of a surgeon for a menace of cancer; yet, till that moment, hope of escape had always been held out to me by the Baron Larrey – hope which, from the reading of the fatal letter, became extinct.' The 'fatal letter', apparently the only one that reached her that year, told of the death of her old friend and landlord, Mr Locke. He had been best man at her wedding and had always been a great support to both Fanny and her husband. The diary suggests that she had hoped to have treatment for her cancer in England, with his support. It seems to have been characteristic of expatriates then, as it is today, to return home if they needed medical treatment for serious conditions. The diary tells us nothing more about the illness or the operation but it shows something of her situation and also how remarkable it is that the letter to her sister was written at all, then reached its recipient (long before the existence of a national postal service), and survived.

Dangers and difficulties of communication such as Fanny Burney encountered were not uncommon. Smaller everyday hazards must often have prevented records from being written at all. Despite this, occasional accounts of the lives and medical problems of women of more humble birth have come down to us, for example, the wife of Thomas Turner who seems to have died from cancer of the womb in the eighteenth century.* Many of the records found and studied so far have been of women in aristocratic, political and intellectual families. This was probably partly because these women tended to be more literate and so more likely to write things down (despite the undoubted fact that many aristocratic families traditionally disregarded formal education, especially for girls, as they still do today). They were also

* Thomas Turner: *The Diary of a Georgian Shopkeeper*, Oxford, 1979.

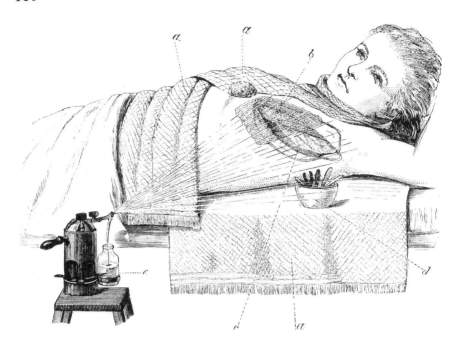

SOME SEVENTY YEARS AFTER FANNY BURNEY'S OPERATION, THE WOUND AFTER MASTECTOMY IS SPRAYED WITH CARBOLIC IN LISTER'S TECHNIQUE BEFORE APPLICATION OF THE DRESSINGS

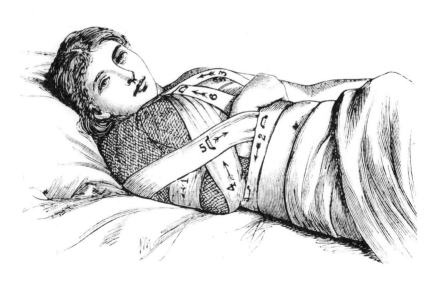

more likely to be well known, or to have well-known relatives and so be deemed to have interesting things to say about themselves or their relatives so that their papers were less likely to be destroyed. An example of this is Mary Gladstone, daughter of the prime minster, who thought her diary should be published, albeit selectively, because it recorded her father's political career and the part she had played in it.* Fanny Burney's editor† opens his introduction by saying that at her birth, 'it seemed highly unlikely that her diary, if she should take it into her head to keep one, would have any interest which arises from the fact that the author has enjoyed the familiar society of the great . . . Yet it is impossible to turn the pages of her diary without being struck by the profusion of great names with which they are studded.' The fact that some of these women believed they had interesting things to record may have motivated some of them to write. Women often, almost traditionally, feel that nothing they might say or contribute would be of interest or value to anyone else. Also, many of the privileged women lived in large houses that remained permanently in the family, with room to store papers and no need of the clearing out that is likely to occur with every move and death. Further, their papers may be kept safely by a family archivist or incorporated into a recognised collection. The historian Jalland explored the lives of women in more than fifty families involved in British politics from about 1860 to 1914, looking at family records, many of them unpublished. I am grateful to her for much of what follows. Most of her evidence comes from the correspondence and diaries of many of these women who were 'highly literate and self conscious even if not formally educated'. Jalland does not set out specifically to explore their medical experiences (except during childbirth, which is largely outside the scope of this book), but she gives us much information about them.

The first impression given by this and other relevant material is its diversity. In the nineteenth century, women were as different and varied in character, circumstances, upbringing and way of life as women are today. The idea that they were virtually all sick, or locked into the home, or uneducated, or anything else, is wrong. They were equally diverse in their experience of health and disease, childbirth and surgery. The women studied by Jalland led lives that were privileged, financially secure and, on the whole, interesting, being in touch with much that was going on in the corridors of power. Doubtless this tended to compensate, as it still does today, for the lack of individual

* P. Jalland: *Women, Marriage and Politics, 1860–1914*, Oxford, 1986, p. 5.
† *The Diary of Fanny Burney.*

professional occupation such as might have worried women with less interest in their lives. On the whole they were healthy. Certainly they did not often regard themselves as sick, though some of them were, and some of them, like women today, used sickness in order to control, improve or escape from aspects of their own lives. Invalidism, though it clearly existed amongst them, was rare, though sickness of some sort was common. For instance, Olive Maxse, daughter of Admiral Maxse, was very preoccupied with her health. She suffered from numerous unspecified illnesses and went on water cures to Germany. Her sister-in-law wrote to Olive's sister, Violet:

> [Olive] is in the state that if amused and interested she becomes perfectly well at once – if with family alone and bored – or with nothing much going on she gets ill at once and will do nothing . . . I know it is a very common form for girls hysteria to take – and the Drs say there need be no alarm – unless she is so bored as to fancy herself really ill – when she might create it. This makes it clear how *fatal* it is for her to be alone with us or your Mother.

Laura Tennant and Edith Balfour both spent the early months of each year at Bordighera on a doctor's advice as a cure for incessant headaches.* In 1885 Laura, soon to die in childbirth, wrote to her fiancé, Alfred Lyttelton:

> I saw the doctor today . . . He said I was tremendously below par – a thing doctors always say . . . and that I had no blood in my body and no pulse and no vitality – He said I had an ulcerated sore throat and that I was to drink port and tonic and put salt into my bath and never to get tired so that when I marry you may not have a little washed out bride whiter than a tablecloth.

How were women affected by the constant emphasis the doctors laid on their delicate constitutions and their inherent sickness? It must have had some effect. Certainly it directed many of the symptoms in 'nervous' disorders and it seemed to justify certain forms of illness. Some writers were sceptical about the increasing 'sickness' of women and indicated that they understood something of what was happening. In *Mary Barton*, Mrs Gaskell tells us that Mrs Carson 'was (as was usual with her, when no particular excitement was going on), very poorly and sitting upstairs in her dressing room, indulging in the luxury of a headache . . . the natural consequence of the state of mental and bodily idleness in which she was placed. Without education enough to value the resources of wealth and leisure, she was circumstanced as to command both.' George Eliot wrote in *Middle-*

* Quoted in Jalland, op. cit., p. 121.

*march*, 'Since she found opinions and intelligence an encumbrance, a wise girl like Rosamund Vincey got rid of them . . . In the process of trying to be what society expected she became unhealthy from lack of exercise and tight-lacing.' By the end of the century the situation was sometimes described more explicitly.

> The more expensive and the more obviously unproductive the women of the household are, the more creditable and more effective for the purpose of reputability of the household or its head will their life be. So much so that the women would have been required not only to afford evidence of a life of leisure, but *even to disable themselves from useful activity.** (My italics.)

It is clear that however much the doctors insisted on the essential sickness of middle-class women and however much they tried to extend the boundaries of disease, health was regarded as very important. As the century advanced, so did ideas about eugenics and 'healthy stock'. There was much discussion about whether those in ill-health had a right to marry and risk passing on their diseases to their children. Echoes of this have returned in modern discussions about 'genetic engineering' and the desirability of eliminating hereditary disease. In the nineteenth century those with diseases thought to be hereditary, like consumption, were advised not to marry, and women were urged not to marry invalids because they could not nurse them and provide for them. It was felt that no confirmed invalid woman should consent to marry, 'The man will naturally tire of being tied to a sickly and no doubt fretful life-companion, while she would suffer from neglect and was liable to leave her young children motherless.' Extreme invalidism was frequently associated with spinsterdom and it is interesting in each case to see and assess the connection between the two.

Some women enjoyed the invalid role and used it as a means to escape from boring chores, social obligations or continual child-bearing. Some found an interest in life by worshipping their doctors. One grateful patient wrote to her doctor, Weir Mitchell, 'Whilst laid by the heels in a country-house with an attack of grippe, also an invalid from gastric affection, the weary eyes of a sick woman fall upon your face in the *Century* of this month – a thrill passes through me – at last I saw the true physician!' Mitchell believed that a doctor, if he had mesmeric powers of will, could become almost godlike.† He used this as an argument against women doctors, saying that they would always

---

* Thorsten Veblen: *The Theory of the Leisure Class*, 1899.
† Burr.

be inferior to a male physician precisely because they could not exercise such tyranny and were unable to 'obtain the needed control over those of their own sex'. He increased his own power by allowing his patients to see no one but him and to talk over their ills and problems with no one else. He tried to cure his patients by restoring their femininity through subordinating them to an enlightened but dictatorial male will. He himself was small and puny, but many of his patients saw him as God. A few saw him as the Devil.

What did most women patients think of their doctors? Those whose records are the fullest or the most accessible were on the whole sophisticated and capable of critical appraisal. Alice James, who was an invalid for many years, saw through the pomposity of the society doctor, Sir Andrew Clark, and recorded it in her diary. Sir Andrew was a physician who looked after many prominent people in London, including Dr Elizabeth Garrett Anderson herself. He seems to have pleased many with his charm. Beatrice Webb (née Potter) wrote in *My Apprenticeship* that he was their 'beloved physician', but not everyone worshipped him. An American who had consulted him some years previously had told Alice James how the great doctor was two hours late for the appointment. As he entered the room and was announced, he immediately added jokingly 'the *late* Sir Andrew Clark'. Alice went to consult him herself, and while waiting for him she predicted to her cousin and friend that Sir Andrew would do the same as he had done with the American. She describes how, no sooner had she said this,

> When hark! the door opens and a florid gentleman enters, and the *late* Sir Andrew falls upon our ears, followed by the same burst of hilarious laughter rippling down to us, thro' all those years. Imagine the martyrdom of a pun which has become an integral portion of one's organism to be lugged through life like the convict's ball and chain. Do you suppose he vainly tries to escape it, or is he passive in its clutches or can it be possible that some memory of the joy still survives which irradiated his being, the first time he heard it fall from his lips in the springtime of his practice?*

Alice, who suffered from multiple complaints including 'neurasthenia', hated the condescension of doctors. She wrote in her diary, 'I suppose one has a greater sense of intellectual degradation after an interview with a doctor than from any human experience'.

In the group of women that she studied, Jalland found that overall the women's negative comments about their doctors outweighed the

* *The Diary of Alice James*, edited by Leon Edel, New York, Dodd, Mead, 1964.

positive and their dominant tone was sceptical. They examined and investigated their doctors before permitting treatment and they exchanged information with each other. They made it clear that they were employing the doctors and were seldom deferential towards them. They did not necessarily believe what they said, and did not hesitate to criticise if they felt like it. One of them referred to 'the not infrequent absurdities of medical advice' in the 1870s. If they thought a treatment had made them or their relatives worse, they told their friends. One described a particular doctor as 'untruthful and quacky', and another said that her daughter's medical treatment was 'abominably organised, wretchedly carried out, and tinged with so much that is ugly and incompetent and revolting.' Yet another said doctors 'normally have a way of fibbing to their patients', they 'think only of their pockets' and their numerous fatal mistakes were 'covered by the earth'. But they also praised doctors of whom they approved, for example, Lady Cowper in 1875 wrote, 'Comberbatch is very attentive and very clever about Chest. Reed *I* think very clever and very safe. Burrows is tip top, but more for kidney disease . . .'

Some doctors were as blunt with their patients as these women were about them. Lady Eileen Elliot, daughter of the Viceroy of India, had attacks of palpitations and feeling faint after her parents forbade her to see a man in whom she was interested. To the dismay of the family, the doctor soon discovered that Eileen had been drowning her sorrows in drink and drugs.

> Eileen has been living on sleeping draughts and stimulants. 2 nights out of every 3 she has taken draughts and also burgundy at luncheon and dinner – no wonder she felt faint. It accounts for everything – ill health, palpitations, hysteria and all.

Many young women, and some young men too, seem to have had some sort of crisis or breakdown, physical or mental, even if they went on to lead full lives. Young Beatrice Potter (later Webb) experienced both. She worried her family sufficiently for them to send her away to school in Bournemouth, where she worked hard on her religious problems. Such incidents are not uncommon today. In the nineteenth century, physical breakdown was probably commoner than it is today. Nowadays, no one is likely to have so many infectious diseases all together and treatment is much more effective. Also, many physical breakdowns in Victorian women were associated with dangerous childbirth, and mental breakdowns were often associated with spinsterdom. Both are rarer, and different, today.

Two of the biggest medical dangers before our own age were

infection and loss of blood. These were particularly likely to happen during childbirth and miscarriage because when the womb expels a foetus the lining is left raw, bleeding, and open to infection. Miscarriage was regarded as even more dangerous than childbirth because part of the placenta is often left behind and becomes a potentially dangerous source of bleeding and infection. Without blood transfusion or antibiotics such complications can become rapidly fatal and out of every thousand babies born alive, on average five mothers died, and this does not include the large number whose babies died too. It also does not include the many deaths where the death certificate gave as cause of death 'disease of the heart' or euphemisms such as 'nervous fever', without mentioning a recent birth. The worst disabling results of childbirth such as fistula, due to incompetent obstetrics, were uncommon in this group of women who could afford the best medical attention available. Nevertheless, Jalland found that the correspondence of pregnant women was 'full of fears and dangers' and there were 'endless sad stories' of women who had miscarriages and stillbirths, often repeated many times. For example, in 1879 Lady Edward Cavendish was 'dreadfully low' because she had 'just had her fourth dead child'.

Even if the sick mother survived, she might have to endure many months of illness or even permanent disability. In July 1886 Gladstone was defeated in the general election following his third period as prime minster. For the next two weeks the lives of his family were hectic, moving back to the family home near Chester with 'such heavy things to carry' and 'rearranging furniture'. Gladstone's daughter Mary, by now Mrs Drew and four-months pregnant, began to bleed.* She became steadily worse, with pain, sickness, bleeding and high temperature. On 29 August her condition seemed to have improved. Her doctor, Dr Burlingham, seemed pleased and gave the impression that it was all over, which it clearly was not. Mary's maid noted 'we have nearly lost my beloved Lady. On September 1st a wee boy was born dead. Lady Grosvenor and Lady Stepney both saw the sad little one before his burial.' Mary's mother told her husband that she had learned 'a great deal': 'yesterday when the doctors supposed all was over, *the* event happened with no *pain* and it moved me very much to see a *well formed* baby supposed to be nearly 4 months!!'

Dr Burlingham seems to have been wrong again and did not realise that Mary had had an 'incomplete' miscarriage, with some of the placenta left inside. She grew steadily worse for two weeks and a

* This case is described with quotations from unpublished diaries and letters by Jalland: op. cit., pp. 165–66.

Dr Dobie, who also seems to have been extraordinarily ignorant, pronounced that it was a 'very mysterious case'. Mary's sister Agnes wrote to her mother that '*either* she was being wrongly treated or the Doctors were not on the right track'. She believed 'there must be something left still – but when Doctors say it is all right one supposes they know best.'

More than two weeks after the miscarriage, Dr Dobie examined Mary for the first time (we are not told how he did this or whether he did an internal examination) and concluded that 'some of the placenta was obstinately adhering' to the uterus and an operation was necessary to expel it. The operation was done under chloroform by a Dr Griffiths and left Mary 'quite prostrate' with sickness.

Two weeks later and a month after the miscarriage Mary feared that she had peritonitis, which turned out to be correct. But Dr Dobie spoke only vaguely about 'chronic inflammation' which merely required time to heal. He asserted that Mary was now safe and the surgeon, Dr Griffiths, sent a 'comforting letter', but Mary was not reassured and suggested sending for Sir Andrew Clark, who came all the way from London to see her twice in October and again in December. He confirmed that there was 'mischief – inflammation in tissues around womb, extending over pelvis'. Mary developed pelvic abscesses and was treated with 'poultices, laudanum, bromide, brandy, quinine, morphia, caster oil, and boiling fomentations' for stomach pains. She thought she was going to die and dictated an informal will. However, she was lucky. After five months of serious illness, she recovered. Two years later she gave birth to a daughter but in May 1890 she had a second miscarriage. She still had enough faith in the ignorant Dr Dobie to call him in and she was lucky to escape a second serious illness.

Mary was both unlucky and lucky. The probability was that three women in every hundred who bore six children (as was the norm) would die in childbirth. The women studied by Jalland provide plenty of personal evidence of this. Nearly everyone had lost a wife, sister, mother or friend in childbirth. Margaret Gladstone became ill with puerperal fever after giving birth to a daughter on 20 July 1870. She had talked of the possibility of dying at the baby's birth and wrote in her journal, 'I felt as if I could leave even this intense and overflowing happiness on earth to be with Jesus'. She was in labour for only five hours, with her husband administering chloroform, but she was 'taken dangerously ill' twelve days after the birth, starting with 'a terrible seizure'. She was prescribed opium, champagne, and brandy and soda every three hours, which shows how little the doctors could do for her. They also ordered a 'lamp bath', which made her mother 'quail at the thought of torturing the poor patient suffering lamb . . . all the applications [that] wore her out and disturbed her so'. The unfortunate patient realised how little the doctors knew and the last time they stood round her bed she whispered to her mother: 'If they would like to learn from my case – let them.' She died on 16 August. To finish the story, the baby, Margaret Ethel, grew up to marry Ramsay Macdonald, Britain's first Labour prime minster, by whom she had six children. She died in 1911, the year after the youngest was born.

It was not only young mothers who died. A woman who had had many previous children, known as a 'grand multip' is at even higher risk. The uterus tends not to function well after many pregnancies and grand multips are at greater risk of complications and bleeding, as well as from disease elsewhere. Gladstone's sister, Mary Lyttelton, died aged forty-four just after giving birth to her twelfth living child. She seems to have died from heart disease, though her husband thought her case was 'an extreme instance of the way in which the doctors withold the truth'. After her previous and eleventh pregnancy, her gynaecologist, Sir Charles Locock, had said that another pregnancy would kill her. Unfortunately he gave this information to her sister and told her husband that 'the mischief was done' only when she was again pregnant.

Alfred, the child whose birth killed Margaret Gladstone, grew up and married Laura Tennant, a girl of small build who became convinced that she would die in childbirth. On 16 April 1886, 'after a time both terribly long and dangerous', she gave birth to a nine-pound boy, whose life was only just saved. She had a forceps delivery, 'a frightful hard business before an hour's work with instruments . . . Almost immediately afterwards a horrid unusual haemorrhage set in . . .' Doctors thought her liver had failed. Sir Andrew Clarke was one of the doctors called in but after five days, she died. Mary Drew, daughter of the prime minister, who was herself nearly to die of childbirth a few months later, described 'the little white bride, inside the coffin, and all the broken hearts around'. Laura's baby survived his birth but died two years later from tuberculous meningitis. Her sister, Margot Asquith, also had a small pelvis and also believed that she would die in childbirth. In May 1895 the doctors had to sacrifice her baby to save her life and Margot had to spend three months flat on her back with phlebitis (inflammation in a vein). Later she lost two more children but also managed to produce a living son and daughter.


Just as some women had brief breakdowns in adolescence or early adult life, so some women had periods of invalidism. Many of these 'illnesses' were actually reactions to circumstances or to personal conflicts and improved when opportunities for a better life arose. In 1838 Harriet Martineau fell ill as a result, she thought, of the strains of coping with her mother. Her doctors diagnosed an ovarian cyst. She concluded that 'a tumour was forming of a kind which usually originates in mental suffering'.* She went to Tynemouth to live on her own with a maid, where she lay in bed for five years. Then she got up and lived for another twenty-eight years. Another example was Elizabeth Barrett who spent several years as an invalid in her bedroom before she eloped with Robert Browning. Sometimes the invalidism was a way of escaping the tedium of the world, either negatively, as an escape, or in order to have time for more important things, as in the case of Charles Darwin and Florence Nightingale. Most, though not all, chronic invalids were women. It enabled them to avoid many things. Nineteenth-century Romantics developed the idea of invalidism as a pretext for leisure and an escape from bourgeois responsibilities. It was 'a way of retiring from the world without having to take responsibility for the decision'. It was encouraged by the 'medicalisation' of life, the conversion of social and political ills into illness.†

There is a woman mentioned in the papers studied by Jalland, who is known only as 'Cecil'. In 1882 she 'feels her nerves very irritable . . . and the swimming of her head hums', so she constantly visited doctors and hydropathic establishments. Cecil's relatives believed that her illness was a sham. She looked 'uncommonly well' and was 'excessively fanciful about her health'. All this suggests that sometimes hypochondriacal behaviour was regarded as abnormal or tedious, just as it is today. Although there were pressures to regard women as inherently sick, such ideas were not necessarily accepted either by the women themselves, by their relatives, or by their doctors.

One of the chronic invalids whose story has come down to us was another member of the Gladstone family, Helen, sister of the prime minister. She was born in 1814, the youngest in the family of six children.§ By the time she was born her middle-aged family had lost

* H. Martineau: *Autobiography*, vol 1, p. 151.
† See Susan Sontag: *Illness as Metaphor*.
§ See S.G. Checkland: *The Gladstones: A Family Biography, 1764–1851*, 1971.

interest in their children except for the clever William, four years older than Helen. Their mother was narrow-minded, evangelical and obsessed with death and suffering and the need for self-discipline to control depravity. She was also a neurotic hypochondriac who gradually became an invalid, continuing to control her husband and family. Meanwhile, the eldest daughter, Anne, died slowly of tuberculosis. Helen herself, though apparently healthy, had been regarded as delicate from birth. By the time she was sixteen she had spasms and bowel problems and frequently visited doctors. The only medicine that helped her was laudanum, a preparation of opium in alcohol which was then used widely. It is still, incidentally, available. In 1835 she rallied in order to nurse her dying mother but soon afterwards she relapsed. She went to live with her ageing father in Scotland and her intake of laudanum increased. She had nothing to do and she lay on her bed for many hours each day. Her brother William tried to make her undergo a rigid regime of self-discipline and prayer. It did not occur to him that she was highly intelligent with nothing to do and that this might be at least part of the trouble. She herself seemed to have no insight into her condition. When her father sent her abroad, she fell in love with a man whose family, like hers, disapproved of the match. She became more and more addicted to opium and more and more desperate, 'I am as a dead branch . . . offering no-one fruit or flower, for I am more beaten down than in any former illness.' She converted to Roman Catholicism, which infuriated her family. Brother William wanted to expel her from the family home but her father refused to do this. She tried to live in Germany, but this ended in hysterical scenes and an overdose of laudanum. Her family tried to keep opium and alcohol away from her but found they could not. She deteriorated and was described with 'clenched hands, locked jaw, and inability to speak except in hysterical outbursts'. In 1848 she travelled to Edinburgh where, after a severe emotional scene, Cardinal Wiseman appeared to perform a miraculous cure with a sacred relic. This received much publicity, which again disturbed her brother William. For the next three years she nursed her father through his final illness. Then she went to Rome and eventually became a nun. She was now much more stable though still addicted to opium. She believed that she was the victim of her male-dominated family, unable to play the role assigned to her as a female, but unable to find a fulfilling alternative.

It is more difficult to know how poorer women viewed their doctors or how doctors behaved towards them. Many never saw a doctor for they could not afford the fees, though many doctors, including the anatomist William Hunter, had consciences and treated them free: indeed, the nineteenth century saw a great increase in free hospitals for the poor. Inevitably, most of the records that come down to us were made by doctors about their patients, not the other way round.

But some remarkable information has survived, though doctors and gynaecology are peripheral to it. In the early years of the twentieth century some women of realistic outlook and strong social conscience were concerned about the conditions under which Britain's poorest mothers gave birth and raised their children. These social reformers formed the Women's Co-operative Guild. In 1914 one of its leaders, Margaret Llewellyn Davies, made a public appeal for direct experiences of childbirth and rearing. She intended to use it as evidence for the Guild's sustained campaign against the Liberal government and local authorities and to improve the virtually non-existent maternal and infant care then available to poorer women. It was shortly before World War I, and the government was more conscious than usual of the 'nation's assets', by which was meant the children of the poor, the future soldiers and workers. People in power were beginning to realise that the neglect of the health of women and infants did not lead to the 'survival of the fittest' but tended to weaken and maim.

There was a wide and interesting response from the wives of manual workers, most of them above average for the lower classes of the time. Typical remarks are, 'I was more fortunately placed than most women', or 'I have not had to go through so much pain and suffering as many poor women have to go through'. Most of the letters were from women who were literate, some remarkably so, despite extreme poverty and deprivation, but some described other women or were written on their behalf. These letters were published in a book that was well received and widely publicised.*

The letters reveal the desperate poverty in which most of the women lived, their inability to control their fertility and, often, the poor standards of medical care that they received. Although the letters are specifically about experiences associated with maternity and none of the questions asked concerned the longterm complications of pregnancy, we get a few glimpses of these. There is much information about poor medical care and careless doctors and midwives (the latter only having been formally registered in England from 1902). Although these letters were written in the twentieth century, many of

* Margaret Llewellyn Davies ed.: *Maternity: Letters from Working Women, collected by the Women's Co-operative Guild, London, 1915*, Virago, 1978.

them describe events that occurred up to forty years before.

Typical remarks are, 'I had to do without the common necessaries to provide doctor's fees, which so undermined my health that when my baby was born I nearly lost my life . . .' '. . .the doctor's bills grew like mushrooms . . .' '. . . I had a midwife this time as I could not afford the doctor's fee . . .', and 'I never had a doctor all the time I was having children. I have had six, one dead . . . We had not many doctor's bills, as our children were all very healthy, and I don't think I have spent a pound on doctoring for myself since I was a baby, for which I am very thankful.'

The women describe exhaustion and starvation. There are descriptions of women still suffering 'inwardly' (probably meaning gynaecologically) after many years, who attribute this to starvation, exhaustion and lack of medical care during pregnancy and childbirth. Many took abortifacients – at a time when what was available to poor women would produce abortion only by poisoning the mother, often leading to her death or serious illness. They also took remedies based on diachylon, a lead substance that caused poisoning. Doctors were not involved in this. As one wrote, 'The news is handed from woman to woman by word of mouth, like any of the other household remedies or "cures" which every woman knows.'

One woman wrote that she had been pregnant continually for fifteen years. Many despaired at the number of their children and feared yet another pregnancy. Many were afraid or had been afraid:

> I had a severe labour lasting two nights and two days. (This was twenty-three years ago) [c. 1880] No effort was made to obtain help for me, although my mother at that time was starting to practise as a midwife, and had all a mother's fears for her daughter in her first labour. At that time it was much more usual to trust to Providence, and if a woman died it only proved her weakness and unfitness for motherhood. My baby only lived seven months.

Many suffered from longterm complications of childbirth. A typical letter refers to women 'suffering from misplacements and various other inward complaints'. One said the cause was 'having to work during pregnancy'. This theme recurs frequently in the book, as does the lack of medical care, along with, in some, a genuine faith in doctors and what they might achieve if only they could be paid. One woman who had lost twins believed

> If I could have had medical treatment, all that suffering could have been prevented, and I might have had a strong child.

Some blamed the doctor for their misfortunes. One blamed her

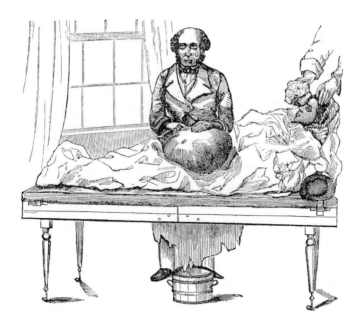

A VICTORIAN SURGEON ABOUT TO OPERATE

doctors for the loss of her babies. One doctor refused to come and the child died. The next time she went into labour the doctor was drinking and sent a midwife instead. Again, the baby died.

One woman wrote that she had kidney trouble (urinary retention) after childbirth and describes yet another who had eclampsia:

> ... falling out of one fit into another, and at last, after her baby was born, she lay two days quite unconscious – in fact they never expected she would recover. She had two doctors, and they gave her every attention, and then when she was getting better her own particular doctor told her that if she had only consulted him before hand he could have saved her a lot of pain ... He said it was some kidney trouble which had been the reason of all she had suffered. In both her case and mine we could have had advice, as far as the expense was concerned, but it was sheer *ignorance*, and the idea that we must put up with it till the nine months were over.

Llewellyn concludes that 'to bear children under such conditions is to bear an intolerable burden of suffering'.

No wonder there were longterm gynaecological after-effects. 'I was in labour thirty-six hours, and after all that suffering had to be delivered by instruments, and was ruptured too badly to have anything done to help me. I am suffering from the ill-effects to-day. This is thirty-one years ago; 1872.' Another, at her fifth confinement, 'was so injured that for nearly ten years I was an invalid'. She attributes this to 'the doctor hurrying the birth, instead of giving nature a chance, and he was rough handling me'. One woman's 'very terrible time' was followed by an ovarian operation. 'After leaving the hospital I was in bed three months, but it was a complete cure . . . Dr — told me I could not have gone through a more serious operation unless I had had my head taken off . . .'

> . . . after the birth of my first baby I suffered from falling womb, and the torture of that was especially cruel at closet, in more ways than I can describe; and quite by accident I learned that other mothers I met were not suffering the same. My baby was ten months old when I told the doctor, who said I ought to have told him before, and he soon put me right. But doctors who attended me never told me anything concerning my babies or myself.

> . . . the baby was hung with navel cord twice round the neck and once round the shoulder . . . [which] caused my womb to come down, and I have had to wear something to hold it up until these late years . . . As my family increased I had to have my legs bandaged.

This woman seems to have had a retained placenta and manual removal of placenta without an anaesthetic: 'I have had the doctor's arm in my body, and felt his fingers tearing the afterbirth from my side.' It is a cause for reflection that at least a generation after anaesthetics came into general use, a woman underwent this operation while fully conscious. Apart from the horrific and painful nature of the procedure, doing it on a conscious patient greatly increases the risk of her dying of shock.

Some, however, seem to get better in the end. After describing a long tale of woe of each pregnancy and confinement, one woman wrote:

> I am now in my forty-sixth year, and seem to be improving in many respects.

# VIII

# TREATMENT

Having examined the state of the profession and glanced at women's lives and illnesses, I shall now look in more detail at the kind of treatment, both drugs and surgery, that women could be expected to receive before anaesthetics were available.

Certainly there was, in one sense, constant pressure towards greater knowledge and more successful treatment, but there is another side to the story. Many women had gynaecological complaints but few of these were serious in the sense of threat to life or health. There were a few heroic operations, mostly done on hopeless cases, but in general pre-anaesthetic gynaecology consisted of local treatment for a range of minor disorders. On the whole it was over these that controversy raged and exploitation occurred.

Women with gynaecological complaints in the first half of the nineteenth century, if they were treated at all, usually had general treatment in the form of bleeding, purges and potions or else local treatment, often in an intensely moralistic atmosphere. These treatments had been handed down from former times. The eighteenth-century French gynaecologist, Jean Astruc, who wrote on 'Disease Incident to Women' in 1743, was deeply concerned with moral aspects of gynaecology, notably 'nymphomania', which he discussed in terms of 'excessive inclination to venery' and 'shameful and immodest disease'. He recommended bleeding, frequent purging with cathartics, and the use of broths or apozemes made from water-lily, marsh-mallows, sorrel, lettuce, hemlock, poppies etc, together with two or three pints of mineral water a day and nine or ten ounces of asses's milk twice a day – 'if the stomach can digest it'. His book contains many pages of mild instructions. Merely following them would have occupied a patient's mind even if it did not heal her body. For local conditions such as 'Inflammation of the uterus', Astruc's recommendations include the 'copious use of oil of sweet almonds', frequent cooling and 'narcotics', by which he means preparations of poppy 'given in very little doses'. But he is not optimistic about the outcome when the ovaries are affected. He tells us 'all diseases of the ovaries are bad' and goes on to recommend the same remedies as before. The one condition for which he recommends an abdominal operation is for a pregnancy in a Fallopian tube. He knew that, without surgical intervention, the condition was almost certain to be fatal so he felt it was worth risking the extreme dangers of an operation.

Time-honoured prescriptions were handed down from pre-scientific days and often dispensed with little or no physical examin-ation and without anything that today we would call a diagnosis. It was gradually becoming more fashionable to examine patients instead of merely listening and questioning, but gynaecology involved special problems of modesty for the patient, ignorance and distaste on the part of the doctor, and prudery in either or both. Many doctors then, as now, had little experience of women's diseases, were embarrassed by them or didn't like the smell.

We have already seen* how strongly the arguments raged about vaginal examination, and when the speculum became widely used this disagreement grew ever more ferocious. The speculum, as its name suggests, is essentially an instrument for viewing. Again, the ancients used it. Those used by Soranus and Paul or Aegina had two flattish blades, rather like a duck's bill, which could be separated by turning a screw. This design is still in use. As is the case today, the instrument was made in different lengths to fit different patients.

In 1801 the speculum was re-introduced into medical practice by a young Frenchman, Récamier (1774–1852). He began to treat ulcers and inflammations of the cervix with local applications, as was already the custom with ulcers and inflammation of the throat. He used a tube about five inches long, through which he could apply his preparations and see what he was doing. He insisted that the speculum was necessary in any gynaecological examination, an idea which provoked criticism and controversy. In Britain it was half a century before the idea began to be widely accepted. One of the first British doctors to recognise its importance was Sir James Simpson, who introduced chloroform to childbirth and wasn't even born while much of the controversy was raging. Even in France the use of the speculum was believed to be a 'serious sacrifice of delicacy', only to be made when it was essential to diagnosis.

The first detailed description in English of a vaginal examination

* In Chapter three.

that resembles those done today seems to have been about 1839.*
With a surprisingly modern attitude William Jones argued that disease
could be effectively treated only when it had been properly diagnosed
and this had to be done by taking into account not only the symptoms
and things visible to the exterior but by observing the internal
alterations that led to them. For instance, trying to cure a vaginal
discharge without knowing the underlying pathological cause was, he
wrote, 'unscientific, empirical and inhuman'.

But morals were often stronger than science in the minds of
gynaecologists and many thought there should be strict limitation in
the speculum's use. Some used accounts of specific horrifying cases as
general arguments against the instrument. For instance, Dr Robert
Lee, Professor of Midwifery at St George's Hospital, cited a case that
occurred about the middle of the century. A middle-aged woman
suffered from paraplegia (paralysed legs). Her physician thought she
suffered from uterine inflammation and, though she had never had any
gynaecological disease, he decided to demonstrate this by using the
speculum. The woman had an intact hymen and, to prevent her
screams from being heard, the doors were closed. A week later her
symptoms returned and she died. At post-mortem she had inflammation at the base of the brain, but no gynaecological disease. Dr Lee
used this shocking story of medical insensitivity and incompetence as
an argument against the use of the speculum.† In the same year the
physiologist Marshall Hall argued in the *Lancet* that it was important
not to damage 'delicacy and purity' and to avoid the 'dulling of the
edge of virgin modesty, and the degradation of pure minds, of the
daughters of England'. He thought the speculum induced a sort of
'mental poisoning' and a 'new and lamentable form of hysteria . . .
*furor uterinus*'. Some of these patients, he said, 'speak of "the womb"
and of "the uterine organs" with a familiarity that was formerly
unknown and which, I trust, will ere long be obsolete.' There was
ribald humour among doctors about 'speculumizers' and how they
would like to perform their art publicly, such as in a theatre,
insinuations that examination by speculum was a form of sexual
intercourse, and advice about how to perform the examination
without 'the slightest exposure'.

Even influential authorities often objected to vaginal examination
or to the use of the speculum, or to both. In the 1835 edition of his
textbook, Fleetwood Churchill barely mentioned the speculum and

---

* William Jones: *Practical Observations on Diseases of Women*, London, 1839.
† R. Lee: 'On the use of the speculum in the diagnosis and treatment of uterine
disease', *Medical-Chirurgical Transactions*, 33, 1850, p. 261–78.

said only, in relation to inflammation of the cervix, 'The diagnosis, with the aid of a speculum, is tolerably easy, but without it, will require great care and a sensitive touch . . .' In the 1844 edition Churchill, in a new preface, states:

> A good deal of discussion has taken place lately as to the use and abuse of the speculum . . . I cannot but regard the speculum as a most valuable instrument in judicious hands but . . . I fear it has often been used improperly, unnecessarily, and from motives which ought not to influence the members of a liberal profession.

He does, however, give detailed description of vaginal examination, including the use of the speculum. He concedes that this has its use:

> if the disease be such as cannot be satisfactorily made out or treated without it, then its use is not only justifiable, but to reject it would be a blameable neglect of the means within our power for the relief of disease.

We have already come across the famous American gynaecologist and teacher, Charles Meigs in Chapter three. He was extreme but not unique in his sentimentality in believing modesty preferable to diagnosis and treatment. A typical British text of the same period, J.H. Bennet's *A Practical Treatise on Inflammation of the Uterus and its Appendages and on Ulceration and Induration of the Neck of the Uterus*, (1850), expressed doubts about the propriety of using the speculum. Another critic, Henry Johnson, thought the speculum had been made 'a piece of gratuitous or unprincipled indecency'.* He expanded his fantasies about the speculum's potential dangers.

> We are told . . . that in France there is quite a furor in its favour, and that ladies of rank write billets to their surgeon requesting him to call and bring his speculum. This may be true and our notions of modesty may be overstrained and out of date. Yet I trust, and I cannot help believing, that some time will elapse before OUR wives and daughters will distinguish themselves in this free and easy style . . .

At the same time Dr Sturt's book, *Female Physiology*, (1851), which intended to give young ladies some knowledge of the structure and function of their own bodies was heavily criticised. The *Lancet* reviewer regarded it as an objectionable work. More than a decade later, in 1863, Dr Edward Tilt published his *Handbook of Uterine*

---

* H.J. Johnson: *Clinical Observations on Diseases of the Genito-urinary Organ*, London, 1851, p. 341–44.

*Therapeutics* for doctors without a section on examination and with no mention of vaginal examination. The book was an enormous success. The *Lancet* praised it and the work was translated into German and Italian. Tilt was then president of the London Obstetrical Society. Only in the fourth edition of his work, in 1878, does he include a chapter on 'Modes of Examination, and Surgical Instruments' and describe (in many pages) the details of vaginal examination.

As the idea of 'diseases of women' developed, so did weird inventions and procedures such as the use of electricity and massage, the extensive use of medicated tampons, various pastes and medicines

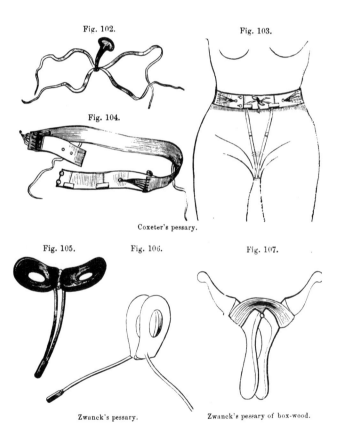

Fig. 102.          Fig. 103.

Fig. 104.

Coxeter's pessary.

Fig. 105.          Fig. 106.          Fig. 107.

Zwanck's pessary.          Zwanck's pessary of box-wood.

A FEW OF THE HUNDREDS OF PESSARIES USED BY THE VICTORIANS, PARTICULRLY
BEFORE SURGERY BECAME RELATIVELY SAFE

and the invention of an enormous and fantastic variety of pessaries, varying from the small and discreet to the enormous and cumbersome. For example, one pessary for prolapse of the womb was huge and whirred round and round rather like a flailing machine; it had to be worn under a skirt with an enormous hoop.* Surgery of all kinds became less likely to be confined to emergencies and much more could be done 'cold'. This led to advances in the field but also to an increase in bizarre and unnecessary operations and procedures.

The increased concentration on women's disorders, often unnecessary, was eventually attacked by W.D. Buck, the president of the New Hampshire State Medical Society for 1866. He referred to the uterus as a 'harmless, unoffensive little organ, stowed away in a quiet place' and 'having no function to perform save at certain periods of life', but furnishing a capital field for 'surgeons anxious for notoriety'. He continues:

> What with burning and cauterizing, cutting and slashing, and gouging, and spitting, and skewering, and pessarying, the old-fashioned womb will cease to exist, except in history. The Transactions of the American Medical Association have figured 123 different kinds of pessaries, embracing every variety . . . They look like the drawings of a turbine water-wheel, or a leaf from a work on entomology . . . I do think that this filling of the vagina with traps, making a Chinese toy shop of it, is outrageous. Our grandmothers never knew they had wombs, only as they were reminded of it by the struggles of a healthy foetus, which, by the by, they always held onto. Nowadays, even our young women must have their wombs shored up, and if a baby accidentally gets in by the side of the machinery, and finds a lodgement in the uterus, it may, perchance, have a knitting needle stuck in its eyes before it has any.†

The eminent Dr Samuel D. Gross of the Jefferson Medical College was also sarcastic. 'At present diseases of the uterus are the fashionable disorders. Not to have an ulcer upon the womb is to be beyond the pale of the sex . . . Doctors and patients alike have a womb on the brain.'§

The usual local treatment consisted of leeching, injections and cauterization.

Leeches had long been used, if not extensively, for disorders of the uterus as well as elsewhere. The indications for their use were

---

* See Ricci: *One Hundred Years*, p. 47. Also Harvey Graham.
† W.D. Buck, *New York Medical Journal*, 1867, 5, 464.
§ Samuel D. Gross: *A Discourse Introductory to the 43rd Course of Lectures in the Jefferson Medical College*, 1867.

expanding, and not just in gynaecology. Leeches were even recommended to be put on the anus, fifteen at a time, to prevent ageing! They had been used in the vagina in Italy at least as early as 1665, each leech being tied to a string. In the eighteenth century Astruc recommended them to draw the blood and relax the uterus. They had become popular for use in general surgery in attempts to control infection and to reduce swelling. In 1831, a paper by J.N. Guilbert read before the Academy of Medicine in Paris proposed that leeches be applied to the diseased cervix. In 1837, Duparcque recommended that they be applied to the cervix as an important part of the treatment of cancer. The treatment was to coincide with 'sanguineous depletion' (bleeding), 'cupping' (the application of a hot and hollow utensil to raise a weal on the skin), purging, starvation (with the idea of starving not the patient but the diseased organ, though how this distinction could be achieved was not made clear), and absolute rest. There was much interest in vaginal discharges during the early nineteenth century: Hollick advised treating white discharge (leucorrhoea) by applying leeches to the labia a few days before a period was expected. Many writers advocated applying them to the vulva or cervix and some at least advised care in doing this. The 1864 edition of Bennet's book advises the doctor to count the leeches as they drop off when satiated, lest he 'lose' some. The author had known leeches to advance into the cavity of the uterus where 'I think I have scarcely ever seen more acute pain than that experienced by several of my patients under these circumstances.'

Altogether, leeches were one of the most popular treatments for both gynaecological and other illnesses. In his chapter on 'Abortions', Meigs even recommended them for toothache in pregnancy: 'If a woman have in her pregnancy an insufferable toothache, you will often cure it by putting a couple of leeches on the gum . . .' In the New York Medical Register during the 1860s there is a list of ten men recognised as 'cuppers and leechers', who were available at any time. There is even a case in 1870 of a congenital prolapse being treated with leeches.

Caustic chemicals such as silver nitrate or hydrate of potassium and the cautery were also used on the cervix. Ulcers of the cervix were often diagnosed and treated in this manner. (We must remember that syphilis was much commoner then than now, even in the 'respectable' classes.) Injections directly into the womb were still popular. They had been done since ancient times; in Greek medicine of the time of Hippocrates, douches flushing the inside of the uterus had been used to wash out bits of placenta and to carry medicaments into the uterine cavity. During the nineteenth century their use increased. Fleetwood Churchill strongly criticised the practice and said it was attended 'with most fatal consequences' and that 'enemata of cold water' would be safer. Since there was no idea of asepsis, both procedures must have been dangerous.

These general and local treatments of women's disorders were ineffective, especially in conditions such as ovarian cyst and other tumours. It must have been obvious that only surgery could alleviate these, yet surgery was too dangerous to attempt except as a desperate remedy. The gynaecological literature of the nineteenth century gives an impression of increasing frustration with current treatments, an increasing tendency on the part of doctors to intervene and a desire for further intervention on the part of both doctors and their women patients.

The breakthrough came with the arrival of anaesthetics, and the change in gynaecological practice was swift and dramatic. What had been slow development over thousands of years became a rush of new treatments by the surgeon's knife. The chance came largely through the ovary. In the eighteenth century Astruc had written 'all diseases of the ovaries are bad', and this had been the experience of doctors through the ages. Henceforth in many cases it would be no longer true. Surgeons would now use the ovary as the basis for the spectacular advances that now took place, advances so dramatic that, one could argue, they went to the head of some of those who brought them about.

The age of advancing surgery and easy operations had begun. This was the new era that critics such as George Bernard Shaw were so much to deplore. As he says through a character in *The Doctor's Dilemma*,

> In my early days, you made your man drunk; and porters and students held him down; and you had to set your teeth and finish the job fast. Nowadays you work at your ease; and the pain doesn't come until afterwards, when you've taken your cheque and rolled up your bag and left the house. I tell you, Colly, chloroform has done a lot of mischief. It's enabled every fool to be a surgeon.

The dramatic changes that took place in gynaecological treatment in the second half of the nineteenth century have excited generations of surgeons and medical historians and, perhaps most of all, those who have been both surgeons and historians. 'Nothing in the entire realm of medicine was more dramatic,' wrote Ricci, Clinical Professor of Gynaecology and Obstetrics at New York Medical College, holder of a number of other prestigious gynaecological appointments and author of several substantial books on the history of gynaecology. He continues, 'For more than two thousand years it had remained medical and stationary and in less than half a century it became surgical and spectacular.' A surgeon with a sense of history might find himself contemplating these events with an excitement that precludes criticism or even appraisal.

Surgical and spectacular! This helps to explain what happened. What had been the dangerous, unknown territory of the abdomen was now accessible to vision, knowledge and skill. For centuries surgeons had waited for the advances that would make their skills widely practicable. Now, at last, they came into their own. Operations that had before been excessively rare, usually fatal or not attempted at all, now became routine. New operations were invented and sought. As before, women were the first recipients of the new developments in the art or science of surgery. It was convenient that the submissive sex had organs inside the abdomen that were liable to give trouble – or were deemed to do so – and which now became relatively easy to reach, repair and remove.

McDowell's life-saving operation on Jane Todd Crawford's ovarian cyst in 1809 was far ahead of its time, but it was soon to become common. Some of the surgical procedures that now became popular had been proposed long before. For instance, in 1823 James Blundell, lecturer in Midwifery at Guy's Hospital, London, read to the Royal Medico-Chirurgical Society of London what Ricci calls an 'epoch-making contribution' in which he recommended removal of ovarian cysts, ruptured and cancerous uteri and repair of ruptured bladders. He showed how it might be possible to open the peritoneal (abdominal) cavity, particularly in cases of disease of the female pelvis. He backed up his argument with details of experiments that he had done on animals.* Although Blundell read his paper to the Society, it was turned down for publication. The author published it himself the same year. He was also the first surgeon in England to remove a cancerous uterus. He was vigorously attacked by anti-vivisectionists to whom he appealed: 'Strike, Gentlemen, but hear! You who would join the laugh at the Egyptians, which will you sacrifice, your women or your cats?'

---

* See his *Principles and Practice of Midwifery*, 1842.

But at that time surgeons were still afraid. The dangers of pain, shock, bleeding and infection were still too great for ovariotomy to be practicable in human beings. Blundell predicted of ovariotomy, 'This operation will, I am persuaded, ultimately come into general use.' He was right and he lived to see it. He died at the age of eighty-seven, having made a fortune from his surgical practice.

Apart from occasional attempts, usually in remote areas, the first gynaecological operations done in America were for pregnancy which had occurred outside the uterus. Known as 'ectopic' pregnancy, this usually occurs in a Fallopian tube and occasionally in the abdomen. It is a dangerous condition because, almost invariably, there is insufficient room for the foetus to grow and so, at some stage in its development, the sac in which it lies ruptures, causing serious haemorrhage from which the mother is likely to die unless there is swift surgical intervention. Ricci says that of the first 500 cases reported, 336 had died.* Surgeons knew that, in order to save the life of the mother, they had to destroy the foetus before it ruptured the sac in which it was growing. As early as 1759 a foetus had been removed and the patient had recovered, but other attempts had been less successful and many doctors experimented with less radical treatment. They tried starving the mother in the mistaken belief that this would starve the growing foetus. They injected drugs such as morphine or poisons such as strychnine to kill the foetus but usually either failed to affect the foetus or else killed the mother too. One surgeon, Robert Barnes, even asked whether infecting the mother with syphilis, known as 'syphilisation' was not justifiable in order to kill the growing foetus, which did not lie in the uterus and so was not accessible to customary methods for procuring an abortion. But none of these measures worked and it was obvious that abdominal surgery was the only hope, if only it could be done safely. In June 1862, at a meeting of the Obstetrical Society of London, the discussion was on whether or not to operate in tubal pregnancy, and the argument continued during the rest of the decade. At first operations were carried out via the vagina (vaginotomy), but success was rare and many mothers died. Finally the pioneer surgeon, Lawson Tait, pronounced:

> Vaginotomy should always give place to abdominal section as being more scientific and less risky.†

Lawson Tait was one of the first to recognise the supreme

---

* Ricci: op. cit., p. 245.
† *Medical Times and Gazette*, 1873, vol. 2, p. 119.

importance of being able to *see* inside the abdomen instead of trying to do things blindly. Abdominal surgery has remained the standard treatment for ectopic pregnancy and to this day is life-saving in what is still a common gynaecological emergency.

The operation that was the most innovative, the most influential and which epitomises most of the questions raised in this book was for the removal of ovarian cysts or, as it came to be known, ovariotomy. All abdominal operations derive from it. So much was learned from doing and practising this operation that it can be argued that all major surgery is based on it. Cysts (which contain fluid) and tumours of the ovaries (also sometimes called 'cysts' and often also containing fluid) were common in the past, as they are today. Anyone who sees gynaecological patients is likely to see many women who suffer from them. Cysts are often found during examination for something else. Some are malignant and need to be removed instantly (the results of this are not good even today). But some cysts and tumours, left to themselves, grow huge, usually because of the accumulation of fluid. They cause mechanical problems in the woman's daily life. No one can lead a fully 'normal' life who carries inside an ovarian cyst the size of, say, a four-year-old child. Nowadays, any woman in whom an ovarian cyst is diagnosed, even a small one, is likely to be advised to have it removed because of its potential dangers. Many are detected on routine physical examination. All are potentially dangerous.

Before the operation for removal of the ovary became practicable, there were many other treatments for the condition. In medicine, when a condition has a number of different treatments, it usually means that no one really knows how to treat it. Previous treatment for ovarian cysts included paracentesis (draining fluid through a hollow tube or needle), internal drugs, incision, deliberately creating a fistula or passage to the outside, injection of the cyst cavity with chemicals, practically all known drugs, emetics, purgatives, mercurials, tonics, applied leeches, fomentations, blistering, electricity, friction and abdominal pressure. None of these treatments were of any use and none prevented the ovarian cysts from growing. Some doctors acknowledged this failure and were disillusioned. The medical literature of the time is filled with therapeutic despair over ovarian cysts.

A French surgeon, Augustine Grisolle, said that the large number of failures stood as a testimonial to the uselessness of drugs for the cure of ovarian cysts. Another, Pierre Lasalle, said: '*Cette maladie est absolument incurable.*' Sir Anthony Paston Cooper, one of England's greatest surgeons, stated that medicine had had but little influence on ovarian cysts. Sir Thomas Watson, after treating a large number of cases with a variety of drugs, admitted that he had not had a single success. Sir James Simpson pointed out that the interior of a cyst had no powers of absorption and so diuretics, used to get rid of the fluid, were ineffective. Many other surgeons were just as pessimistic and there were reports of cysts bursting spontaneously inside, usually accompanied by death. Some surgeons tapped large and disabling cysts and let out the fluid. This had been done occasionally since 1701, when Robert Houston in America introduced the practice of treating 'ovarian dropsy' by tapping. William Hunter had been one of the first to propose tapping ovarian cysts and he was probably the first to

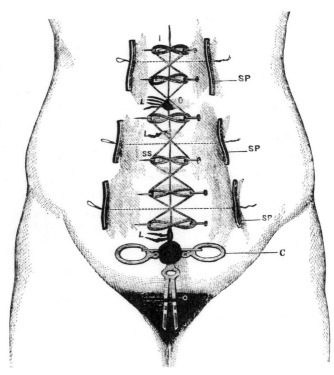

HOW SOME SURGEONS CLOSED THE WOUND AFTER OVARIOTOMY

propose excision, in 1757. In the same year he recommended that a cyst be tapped before it had reached a critical stage. However, the technique was dangerous and for the most part ineffective because the fluid soon accumulated again.

From the middle of the nineteenth century, the operation for removal of an ovary was called, incorrectly and with hybrid etymology, 'ovariotomy'. Later 'oöphorectomy', a more accurate description, appeared, though initially this was used to refer to the removal of *normal* ovaries and only later referred to what it actually describes, the removal of an ovary. Today much more is known about endocrines, hormones and the *functions* of the ovary and every attempt is made during operations to conserve as much ovarian tissue as possible so that the operation is often a partial oöphorectomy, often combined with hysterectomy, or removal of the uterus.

After Ephraim McDowell, more ovariotomies were done, even before the use of anaesthetics, especially in America. Pioneer patients such as Jane Todd Crawford realised that surgery was their only hope. McDowell sent a manuscript containing an account of this operation to Edinburgh to his old teacher, John Bell, who, it so happened, was seriously ill and died soon afterwards. The manuscript fell into the hands of John Lizars, who tried the operation on four cases and published the results.* These were not encouraging for those eager to extend the boundaries of surgery.

In the first case the diagnosis was wrong; there was no ovarian tumour but only 'tympanites and obesity'. In the second case the tumour was in the uterus, not the ovary, and Lizars left it where it was. In one of the remaining two cases, the patient died. This sorry tale is indicative of the difficulties our forbears had not only in doing these operations but in making the correct diagnosis before doing them.

McDowell also sent a report of his operation to Philip Syng Physick, Professor of Surgery at the University of Pennsylvania – the professor was not an innovator and he ignored it – and to Thomas Chalkley James, the first professor of midwifery in Pennsylvania: with it he included accounts of two more cases of ovariotomy, but no one seemed interested in him. Then Emiliani of Faenza, Italy, did the operation successfully in 1815 and Nathan Smith performed the operation in Vermont in 1821. It was first performed in England in 1836 by William Jeaffreson of Framlingham in Suffolk and he was followed by West of Tunbridge Wells. But there was no successful case

* J. Lizars: *Observations on Extraction of Diseased Ovaria*, 1825.

in London until 1842, when Isaac Baker Brown, having failed in his first three attempts, operated on his sister.

The enthusiasm of surgeons continued to increase and the operation was done with increasing frequency and success, though not without opposition. The first operations were nearly all for severe cases, mostly with cysts so large that they seriously hampered movement and everyday life. In fact 'more than twice the size of a boy's head' seems to have been regarded as the minimum size for operation on a cyst and many were much larger. But even these operations had their critics. In 1836 Professor H. Hevin classified ovariotomy as downright murder. Two years later he reviewed the history of ovariotomy and came to the same conclusion. In 1843 a pioneer surgeon, Alexander Dunlap of Springfield, Ohio, sent a case report of his first ovariotomy to the *Western Lancet*, which was edited by one of his former professors. They refused to print it and returned it saying they could not publish a case of such an unjustifiable operation. In Britain the chief opponents were Robert Liston and Robert Lee of London and J. Matthews Duncan of Edinburgh. In 1844 Liston, a prominent surgeon, stigmatized all ovariotomists as 'bell-rippers'. In the same year Samuel Ashwell wrote of his reluctance to do the operation. In America, Professor Meigs was against the operation for his 'dear little ladies' and, in a lengthy article, was accused by Rogers of having entered the field with 'quite as little to offer in behalf of the women, and with partisan zeal set his head against all who would think to do otherwise'. Rogers continues, 'he must indeed be a madman who under such circumstances would neglect anything in his power to secure the chances such an operation would afford of saving the life of the patient.'* Meigs replied 'with characteristic zeal in the art of reactionary tendencies' that 'such a diagnosis would not lead to any hopeful therapeutic or chirurgical intervention, for nothing is to be done in these melancholy cases beyond the adoption of mere palliative measures . . . No man would be mad enough under such diagnostics to perform a gastrotomy operation.'

After about 1840, though it would still have to be done without an anaesthetic for another decade, the operation of ovariotomy became increasingly popular, and still more popular after the mid-century, as anaesthetics became available and techniques improved. But it did not happen without controversy. Questions were asked; were attempts to treat diseased ovaries by surgical operation to be encouraged without danger to the character of the profession? The

* Rogers: *Trans Am. Med. Ass.*, 18, 1865, p. 85.

New York gynaecologist, Peaslee, rebuffed Lee, an opponent of ovariotomy, by stating: 'He is merely an obstetrician, but not an obstetric surgeon, and therefore has no special claim to be heard on the question.' In France there was strong opposition. One surgeon said it might be justified sometimes but *'une audace américaine'* was necessary in order to do it. The surgeons replied that it was better to operate than to abandon patients to a certain death.

In England the most successful early ovariotomists were Charles Clay of Manchester, and Thomas Spencer Wells, who practised in London. Clay began to do ovariotomies in 1842 and by March 1863 he had done 108 operations with seventy successes. In 1854 Isaac Baker Brown published his highly original book *On Some Diseases of Women admitting of Surgical Treatment*. It was the first gynaecological book devoted purely to surgery. Hitherto gynaecological diseases had been classified according to whether they affected virgins, married women, widows or old women. Brown simply divided them into two groups: those resulting directly or indirectly from labour and those arising without reference to labour.

Spencer Wells did his first successful ovariotomy in 1858 and had soon had hundreds of successes. This was before the work of Pasteur and Lister, and nothing was known about germs in infection, but Wells knew that cleanliness was important. He worked hygienically and became well known for his generous use of soap and water. He also introduced the haemostat, an instrument that grips cut blood vessels and so controls bleeding. To this day operating theatres are full of 'Spencer-Wells forceps', the type invented by Wells for this purpose.

The operation of ovariotomy gradually became accepted as *the* operation by which a surgeon's skill and worth were assessed. Almost any description of a surgeon in the second part of the nineteenth century informs the reader of the date when he 'did his first ovariotomy'. Clearly it was regarded as an important milestone in a surgeon's career.

Once anaesthesia was established, many of the restraints on surgery seemed to vanish. Knowledge and experience increased rapidly as did the number of operations performed. The indications for doing them became less stringent and the number of operators increased. One of the most successful of these surgeons and in some ways the most courageous and successful of them all, was Lawson Tait of Birmingham, whose patients did much better than those of most other surgeons. Not only was he a brilliant operator but, like Spencer Wells, he was meticulous in choosing suitable patients and in operating on them conscientiously and with great cleanliness. Gradually he grew bolder and began to advocate exploratory incision. In the fourth edition of his *Disease of the Ovaries* (the edition he dedicated to Sims), he wrote, '. . . I venture to lay down a surgical law that in every case of disease in the abdomen or pelvis, in which the health is destroyed or life threatened, and in which the condition is not evidently due to malignant disease, an exploration of the cavity should be made.'

There were still opponents who disapproved of the operation. In 1862 Edward Tilt, a gynaecologist much praised in the *Lancet* for his up-to-date knowledge, published his book *On Uterine and Ovarian Inflammation* in which he made no mention of ovariotomy. French surgeons also remained hostile. One said that ovariotomy was 'a frightful operation which ought to be forbidden.' Another said it 'should be placed among the prerogatives of the executioner.' At the same time the chief opponent of the operation in England was Dr Robert Lee. He admitted that he had seen Wells operate and 'a most horrible sight it certainly appeared, the bowels rushed out of the wound' and reminded him of the fate of Judas Iscariot. But he admitted that the patient recovered. The following week a *Lancet* editorial commented:

> Thanks in no small measure to the indefatigable and restless opposition of Dr. Robert Lee, ovariotomy, which had for some time been one of the most successful and important of the great operations, has become the most illustrious and renowned. Opposition is the touchstone of truth; and the repeated onslaughts of Dr. Robert Lee have in each case brought down statistics so full and triumphant . . . that the case in favour of the operation has long since been thoroughly established . . . It is astonishing that any voice should be raised to carp at an operation which has been practised with results so triumphant.*

The New York gynaecologist, E.R. Peaslee, said that when he read his monograph on ovariotomy before the New York Academy of Medicine in 1864, there was not a single surgeon in the audience who would defend the operation. Meigs was one of the opponents. This eminent professor from Philadelphia began his own lecture with:

> Gentlemen, it is my painful duty to announce to you that a respectable lady who, a few days ago, came from New York to this city with an ovarian tumour which was removed by Dr Atlee, returned to that city today, a corpse.

By 1886, Sir Frederick Treves in his *Textbook of Surgery*, was

---

* *Lancet*, March 14, 1863, p. 303.

writing that ovariotomy should be done as soon as an ovarian tumour has been diagnosed:

> The mortality after the operation is now so low that the patient will run greater risks by retaining an apparently quiescent tumour than by subjecting to its removal by the knife.

Once ovariotomy was accepted, the way was open for the development of many other operations. In August, 1879, Lawson Tait did his first cholecystectomy (removal of the gall bladder). It was the first successful one done in Britain and the second in the world. His counterpart in America, leading the field in gynaecology, was first Sims, then Emmet, then Kelly. Comparing their textbooks shows how fast and far operative gynaecology had developed. Meanwhile other operations were developed, too. Surgeons began, among other things, to remove large fibroids and to tackle cancer.

Fibroids had not been fully understood until the end of the eighteenth century. It had taken a long time to distinguish these benign but often large tumours of the uterine muscle from cancer. For many years they were treated with bromine and iodine compounds, often administered for months and years in combination with mineral spring waters. Attempts were made to get them to disappear, disintegrate or be absorbed, also to remove them through the vagina. None of these remedies was successful. Removal of the tumours by surgery was not approved. Unsuccessful attempts to do this were made in both England and America. The first successful operation was done by W.L. Atlee in America in 1844 but, as with other operations, it was a long time before the operation was accepted.

Cancer was another big problem, both in the cervix and deep in the body of the uterus. For a long time it was confused with fibroids. In 1812 John Clarke described a peculiar type of degeneration of the cervix which, because of its appearance, he called a cauliflower excrescence. Gradually the nature of the condition was understood, although treatment continued to consist of such ineffective measures as leeches applied to the cervix, starvation to prevent nourishment of the diseased organ, purgation and violent vaginal irritation. Even as late as 1878 some gynaecologists were recommending that cancer of the cervix be treated by electrical stimulation. In that year the first total hysterectomy was performed through the abdomen. 'Radical' abdominal hysterectomy, in which the glands and surrounding tissues were removed, was not done until 1895. By 1882 it was possible to collect ninety-five cases in which the uterus had been totally *extirpated* (the rather drastic word used by the surgeons of the time). Meanwhile,

in 1883, Lawson Tait, ever a pioneer, operated successfully on a
ruptured pregnancy and in 1891 it was shown convincingly by
Schauta that prompt operation reduced the mortality-rate in ectopic
pregnancy from 86.9 per cent to 5.7 per cent. These figures indicate the
increasing safety of surgery at this time, which encouraged the
profession to do more of it.

There was no doubt about it, the golden age of surgery had begun.
There seemed no limit to what might now be achieved. The surgeons,
now widely known as 'the ovariotomists' because of their prowess in
that operation and the extent to which they did it, were jubilant,
pressing foward to conquer new fields.

Again, it was largely women who submitted to the experiments
that were necessary for progress. But not all women were submissive.
Some were becoming wary of undergoing such dangerous operations,
and a few cases are recorded of women who refused a proposed
ovariotomy.

But many conditions from which women suffered could be
alleviated only by surgery. Huge and growing ovarian cysts, gaping
fistulae leading to distressing incontinence, disabling tumours – such
things still begin to develop under modern conditions but treatment
prevents them from progressing or deteriorating as they did a hundred
years ago. Surgery is truly life-enhancing for those who develop such
conditions.

In the nineteenth century, it became fashionable for surgeons to
operate on a supposed gynaecological disorder, 'malposition' of the
womb. In most women who are not pregnant the womb lies deep in the
pelvis and is both tilted and bent forwards. If it is straight or points
backwards, as it is in a large minority of normal women, it is known as
'retroverted' or 'retroflexed'. If it slides downwards into the vagina, it
is known as 'prolapsed'. Prolapse of the uterus or womb has been
known since ancient times as a source of discomfort and disability.
When the womb descends to a certain level the woman feels
uncomfortable, with a dragging sensation. When it descends still
further, she can feel it, like a foreign body in the vagina. Sometimes it
descends so far that the whole organ hangs outside the body in a
condition known as 'total procidentia', which is extremely uncomfortable, interferes with normal daily life and makes sex impossible. Prolapse was said to be one of the female ailments described
by Cleopatra, who prescribed an astringent solution to be applied
internally.* Hippocrates was the first to attribute infertility to it and

---

* According to Bernutz & Gurpil in *Diseases of Women*, 1866.

suggested that wet feet, excessive exertion, fatigue and sexual excess, especially soon after childbirth, were the causes. He treated persistent prolapse by tying the patient to a ladder-frame, then tipping her upside down and moving the ladder up and down rapidly for several minutes. This is not one of the most impressive Hippocratic treatments but it does indicate how little could be done for the condition. Meanwhile some of Hippocrates's contemporaries would insert a piece of beef into the vagina to hold up the uterus, which of course it didn't. It seems that procidentia was the condition that gave the ancients the idea that hysteria was caused by the womb wandering inside the body.

Until the fourteenth century a popular treatment for prolapse was to block the vaginal canal. Sometimes pomegranates were used as pessaries. During the sixteenth century it became popular to do hysterectomy, cutting out the womb via the vagina. The surgeon placed twine round the prolapsed uterus and tightened it a little each day until it fell off. The stump was then treated with a mixture of wine, honey and aloes. Then soft rubber rings were used as pessaries but they produced irritation. Later it was found that hard rubber or porcelain was more suitable for supporting the falling uterus.

By the nineteenth century there was already concern and discussion about what was and what was not normal and there was disagreement about minor conditions of displacement such as retro-version. In 1838, in *Traité des Maladies des Femmes et de l'Hygiène spéciale de leur sexe*, Colombat pronounced on the subject of displacements: 'Those inclinations that take place in the non-gravid womb require no special treatment.' This was echoed in the *Lancet* of 1856, where Tilt referred to the 'innocuous displacement' of the womb. But it was not long before some surgeons were behaving as though the normal variation of a backward-facing womb was a dire condition demanding major surgery. It was also noted that disabling prolapse of the womb was much commoner in the lower classes, who were more likely to be subjected to unskilful midwifery and traumatic deliveries. A doctor in Louisiana in 1859 expressed astonishment at how common it was in slave women. He had seen cases where 'the uterus protruded nearly as large as a coconut' and attributed it to the 'ignorance and obtrusive interference of our plantation accoucheurs and "nigger midwives".'*

Meanwhile other surgeons were busy inventing operations to 'correct' any 'malposition' of the womb, particularly for the upper classes. Since about one third of all women have wombs that tilt

* Quoted by Shorter: *A History of Women's Bodies*, p. 273.

backwards, this was a rich field in which to learn surgical techniques and a lucrative trade for those who wished to make money. In vain Edward Tilt inveighed against the 'Displacement theory', which, he wrote, was 'founded on the most fallacious assumption' and was ' an absolute fallacy'.*

During the 1870s and 1880s there was increasing interest in surgery for 'displacements' and many operations were invented. Most of it was ineffective because it was surgery on normal variations of human anatomy for symptoms that had nothing to do with it. Any apparent benefit was psychological. This period is often named the golden age of surgery, but has also been called 'the dark ages of operative furor'† in which the idea became firmly established that a backward-facing womb was an abnormality, made women ill and required immediate correction. One of the advantages of the operation for the surgeon was that during the operation no tissue was removed and so there was nothing to send to the pathologist for examination and analysis. Thus the danger that nothing abnormal would be discovered was averted. Another advantage was that the weeks resting in bed after the operation nearly always gave some relief or made some change in the patient. At a major conference in 1895, Theilhaber, a German surgeon, declared that in his opinion the symptoms ascribed to retroversion of the uterus (backache, abdominal pain, haemorrhage, leucorrhoea, bladder disturbance, nervousness, difficult periods and sterility) were actually due to other conditions. He stirred up enormous anger and hostility from the other gynaecologists. He was not the only critic, but the number of operations performed continued to increase. The idea that a backward-facing uterus required urgent surgery became part of the conventional wisdom of the profession and was accepted unquestioningly by those at the top of the profession.

The Alexander-Adams operation for suspending the uterus became extremely popular and innumerable variations were tried. By 1925, 110 modifications of the original operation were recorded in one textbook§ and these continued to increase. The operation was done hundreds and thousands of times.** The same period saw an increasing number of operations on tonsils, appendices and ovaries. In 1911 Alexander, the American inventor of the operation, was asked to

---

* E.J. Tilt: *A Handbook of Uterine Therapeutics*, 1863, p. 170–71.
† Frederic C. Fluhmann: 'The Rise and Fall of the Suspension Operations for Uterin Displacement', *John Hopkins Medical Journal*, 1955, p. 96, 59–70.
§ H.S. Crossen: *Operative Gynecolgy*, St. Louis, Mo., 3rd edn., 1925.
** For some details of this see Fluhmann, op. cit., p. 64.

perform his operation for suspension of the uterus in front of some visiting surgeons in Liverpool. He had four assistants whom he sent 'into the north, the east, the west, and the south of Liverpool, and after an ardous search' they returned 'with the report that they had been unable to find one woman in that great city who had not had the Alexander operation performed upon her.'*

The apogee of surgery for prolapse was the operation invented by Donald and Fothergill which came to be known as the 'Manchester operation'. This was effective 'correction' of the 'malposition' which was welcomed after so much ineffective surgical meddling, but the reasons for which it was done were often doubtful. Operations of dubious value, done with dubious indications including minor displacements, were still done and are still done today.

Enthusiasm for major gynaecological surgery increased and at times the idealisation of surgical advance and surgical practice reached almost lyrical heights, even in the most prosaic of circumstances. Dr Robert Barnes, whose views on women we have already encountered, wrote in 1890:

> Gynaecology is largely surgical, and the true solution of its most important problems is revealed by direct appeal to surgery . . . It is vivisection of the noblest kind . . . The surgeon learns, the subject gains life in health.†

Barnes refers to a Professor Coste who 'had brought together in the Musée de France a fine collection of uteruses and ovaries taken from women of all ages who committed suicide during menstruation.' Even more extreme were the praises of extreme surgery which a London doctor, a professor of Forensic Medicine, recorded in a pamphlet which he had privately printed in 1857.§ Contemplating the recent increase in mutilating gynaecological operations, he compared the surgery with the deeds of Christ and wrote 'for eighteen hundred years and a half and more, the divine truth was unregarded'.

It is clear that the mutilation of women by surgery, carried out in the interests of conformity, was regarded by some as a fine thing to do.

---

* J.G. Clark: 'The operative treatment of the retroverted uterus,' *Surg. Gynec. and Obst.*, 20, 1915, p. 597.
† Robert Barnes: 'On the Correlations of the Sexual Functions and Mental Disorders of Women', *Brit. Gyn. J.*, 6, 1890–91, p. 391–402.
§ John Scoffern.

# IX

# *MUTILATION*

To mutilate is to damage or destroy something healthy. An honest doctor who mutilates a patient needs to know or believe that the patient will benefit. Few Victorian surgeons seem to have doubted their knowledge or understanding of women's needs, either physical or psychological. Amid the excitements of being able, at last, to operate on unconscious patients and to avoid most infection, many surgeons concentrated not so much on how women's bodies or minds worked or even on what satisfied or hurt their women patients, as on inventing new operations and learning how to perform them skilfully and safely. They showed no interest or concern in women's health in general or in preventing the 'diseases' that they so eagerly sought to cure. Certainly they hoped to relieve suffering, but many of them saw this as helping women to comply with the expectations of men, particularly their husbands. Surgeons, who shared the prejudices of the age, began to apply their growing skill in excising women's reproductive organs for symptoms or complaints they did not understand and which often did not relate directly to the organ. Increasingly, they operated on women not only for gynaecological symptoms but for conditions we would now regard as psychological. They justified this not through scientific evidence, of which none existed, but through prevalent beliefs and fantasies about women which they liked to think were scientific.

The fashion developed for removing ovaries not because they were diseased and dangerous but in order to modify or control symptoms. These symptoms often related to the genital organ, but increasingly they did not. Once surgery was regarded as reasonably safe and painless, surgeons began to look at behaviour, especially overt sexual behaviour such as masturbation and 'nymphomania', as suitable for surgery. This was widely and not always critically described as 'castration' or 'spaying'. It became known as 'Battey's operation', named after the surgeon Robert Battey, who pioneered it.

The removal of normal ovaries has an ancient history. When Battey's operation was fashionable, surgeons often justified it by pointing out that women were castrated in ancient Lydia and that castrated women with male singing voices were entertainers in nineteenth-century India. This reflects the way in which our forbears thought about women. More recently in 1756, Percival Pott removed normal ovaries which had slid into a hernial sac; he probably performed this operation because of severe pain. The great eighteenth-century surgeon John Hunter had even written that he could see no reason why a woman should not suffer spaying safely, as did other animals.

Robert Battey, like many pioneers in surgery, was an American Southerner and a highly skilled surgeon. During the four years of the American Civil War he was surgeon to the Confederate Army and, in one of the bloodiest wars in history, gained enormous experience. An intelligent, serious and well-intentioned man, Battey thought long and seriously about the suffering endured by some of his women patients. At this time he was one of the leading surgeons in the South having resumed his practice in Rome, Georgia, after the Civil War. In the South there were fewer restrictions on operating and also far less bureaucracy than in the big medical centres of the northern United States and Europe. In 1869 he performed his first ovariotomy, in which he removed a cyst weighing thirty pounds from the wife of a physician. He set up his own hospital with his wife, who assisted him in his work. For two years he was Professor of Obstetrics at Atlanta Medical College, but he preferred private practice. He was a founding member of the Georgia Gynaecological Society.

In 1872, after much doubt, thought and consultation with his colleagues, Battey removed the ovaries of a woman because he believed that, though apparently normal, they were the cause of her symptoms. This deliberate and seemingly well-meaning incident heralded an extraordinary period in the history of medicine and gynaecology.

In 'Battey's operation', the ovaries were removed not because they were perceived directly to be diseased but in order to relieve other symptoms by producing an artificial menopause. At first these 'other symptoms' for which ovaries were removed were gynaecological, for example 'excessive' menstrual bleeding, but surgeons soon extended the operation to women who were 'insane', hysterical, unhappy,

difficult for their husbands to control, for example those who were
unfaithful to their husbands or disliked running a household. It
seemed to them logical and justified to treat these women as abnormal
and attempt to make them conform to the 'normality' of obedience,
submission, diffidence and running their households in ways that
pleased their husbands. It is misleading simply to talk of 'oppression':
'oppression', particularly the oppression of women by men, is another
ideological concept and can divert attention from the facts. The
history of Battey's operation demonstrates how the medical profession could adopt untested procedures and unproven theories that
fitted the beliefs and prejudices of established doctors and society at
large. Moreover, they must have persuaded the patients that they
needed these operations and have given them enough confidence to
submit to them. It also shows how some medical treatments, even
those involving radical changes in body function and human life, can
be enormously popular in one era and virtually extinct a few years
later. The history of the medical profession contains many such sagas
and we can learn from them. Not least we can learn from what became
another characteristic of Battey's and other mutilating operations: the
tendency, once the craze was over, to gloss over it, conceal it and make
it difficult to study.

The patient who first engaged Battey's interest in this way had
never menstruated and turned out not to have a uterus. At monthly
intervals she suffered from 'violent perturbations of her nervous and
vascular system' with bouts of extreme mental and physical suffering.
She was also said to have an enlarged heart with inflammation
(endocarditis) and was 'in the bloom of early womanhood – gifted
with charms beyond the lot of the majority of her sex'. Battey
rationalised in terms of her 'molimen', a quaint word first used about
1865 and derived from the Latin *moliri*, meaning 'to make an effort'.
Used medically, it came to mean 'an effort by which the body strives to
perform a natural function', especially 'the straining to produce
menstruation'. Thus the word reveals something of how doctors
thought about women and their functions. Battey reasoned that 'if she
could be relieved of her ovaries . . . the menstrual molimen would
cease; the violent strain upon her heart would be at an end; there might
be hope for her.' It was pure theory, a personal fantasy. He tried to find
a precedent – a record of a similar case who had been cured by
ovariotomy – but he was unsuccessful. Meanwhile, without his having
carried out the operation, the patient grew worse and died. Battey was
very upset and resolved that 'another such case should not perish in my

keeping without reaching out a friendly hand in the hope of rescue'.*

Meanwhile he was consulted by another patient, Julia Omberg, aged twenty-three, who had had only two 'normal' periods in her life. While menstruating she suffered from convulsions which left her semi-comatose. She also suffered from multiple haemorrhage, severe 'rheumatic' pain and a pelvic abscess. Battey reported later that 'her sufferings were most intense . . . [she] felt there was no future for her in this life, and that death would be a relief.' She was also dependent on morphia of which 'her usual dose [was] a full grain of the sulfate' (60mgms, a substantial daily dose, indicating substantial addiction). Clearly Battey also saw in Julia a molimen striving towards menstruation. In 1872 he had an idea, which he described as 'the creature of my own thought'. It was that 'a normal ovariotomy' would bring about her 'radical cure'. He had reservations about doing something so new and dramatic. He wrote to several distinguished gynaecologists asking for advice. The Gynaecological Society of Boston discussed his enquiry at its meeting of 4 June 1872.

Finally, after much consideration and thought, Battey operated on 17 August 1872, in his own house. He removed both ovaries, which appeared to be normal. He admitted that he was so nervous about the outcome that he didn't leave the house for ten days, 'even for a change of linen'. He said that his colleagues held nightly meetings 'awaiting [the patient's] demise with anxious longings in order to institute proceedings in our court and put me before the bar as a criminal.' The patient developed peritonitis but recovered. Probably the infecting organism, coming from a private house, was less virulent than hospital germs. A few weeks later Battey published an account of the case and followed it up by reports on her progress over the next seven months. After the operation her 'menstrual molimen' disappeared along with the nervous symptoms, convulsions, pelvic inflammation, abscesses and internal bleeding. A colleague observed that Miss Julia presented 'all the evidence of perfect health'. It sounded almost miraculous.

Battey, like many successful surgeons, seems to have had a charismatic personality, attractive to women, which doubtless aided his 'success' in this case and also in others. One cannot help wondering whether his success in making accurate diagnoses was as great. One of the problems was that he was so enthusiastic about the operation that he tended to concentrate on its success without ever defining his reasons

* R. Battey 'Normal Ovariotomy – Case', *Atlanta Medical and Surgical Journal*, 10, 1872, p.6. This was Battey's first report on his operation of removal of normal ovaries. Others followed.

for doing it. However, he did at least remain cautious. At the International Medical Congress of 1886 he protested at the abuse of the operation by other surgeons and said that up to that date he had met only fifteen cases in which he believed the procedure was justified. He always insisted that he never did it other than for gynaecological disorder and, unlike some other surgeons, he never removed the Fallopian tubes or the clitoris. What he aimed to produce was an artificial menopause. He wrote:

> I have hoped, through the intervention of the great nervous revolution which ordinarily accompanies the climacteric, to uproot and remove serious sexual disorders and reestablish the general health.*

Battey continued with his 'successes', though he was criticised for 'spaying' and 'castrating' women. In spite of having called his initial report 'Normal Ovariotomy', by 1876 he denied that he was doing 'normal ovariotomy' because, he said, the ovaries must be abnormal because they were producing the symptoms which he was curing. These symptoms, he said, might include insanity or epilepsy caused by uterine or ovarian disease. He found it necessary to defend himself and change his stance. He wrote, 'In my opinion the removal of the functionally active ovaries is indicated in the case of any grave disease which is either dangerous to life or destructive of health and happiness, which is incurable by other and less radical means, and which we may reasonably expect to remove by the arrest of ovulation or change of life.' Later he narrowed these conditions somewhat.

An essential part of surgical theory and practice is to define the 'indications' for doing any operation and, when it is performed, to know precisely why it is being done. One of the problems about Battey's operation was that the indications for doing it were never well-defined. He recommended the operation for 'menstrual pain' as well as for more serious symptoms. For the next fifteen years he continued to publish reports of his successes, and some of them seem to have been remarkable. To the more cynical modern eye, this doubtless reveals the power of fantasy, of the placebo effect and, probably, also of the personality of a charismatic doctor. Certainly, modesty about his achievements was not one of Battey's characteristics and neither was a questioning attitude towards what he was doing. In later publications he cited many successes, for example the 'entire cessation of the epileptiform and at times cataleptic, convulsions'. He refers to 'gratifying improvement in general health',

---

* R. Battey: 'Battey's Operation: Its Matured Results', *Transactions of the American Gynaecological Society*, 12, 1887, p. 253–274.

'good and satisfactory cure'. One patient, who had been bedridden and 'requiring the constant use of opiates to allay her pain . . . bounced like an India rubber ball at once into a state of perfect health and comfort'. He had followed her up for twelve years. There was Case 5, a housemaid who was 'wholly unable to earn her support' through 'oöphoro-epilepsy' (another term derived from contemporary attitudes towards women which has become obsolete). The operation resulted in 'complete cure'. Case 16, bedridden for four years, 'made gratifying improvement'. Case 29 'was a great sufferer'. After the operation she still had 'slight nervous disturbances' but 'the contrast in her condition is so great that the case may well be classed as a complete cure'. Interestingly, Battey noted that the operation did not cure drug addiction. His self-deception did not extend that far. His wishful thinking may have led to exaggeration, but he was not a conscious liar and seems honestly to have believed what he wrote.

Descriptions from the patients themselves are hard to find, but one is recorded as having written:

> No pen can write the sufferings I endured in the five years previous to my operation. At times I became almost desperate enough to take my own life and end my sufferings . . . My life now seems a new one, and I am getting along splendidly . . . I am now a well, happy, and cheerful girl and do not feel like the same person at all.*

Battey tried hard to think things through. He was always thoughtful, despite the limitations in his thought. He also tried to analyse his own motives and referred to his 'feeling of dissatisfaction and unrest when foiled in my attempts to relieve suffering women through the orthodox means.' He called himself 'an earnest seeker after truth and wisdom' and continued to insist, as did so many of his contemporaries, that 'Insanity is not very infrequently caused by uterine and ovarian disease.'

Some surgeons were less careful. The diagnosis of *ovariomania* was becoming increasingly popular. It described symptoms or behaviour that were, according to the beliefs of the time, thought to be caused by the ovaries or which could be used to justify surgery. The word provided a seemingly solid foundation and justification for mutilating operations. There now began a period of intense surgical activity in which increasing numbers of gynaecologists removed more and more ovaries for symptoms whose severity decreased as the indications for the operation became ever vaguer. The situation was

* Quoted in Lawrence Longo's 'The Rise and Fall of Battey's Operation: a fashion in surgery', *Bulletin of the History of Medicine*, 1979, p. 256.

worse in America than in Europe because medical practice there, like medical education and training, was less regulated and less supervised and it was easier for doctors to 'qualify' and then learn the craft of surgery by practising on living patients.

This led to some gynaecologists being anxious to ensure restraint. Tilt wrote in his *A Handbook of Uterine Therapeutics* that the operation of ovariotomy 'should never be thought of, so long as there is some better plan of treatment'.* In 1879 Thomas Emmet, an eminent New York gynaecologist, criticised the operation in his textbook. In 1886 Spencer Wells, who had done the operation himself many times, declared explicitly in his *Diseases of the Ovaries*, that it should not be done for 'nymphomania', insanity or any other form of mental disease. Then surgeons tried to operate on the ovaries in a manner that they hoped would retain their function. This was a way of continuing to operate while taking account of the increasing knowledge of female physiology. Also in 1886, the great surgeon Treves (of 'Elephant Man' fame) wrote a section in his *Textbook of Surgery* on 'Oöpherectomy; Battey's operation; spaying, castration of women', 'the removal of ovaries that are either apparently normal, or that present other structural changes than those of a new growth'. He wrote, 'It may at once be said that in the great majority of the operations already performed, the ovaries have presented some evidence of structural disease' and that the indications for it 'have not yet been very distinctly formulated, and considerable difference of opinion exists as to the propriety of performing oöpherectomy for certain of the conditions for which it has already been adopted.' He gave indications for doing the operation, 'keeping as far as possible to structural changes'. However, he could not detach himself too far from the prevailing view that the ovaries caused mental trouble, and his indications include, 'some cases of mania, epilepsy and hysteria'. He believed that under this heading, 'the application of the operation is exceedingly questionable. Indeed, so far as practice has at present proceeded in this direction, it would appear to be unjustifiable to remove the ovaries in these cases unless there is evidence that they are diseased, are beyond the reach of other treatment, and are the principle cause of the nervous or mental disorder.' He recommends the rest treatment of Weir Mitchell. 'In actual insanity, also, the indications for this operation are by no means clear, and the same applies to epilepsy, and even to that form of epilepsy in which the attacks are coincident with the menstrual period.' His painful ambivalence and

* Tilt: op. cit., p. 284.

indecisiveness are clear, as is his honesty and his inability to break from his received beliefs about neurotic women.

But many were not so cautious. Battey's operation was hailed as 'one of the unequalled triumph(s) of surgery'. Like most medical treatments which spring from the popular beliefs or conventional wisdom of their time, it was openly abused and not only by surgeons. William S. Stewart of Philadelphia described 'A remarkable case of Nymphomania and its cure'. William Goodell, professor of Obstetrics and Gynaecology at the University of Pennsylvania advocated Battey's operation for all cases of insanity. He even tried to make sure that his ideas were 'successful', even if his treatment was not.

> If the operation be not followed by a cure, the surgeon can console himself with the thought that he has brought about a sterility in a woman who might otherwise have given birth to insane progeny. In fact, I am not sure but that, in this progressive age, it may not in the future be deemed sound political economy to stamp out insanity by removing the ovaries of insane women.*

Here the story becomes even more sinister. Goodell believed that an insane woman was liable to transmit the 'taint' of insanity to her descendants. His idea of sterilising insane women became popular. Many of the women regarded as insane would now be regarded as suffering from 'tension states' or hysteria. This was a time of anxiety about the decline in quality of the population, the tendency of 'inferior' races to breed more than did the 'superior races', and the fear that white America was being swamped by huge influxes of immigrants of 'inferior' quality. The idea was growing in many people's minds, including Battey's, that the unfit should be sterilised. It led, especially in America, to enthusiastic and widespread removal of ovaries. The idea grew that it would help to ensure purity of race. Many psychiatrists thought that all cases of female 'insanity' were sexual in origin and would be improved by 'extirpation' of the ovaries.

It was probably the use of the operation by psychiatrists that, more than anything else, led to its downfall. Even in an age that believed implicitly in the power of the ovary over a woman's whole being, there were limits to what was regarded as tolerable interference. As early as 1874 the Medical Board of the Women's Hospital in New York opposed Sims in his practice of removing normal ovaries. The operation was brought into serious disrepute by its almost wholesale

---

* *Transactions of the International Medical Congress*, Seventh Session, London, 1881.

use in Maryland in the treatment of convulsive disorders and insanity. There the indications for the operation came to include melancholia, 'simple' mania, puerperal mania, hysterical mania, hystero-epilepsy with mania, and epilepsy. The surgeon, George H. Rohe, tried to justify himself by insisting that an insane person 'having lucid intervals could give a valid consent to any operation during said interval, being at that time considered by the law as sane.' At a state hospital for the insane in Pennsylvania a separate annex ward was established for women to have the operation. The surgeons began to operate and fifty more patients had been 'marked for operation' when the committee on lunacy of the Pennsylvania State Board of Public Charities investigated. For the first time medico-legal considerations were taken into account. The committee stated, 'The zeal of the gynaecologist is being carried to an unusual extent when it proposes to use a State Hospital for the Insane as an experimental station, where lunatic women are to be subjected to doubtful operations for supposed cures.' It was felt that if the operation was permitted on forty or fifty patients, 'it might be well to practice [sic] the experiment upon the entire lunatic population, so that the gynaecologist may have the large opportunity he doubtless craves to see just what would happen.' He could then 'read his conclusions learnedly to his gynaecological brethren, with the resultant added forward movement up his ladder of fame.'

The committee concluded that the operation was 'illegal . . . experimental [in] character, brutal and inhumane, and not excusable on any reasonable ground.' Supporters of the operation opposed this strongly, but it was losing its popularity in both America and Europe.

Senior surgeons were also becoming worried by the extent to which the operation was done and by the psychological 'indications' for doing it. Britain was seldom as extreme as the United States in its medical excesses, but the operation had also been popular. It was now losing the support of some of the prominent men who had performed it many times. The great Sir Thomas Spencer Wells himself, who had practised Battey's operation extensively, began to feel critical. He referred to his colleagues as 'rash, inconsistent, thoughtless partisans, whose failures do not reflect so much discredit on themselves as on the operation they have performed in unsuitable cases.' He warned of the discredit that would be likely to follow 'indiscriminate support of zealous but injudicious advocates', and now this was coming to pass. Wells later prophesied, 'gynaecologists will never empty the lunatic asylums'.

By the end of the century the operation had so fallen into

disrepute that it was not even mentioned in many of the textbooks. Textbooks exist to give the *current* state of knowledge on a particular subject for those who wish to learn from it. What is outmoded tends to be omitted, regardless of whether it is disreputable or not. What is interesting about Battey's operation is the way in which it disappeared not only from the textbooks but also from most of the history books.

However, it is easier to find information about Battey's operation than about some other operations which fell into disrepute. This is because it was performed on a large scale for so many years and on both sides of the Atlantic. As a result the journals of the time are full of references, descriptions and comment – and the contemporary literature on the subject is vast.

Until recently historians, particularly those who were themselves surgeons, seldom questioned even the most dubious operations. Standard works and surgeons who take up the study of history seldom discuss the possibility that this new rush of operations might not always be beneficial or mention that they came to be regarded with distaste or opprobrium. Despite the large quantity of material about Battey's operation and the popularity of the operation during the last decades of the nineteenth century, many medical historians and reference books on medical history have been reticent about describing Battey and his operation. The subject is frequently omitted altogether, mentioned only in passing, or tucked away somewhere else. Garrison's widely used reference book praises the 'ovariotomists' warmly and lists Battey as one of the most distinguished, without even mentioning, let alone discussing, his particular operation. Ricci's monumental *One Hundred Years of Gynaecology* contains a substantial section on ovariotomy that does not even mention Battey's operation; instead Ricci created a different section which he describes as 'Ovaries, extirpation of normal' in an obscure chapter called 'Miscellaneous Data (Ovarian)'. It seems that he was too honest to omit it altogether but wished to give it as little prominence as possible. Others are more disingenuous. Munro Kerr's important review of the history of British obstetrics and gynaecology with contributions from its most distinguished practitioners describes ovariotomy only in the most glowing terms and does not mention Battey (who was, of course, American, but his operation was popular in Europe). The book refers to 'the first battlefield whereon abdominal engagements were fought and won . . . it was in ovariotomies that the first triumphs were gained' and praises uncritically those surgeons who, 'when prejudice against operation had been overcome . . . first began to observe disease in its early stages rather then wait for those complications which hitherto had brought patients so frequently to the post-mortem room.'

However, not every surgeon-historian was so laudatory. Jameson wrote that Battey started 'an evil practice - which has not yet been entirely eradicated. The ill-effects to which "Battey's operation" gave rise are only now becoming appreciated . . .'*

During the period when Battey's operation was popular on both sides of the Atlantic, many thousands of women were castrated. It was estimated that by 1906 about 150,000 women had had the operation, though we are not told how this calculation was made.† Most of these women were young; the average age was thirty. Some surgeons even accused colleagues of inhumanity, cruelty and criminal neglect if they failed to perform it. Some produced tortuous reasoning to defend it. Lawson Tait in a letter to the *Lancet*, criticised the journal for confusing 'spaying' – done on animals before puberty to improve the food supply – and 'removal of the human uterine appendages' – done after puberty with 'no other purpose than the saving of life and the relief of suffering'. The two operations 'have therefore no conceivable resemblance' and to talk of 'spaying' women is to display ignorance and 'indulge in wilful misrepresentation for purposes of giving offence'. But such arguments could not resurrect one of the more disreputable practices in the history of gynaecology.

By the twentieth century Battey's operation was largely discredited, but many maintained that it contributed to an understanding of gynaecological disease and the advancement of pelvic surgery. Certainly it taught many surgeons to find their way through the normal female genital tract and it probably contributed to the increasing popularity of general abdominal surgery. It also gave doctors an idea about hormones even before these were discovered. Battey knew, without being able to explain it, that the ovaries controlled menstruation. It is also a sorry tale, though; one of the occasions when virtually an entire profession, albeit sometimes cautiously, embraced with enthusiasm a theory that had no scientific basis and put into practice a dangerous and mutilating treatment which was certainly safer than it would have been a few years before, but which turned out to be unnecessary and meddlesome, diverting attention from a fruitful search for methods of truly helping the women who suffered.

* Jameson: *Gynaecology and Obstetrics*, 1962.
† E. van de Warker: 'The Fetich of the Ovary', *American Journal of Obstetrics and Diseases of Women and Children*, 1906, 54, 369.

Removing normal ovaries (Battey's operation) is internal mutilation. The surgeons of the new age invented other mutilating operations and were quick to justify them. Some of these operations were designed to alter behaviour, particularly the behaviour of women. Some operations were more general, such as Dieffenbach's hemiglossectomy, cutting out half the tongue as a cure for stuttering. Such operations were not confined to women – indeed, stuttering is commoner in men – but they were uncommon. We also know that 'glossodectomy' or removal of the tongue, or perhaps part of it, was done on women who were considered too talkative. There is no record of this having been done on men. In most mutilating operations, especially those of the reproductive organs, the patients were women.

To their credit, most senior gynaecologists disapproved of the more bizarre of these operations. They were often uncertain about them, ambivalent or critical, even though they did little or nothing to discredit them and most seemed to think it normal that such operations should be performed even if they sometimes disapproved of the way in which they were done.

In 1876 there appeared a small book, a paean of praise to Isaac Baker Brown, the pioneering surgeon who was busy inventing and performing these operations. The book was written by Dr John Scoffern who was 'formerly professor of forensic medicine and Chemistry at the Aldersgate College of medicine'.* Scoffern seems to have regarded Baker Brown as a kind of second Christ. Having quoted Jesus, 'If thy right hand offend thee, cut it off', he writes that 1850 years after Christ's death, 'It remained for Mr Baker Brown to give the precept effect'. Scoffern emphasises 'the connection between sinning and the organic cause of sinning; the alliance indicated by Christ . . . If a tongue resolutely bent on evil speaking be excised, that tongue can speak ill no more.' This is 'the "glossodectomie" method'. He admits that literal glossodectomy, cutting out the tongue, is too barbarous to be done in England, and so 'the triumph of psychological surgery is seen in this, viz.:- mild, peripheral, and subcutaneous operations are made to produce the results aimed at, instead of amputation.'

The book reveals some bizarre fantasies, apparently not limited to a small medical fraternity but supported by 'some of the chief personages in the land', who included bishops, princes and princesses. He praises 'the masterly treatment of Mr. Baker Brown' and his amazing effect on his patients:

* J. Scoffern: *The London Surgical Home and Modern Surgical Psychology.*

They go in, those patients to be operated upon; they come out cured, few but themselves the wiser for what has happened: to so high a pinnacle of excellence is the eliminative surgical method carried in these days.

He then tells us that women who talk too much, tend to appropriate what does not belong to them or who are overkeen on dancing may be cured or returned to normality by simple surgery. A 'lady of voluble speech and evil tongue' may undergo the operation of 'glossodectomy' which, he explains 'in plain English means a surgical operation upon the tongue, whereby its abnormal volubility is tempered'. The aim of the 'glossodectomie' operation for talking too much was 'to modify the development of the lingual muscles' such as 'promotes rapidity of motion'. It was thought that 'the mere inability to speak much without languour often ensures peace when the desire of war is present.' The idea was to 'reduce a woman's power of utterance' to a normal state by partially dividing some of the muscles of the tongue. There are clear sexual, mainly phallic, undertones in the description.

> The patient being under the effects of chloroform, a very fine knife is run quite through the tongue and rapidly withdrawn. The result is that certain muscular fibres are cut; the mobility of the organ is in some measure impaired, – to the extent, namely, of making continuous and violent objurgation impossible, but not of interfering with any temperate conversation.

But he admits:

> The tongue, even in its tempered state, is always a mobile organ. Perfect quietude of this member is impossible to attain, however much the patient may be willing.

The author emphasises that the operation does not interfere with 'the normal and legitimate limits of temperate conversation and agreeable singing.' In other words, the claim is that the operation forces the patient to conform to the behaviour expected of a woman by making it impossible for her to do anything else.

With similar logic an operation was devised for 'kleptomania', a condition characterised by a 'thief-like' deed and which seems to have existed only in 'ladies', since the working class were merely thieves. Stealing from the new, improved shops, full of the manufactured goods of the industrial revolution, was becoming a new social problem. The intellectual discovery of 'kleptomania' was dominated by medical beliefs about female inferiority and weakness and it must have seemed natural and desirable to find medical and, even more, surgical solutions. A kleptomaniac who had been a patient in Isaac Baker Brown's hospital 'may have undergone treatment whereby the thief-like deed is made impossible henceforth'. This consisted of an operation 'partially dividing' small muscles and tendons in the hand with 'a fine, small knife, passed under the skin'. The idea was to prevent legerdemain and thus 'the misappropriation of small objects' without detectable movement of the hand.

The other condition described and discussed is 'gyromania' with which it seems some young ladies were afflicted. It was a woman's 'morbid desire to spin round and round, her waist encircled by a male arm. In such a case a mild subcutaneous operation is all that has to be done.' Scoffern describes a case of Miss –, who 'had a disordered rage for waltzing'. He refers to this as an 'emergency' in which a bishop was consulted. He recommended surgery. Miss – underwent 'a mild peripheral operation'. Again, a narrow knife was inserted and, after 'division of a few fibres of the glutaei and gastrocnemii muscles [in the buttocks and calf], no more', the patient was cured. She left the surgical home 'as complete an ornament to her sex as any charming woman can well be'.

One of the most interesting mutilations in the early decades of anaesthetics was clitoridectomy, the removal of the clitoris. The operation was an old one but now enjoyed a new vogue in both England and the United States. Far fewer clitoridectomies were done than oöphorectomies (the name by which the surgical removal of normal ovaries came to be known), but the operation has a special place in the history of surgery on women and a particular significance in the history of sexuality in the nineteenth century. While the ovaries were invisible and symbolically connected with reproduction, the clitoris was palpably part of women's sexuality, especially her appreciation of sexual feeling and her enjoyment of sex. In the climate of feeling and opinion then prevailing, the clitoris was regarded as a source of psychological disturbance and as such, came under the surgeon's knife.

Mutilating operations on the clitoris have a long history during which they have varied in both intention and techniques. They have been, and still are, part of a long tradition of religious ritual, mostly in muslim parts of Africa. In Europe, until the new craze of the 1860s, the operation was done only for tumours or visible physical disease such as syphilis. Only in the second half of the nineteenth century did clitoridectomy become, for some doctors, a common practice and even an ideological crusade.

The clitoris is the female organ that corresponds to the penis. Though much smaller, it is composed of similar tissues and is erectile and sensitive to sexual feeling and stimulation. 'Clitoridectomy' is a word often used loosely to cover several different operations. An operation on the clitoris may be a true clitoridectomy, in which the entire organ is removed. This may even be part of a 'vulvectomy', in which the labia are excised. In Victorian times a popular word for this was 'extirpation'. Sometimes the operation done was actually circumcision, the removal of the hood of tissue that surrounds the organ, and sometimes it was infibulation, which is removal not only of the clitoris but also of the front parts of the labia, done to leave raw parts which are then sewn together. In Europe and America the thinking behind the operation was not religious, but rather that what was regarded as a source of trouble, or a potential source of trouble, should be removed. This kind of thinking can still be detected among some surgeons today, particularly in relation to organs such as the uterus and appendix.

Standard reference books give little information about clitoridectomy in Europe or America. The subject, which became a source of deep shame to an emerging profession, is concealed even more than Battey's operation. It was easier to conceal because the operation was not so fashionable and less was written about it. Modern gynaecological textbooks do not mention clitoridectomy and many of them refer to the clitoris only in the anatomical description. More surprising until one understands the process, many otherwise comprehensive history books do not mention it. The only reference to the clitoris in Garrison's monumental history of medicine is in the section on ancient Egypt, which refers to a plaque recording a suit for the recovery of costs for a clitoridectomy. The dramatic history of the operation in Victorian Britain and America is not even mentioned.

Until the mid-nineteenth century, clitoridectomy was a rare operation occasionally performed for severe disease of that organ. Many old textbooks and reports describe its physical disorders and the indications for removing it. Some of these contain striking pictures of tumours of the clitoris weighing several pounds and describe techniques for removing them. These accounts with their lurid, hand-drawn illustrations are a salutary reminder of the painful, disabling and embarrassing medical abnormalities which can develop unchecked in those without access to modern surgery. It is difficult to envisage someone in the twentieth-century industrial world, or even in the Third World, burdened with a tumour of the clitoris weighing several pounds.

Such gruesome pathological conditions were only a small part of a surgeon's practice. There was no question of a surgeon operating on a clitoris simply because the woman masturbated or was psychologically disturbed, though such an operation had sometimes been suggested as a theoretical possibility. Already in the eighteenth century masturbation had been considered to be a disease and this idea grew stronger during the nineteenth century, though not all surgeons liked it. Typical of many surgeons was Fleetwood Churchill, a respected authority, whose textbook contained bizarre pictures of enlargement of the clitoris and described 'cauliflower growths'. Churchill denied that enlargement was sexual and said that most cases were due to syphilis. He also described a clitoris eight inches long which developed after a course of mercury for syphilis. He insisted that if the condition was not too severe or inconveniencing, treatment should be 'cooling or astringent lotions or the application of caustic to the part'. He advised 'amputation' only 'if the enlargement be so excessive as to occasion physical inconvenience, or so sensitive as to give rise to sexual excitement.' He showed none of the sentimentality about women that was beginning to afflict some of his colleagues.

Nevertheless, for many the clitoris was acquiring a new significance and was included, along with many minor gynaecological conditions, in the increasing involvement of surgery in the idealisation and control of women. This gradual sexualisation can be traced through the textbooks and medical literature of the time. Some surgeons were strongly affected by it, others much less. In 1844 Samuel Ashwell, member of the Royal College of Physicians and Obstetric Physician and Lecturer to Guy's Hospital wrote:

> Sometimes an enlarged clitoris is marked by exquisite sensibility of its mucous membrane . . . it frequently gives rise to sexual passion, and subdues every feeling of modesty and delicacy . . . the health soon becomes impaired, constant headache . . . sometimes frequent attacks of hysteria. The mind loses all discipline, and the thoughts and expressions assume a sentimental and amatory character, while compassion and pity are sought to be elicited from the attendants . . . If the growth is insensible, and relief is sought for its mechanical annoyance . . . the best way is to excise it . . . Excision also is required when the growth is attended with undue sensibility . . . A few leeches may be applied near the part . . . Hydrocyanic acid in solution, will be found very efficatious as a lotion.*

* S. Ashwell: *A Practical Treatise on the Diseases Peculiar to Women*, p. 708.

Psychiatry was one route by which disorders of the clitoris expanded in the thoughts and fantasies of doctors to encompass sexuality without any need to find local pathology. The idea spread that insanity in females was caused by uncontrolled sexuality, particularly masturbation and 'nymphomania'. This was strengthened by the observation that many lunatics in asylums (presumably having little else to do), masturbated freely and made overt and indiscriminate sexual advances.

The nineteenth-century obsession with masturbation has been fully chronicled in many books, for example Alex Comfort's *The Anxiety Makers* and Steven Marcus's *The Other Victorians*. Disapproval of the practice can be found in many ages but nowhere did it arouse such passion and therapeutic zeal as in nineteenth-century Britain and America. The answer that seemed obvious to many was local treatment and thus the gynaecologist came to be regarded as the 'expert' and spokesman in sexual matters. Many different treatments were prescribed, most of them unpleasant. There were hot-water enemas, leeches applied to the vulva and cauterisation of the clitoris. The 'obvious' solution, clitoridectomy, or removal of the organ, had been advocated by various gynaecologists for many years but it struck one of Britain's most skilful, intelligent and original surgeons so forcibly that he proceeded to practise it in a big way, as demonstrated by the number of articles in the Surgeon-General's Catalogue.

The surgeon was Isaac Baker Brown of London, whom we have already met several times. Born in Essex in 1812, the son of a 'country gentleman', he was the grandson of the Reverend James Boyce, who had been master of the Bluecoat School when Samuel Taylor Coleridge and Charles Lamb were pupils. He distinguished himself as a student at Guy's Hospital, won many prizes and trained as a surgeon. He was an enthusiast for the new operations and was the first to use the term 'ovariotomy' in place of the customary rather gruesome expression 'extirpation of the ovaries'.

Baker Brown was prominent in the close group of London doctors at the top of the medical profession that nowadays would be called the medical establishment. A skilled and original surgeon, he was one of the founders of St Mary's Hospital in London, a great teaching hospital. The first meeting for its foundation took place in his dining-room and he became the hospital's surgeon and accoucheur. In 1854 he published an innovative book, based on his personal experience. Called *On Surgical Diseases of Women*, it was probably the first text ever written that dealt solely with surgical treatment for diseases of women and it was well received. His obituarist in the

*British Medical Journal (BMJ)* wrote in 1873 that it 'established his celebrity as an operator at once bold, ingenious and successful, and of itself will ensure his memory.' In 1854 the *BMJ* said 'his operating theatre is one of the most attractive to the professional visitor in all London'. One of his distinguished guests was the French surgeon, Auguste Nélaton, who watched him perform three ovariotomies in one afternoon in 1861. Nélaton, who was staying in Baker Brown's house at the time, also visited other Baker Brown patients who were recovering from ovariotomy. Impressed by what he saw, he returned to France and encouraged the operation there.

Baker Brown is chiefly remembered today for clitoridectomy, which he popularised in England and introduced to the United States, where it was practised on a substantial scale long after it had been discredited in Britain. The popularity of this operation may have been due to the fact that it was a logical development from the increasing anxiety about female sexuality and auto-erotic activity that could be traced back for many centuries but which, at this time, was creating unprecedented anxiety and dominating the thoughts of many people, especially doctors, educators and parents. The clitoris was held to be the cause of female masturbation, a practice held to be dangerous and a common cause of debility and insanity. The clitoris symbolised the aspect of women that men could arouse but not control. Uncontrollable, unconforming women seemed to threaten men and aroused intense anxiety in many, as they still do today. Clitoridectomy was the surgical expression of an ideology that restricted female sexuality to reproduction. The removal of the clitoris eliminated the woman's sexual pleasure. Baker Brown, like many of his contemporaries, believed that masturbation, which he coyly called 'peripheral excitement', was the cardinal symptom, perhaps the essence, of female insanity.

In 1858 Baker Brown opened a private surgical clinic at 16 Stanley Terrace, Notting Hill. He called it 'The London Home for Surgical Diseases of Women'. It had twenty beds. He advertised it in the 'London and Provincial Medical Directory'. The following January he resigned from St Mary's Hospital. The next year he changed the name of his clinic to the London Surgical Home for Diseases of Women, and it grew over the next three years to thirty-four beds. The following year, 1865, he was elected president of the Medical Society of London, a distinguished institution that still exists. The clinic was largely, though not exclusively, for the performance of clitoridectomy.

Baker Brown was at the height of his success but was already being criticised, particularly for his self-promotion. However, this criticism seems not to have worried him. In 1866 the London and Provincial Gazette carried the largest and most elaborate advertisement for the home, which was now called simply the London Surgical Home. An editorial in the *BMJ* in January 1866 remarked, 'We doubt whether the profession will approve of the way in which this particular institution is brought before the public . . . A superfluous amount of self-laudation is not always a real recommendation.' The editor then reported Isaac Baker Brown's own words, 'I thought we had discovered a model of curing a class of cases hitherto perfectly incurable – I mean cases of epilepsy, sometimes including insanity and hysteria.'

The *BMJ* was complaining about an article that had recently been published in the *Standard*, written by a distinguished member of the Press to show his gratitude to the home for the care of his wife. The article said that Baker Brown had provided not only 'ordinary and known' treatment, but had 'actually succeeded in accomplishing with success operations never before performed in England; in one class of cases at least, never, we believe, previously done anywhere.'

The 'class of cases' referred to consisted of women and girls of whose behaviour middle-class males disapproved. No criticism was made of the clitoridectomies that Baker Brown was performing on them. At this stage the *BMJ* objected only to the publicity, not to the operations. Ever since the British establishment organised itself, it has tended to be uncritical about the way in which doctors of whom it approves treat their patients, but it has been strongly opposed to any form of self-advertisement. Baker Brown protested his innocence but it looked as though he had engineered the adulatory article, or at least condoned it. The editor of the *BMJ* clearly thought he had and was hostile. Baker Brown was making enemies, perhaps arousing envy of his daring and his success.

A few weeks later, in March 1866, a book by Baker Brown was published. It was called *The Curability of certain forms of Insanity, Epilepsy, Catalepsy, and Hysteria in Females* and was very different from his previous tome. It was a handsome book that has been described as 'a slim red volume, with its author's name and title inscribed in clear gold letters'. It was to cause one of the biggest medical rows of the century.

# X

# EXPULSION

The book that caused so much trouble was a report on forty-eight cases of 'peripheral excitement' (the word masturbation is not mentioned though that is what the book is about). To justify his actions Baker Brown liked to quote distinguished medical men, often giving their words new meanings. He had read the lectures which the distinguished neurologist Charles-Édouard Brown-Séquard had given before the Royal College of Surgeons and published in the *Lancet* in 1858. He wrote:

> I was struck with a fact much insisted upon by the learned physiologist, namely the great mischief which might be caused in the system generally, and in the nervous centres especially, by peripheral excitement.

Brown-Séquard had made general statements about 'peripheral excitement' in the sense of general nerve stimulation, but Baker Brown transposed the idea to the female genitalia, concentrating on the pudic nerve (which runs to the clitoris) and found that this 'threw a new light' on to some cases in which he had failed. It made him think that these cases 'depended on the peripheral excitement of the pudic nerve'. He 'at once subjected this deduction to a surgical test, by removing the cause of the excitement'. This is a typical rationalisation of action through belief. Later Brown-Séquard complained that Baker Brown had used his work out of context.

Baker Brown also supported his actions by quoting from another authority, Handfield-Jones, who had written, 'it is abundantly clear that the great majority of disorders we have to treat at the present time show more or less marked indications of failure of nervous power'. Baker Brown gives neurological explanations, all pointing towards the 'logical' solution of clitoridectomy. He quotes Sir William Gull, who wrote up a case of 'complete paraplegia induced by sexual excess', then cites a case of epilepsy originating in bad teeth and one in which bad teeth cause paraplegia. He came to the conclusion that many diseases of females 'depend on loss of nerve power, and this was produced by peripheral irritation, arising originally in some branches of the pudic nerve, more particularly the incident nerve supplying the clitoris, and sometimes the small branches which supply the vagina, perinaeum, and anus.'

It would be difficult to find a better example of pseudo-scientific rationalisation. Baker Brown continues by describing the 'disease' for which he has now found a 'cure'. The description is typical of much that the Victorian age produced in belief or invention. He describes the disease as going through eight stages – hysteria, spinal irritation (with reflex action on uterus, ovaries etc), and giving rise to uterine displacements, amaurosis (blindness), hemiplegia (paralysis down one side), paraplegia (paralysis in both legs), epileptoid fits of hysterical epilepsy. Other conditions held in these systems of belief included cataleptic fits, epileptic fits, 'idiotcy' [sic], mania and death.

He justifies the inclusion of 'death' by describing a case of a nineteen year-old girl who suffered from acute headache and blindness. 'She was found dead, and with every evidence of having expired during a paroxysm of abnormal excitement.' He does not give the evidence for this statement. Again he appeals to the great Brown-Séquard, who, he said, agreed that 'destruction of the nerve causing irritation was the only effective cure'. He thought it was more humane to operate than to use the cautery. He admitted that he had received objections (and some of them were as illogical as his own arguments) about unsexing the female, preventing normal excitement in 'marital intercourse', causing sterility and so on, but counters the moral criticisms by saying:

> I am here at a loss how to give an answer, for I can scarcely conceive how such a question can be raised against a method of treatment which has for its object the cure of a disease, that is rapidly tending to lower the moral tone, and which treatment is dictated by the loftiest and most moral considerations.

He adds that he always had his diagnosis 'confirmed' by the patient or her friends. It first appeared at puberty when girls became 'restless and excited' and 'indifferent to the social influences of domestic life'. Other symptoms and signs were depression, loss of appetite, 'a quivering of the eyelids, and an inability to look one in the face'. One sign of the disease was that sufferers often wished to leave home, work and become nurses or sisters of charity. This failure to conform to what was expected of women was important in diagnosis.

He described the case of a twenty-six year-old dressmaker who for the previous five years had been 'so ill as to render her unable to do any work'. (It was all right for lower class women to work. Indeed they were expected to do so.) 'Her physiognomy at once told me the nature of the case.' She was, he tells us, 'much attenuated', sick with pain after meals, had 'constant acid eructations', was so weak that sometimes she could not cross the room, and complained of burning aching pain with great weakness in the lower back. Her periods were irregular with heavy leucorrhoea (white discharge) and costive bowels. He says nothing else about her condition. He refers to no gynaecological abnormality. He does not mention that he even examined her. He admitted her to his clinic and 'divided the clitoris subcutaneously'. Two months later, she was well.

In other cases he also describes 'evidence of peripheral excitement' and he says repeatedly, 'I performed my usual operation'. 'The patient made a good recovery; she remained quite well, and became in every respect a good wife.' In five of his cases part of the 'illness' was a desire to obtain a divorce under the new divorce act of 1857. Each one of these, after removal of her clitoris, became docile and returned to her husband.

He removed the clitoris of a twenty year-old woman because she 'was disobedient to her mother's wishes', sent visiting cards to men she liked and spent 'much time in serious reading'. Within two years of the operation she was married with a baby and was again pregnant. Many of his patients became pregnant shortly after their operations.

Another young woman who underwent his operation had been angry and uncooperative, going for long solitary walks and addressing her mother as 'monsieur le diable' and her father as 'God'. After the operation she 'moved in high society' and was 'universally admired'. Yet another girl 'had been confined to a spinal couch' for six years and 'had also supposed to suffer from retroversion of the uterus'. 'She had worn a spinal apparatus, attached to which was a steel spring, pressing on sacrum and pubis, and intended to support the perinaeum, and keep the uterus in position.' Baker Brown 'found the uterus normal in position and healthy in appearance' (presumably he looked only at the cervix, the only part of the uterus visible from the outside), but:

> On further questioning and examination, I diagnosed peripheral irritation of the pudic nerve. My opinion was strongly contested, as I was told that the young lady was very religious; but, as I explained, her

illness was to be attributed solely to a physical condition, and was not necessarily immoral . . . Ultimately I performed my operation in the usual manner.

Baker Brown operated on a wide range of cases and treated them all in much the same way. There were girls as young as ten years old, severe hysterics and women with eye problems. He made no mention of unsuccessful cases. It seems that the apparently milder cases were all cured or greatly improved. In more serious stages of the disease, Baker Brown says that there was 'great temporary relief but not permanent benefit'. Even in these cases, all were benefited and the insane were cured. It is as if Baker Brown had not only enormous conceit but also superhuman powers.

The reason I have discussed the book at such great length is because it led to one of the biggest rows the medical profession has ever experienced. It was clear that Isaac Baker Brown was not representing the views of the majority. Most of the British medical profession was opposed to clitoridectomy when it was done for psycho-social reasons, though most doctors seem to have approved of it for 'nymphomania'. The rows and arguments that followed publication reveal much about the feelings of the age.

Had opinion been undivided there could not have been such a rumpus. But, although many surgeons and other doctors were appalled to discover what Baker Brown had been doing, he was a respected and popular figure who, to many, was re-establishing the natural order of things and doing what needed to be done. In March 1866, the month of publication of the infamous book, the *Lancet* reported that their Highnesses the Prince and Princess of Wales had sent twenty-five guineas each to the London Surgical Home. This was a period in which royal patronage of good causes was becoming increasingly important to institutions connected with health and medicine. The book seemed to be well received at the heart of the establishment. There was a laudatory paragraph in *The Times* saying that Isaac Baker Brown had 'successfully brought insanity within the scope of surgical treatment'. The *Church Times* on 29 April 1866 was enthusiastic about the book and urged the clergy to promote clitoridectomy.

> We desire to call the attention of the clergy especially to a little book, which will enable them to suggest a remedy for some of the most distressing cases of illness which they frequently discover among their parishioners. Epileptic conditions have been long considered usually incurable. Mr Baker Brown, FRCS, the eminent surgeon, has discovered and applied with great success, at the London Surgical Home for Gentlewomen, and elsewhere, a remedy for certain forms of

epilepsy and kindred diseases. He has published . . . a little volume of cases, which prove incontestably the success of the treatment, and which the clergy will be doing a service, especially to their poorer parishioners, by bringing under the notice of medical men, any of whom can, if possessed of ordinary surgical skills, perform the operation with but slight assistance.

This enthusiastic review in the *Church Times* was reported in the *British Medical Journal* under the heading 'Spiritual Advice'.

At least the medical profession was more cautious. One fellow of the Obstetrical Society, Dr T. Hawkes Tanner, asked questions about the excision of the clitoris as a cure for hysteria.

Is the operation of clitoridectomy likely to prove a valuable addition to the means which we possess for the cure of hysteria, epilepsy, and insanity?'

He said he hoped to obtain opinions rather than impose his own. Was the profession preventing patients from having valuable treatment or were they encouraging them to accept erroneous treatment? He pointed out that there is no proof of the soundness of the theory on which opinion was based. He described patients 'tortured by lascivious dreams', who 'confessed to the long-continued practice of masturbation', were 'suffering from bad health' with 'burning pains all down the left side of the stomach'. He described a number of cases, some of whom had obtained temporary relief from clitoridectomy and some with none.

On 28 April 1866, The *BMJ* continued its attack on Isaac Baker Brown by publishing a vitriolic, three-page review of his new book. Much of its criticism was repeated later and helped to form the charges that were subsequently brought against him. The reviewer was about as hostile as a reviewer can be. He began with a sneer:

We do not propose to attempt a criticism of the operation recommended in Mr Baker Brown's book; for we confess that it is beyond our knowledge. Mr. Brown proposes a cure for 'epilepsy etc.', in females, which is entirely new to us. We have heard of cases of epilepsy in which the testicles have been removed by way of cure; but of the excision of the clitoris and nymphae as a cure of that disease, etc., in females, we know nothing, except what we learn from Mr. Brown's book.

He continues in this style for many paragraphs laden with irony and sarcasm and demands more evidence to justify Baker Brown's claims, attacks the London Surgical Home and deplores the appearance of the book.

We have not space to discuss Mr. Brown's theory of 'peripheral excitation'. We do not consider it well-founded in physiology or pathology . . . But we can afford to pass by a theory of a diseased state, if we only get a cure for it. And we trust that the further experience of the profession may confirm the statement that excision of the clitoris is capable of curing any of the forms of catalepsy, epilepsy, or insanity.

. . . While admitting that . . . the operation may be of value in certain forms of nervous disease, we cannot help suspecting that Mr. Brown has considerably exaggerated its value. Indeed, anyone who has read the last Annual Report of the London Surgical Home, will not have failed to note that a regrettable spirit of exaggeration attaches generally to the doings of its medical officers.

We feel bound also to observe that a serious medical work on the subject of Female Masturbation should bear on its outward *facies* none of those characters which belong to a class of works which lie upon drawing room tables. There was surely no necessity that this little book should not only bear its title with the author's name on the back, but also have a sort of title-page in gilt letters also with the author's name spread over its side. Mr. Brown is not responsible for the doings of his publisher, but still he will, we hope, in future have the objectionable feature to which we allude removed.

It is interesting to note that, hostile as the reviewer is, he accepts that masturbation can cause epilepsy, demanding only 'wider information on the subject'.

After this attack, the criticism increased. The next issue of the *BMJ* contained a letter on 'Mr Brown's Operation' from 'A provincial F.R.C.P.' who complained that the annual report of the London Surgical Home had been sent to 'half the nobility in the kingdom' and hinted that Brown was not the only doctor who mingled professional with sexual activity. Referring to Brown's book 'and the subject to which it really relates', he wrote:

> There is one question which must occur to everyone, and I put it with all professional propriety: What is the value, *in toro nuptiali*, of a woman on whom 'the operation as usual' has been performed? I have heard of bachelors fighting shy of young ladies who are known to have consulted a certain celebrated physician who insists in [sic] a 'digital exploration' in every case of illness, but this! . . .
>
> I had already been astounded by the notice in the *Church Times* . . . Fancy some innocent curate going about recommending his easy little operation for 'distressing cases of illness'.

More letters on the subject were published during the next few weeks, most of them anonymous. Precedents were quoted, going as far back as the seventeenth century. One letter from Thos. Littleton, FRCS, quoted, 'What is sauce for the goose is sauce for the gander' and asserted that to be consistent, Baker Brown should extend the advantages of his operation to both sexes. On 2 June, the editor of the *BMJ* again attacked him, largely for self-advertisement; for 'spreading the fame of his operation throughout the world' and pretending that the praise came from other than himself.

On 9 June the *Lancet* published a critical letter from a Dr Gage Moore of Ipswich concerning 'the very questionable operation performed by Mr Baker Brown for the cure of epilepsy'. The writer asked his 'professional brethren' 'not to persecute Mr Brown and his followers or to speak too disparagingly of their knowledge, either for or against.' He suggested that very few patients would be found to be permanently cured and he cited a case of a patient who was not helped at all by the operation. A reply came from Dr Geo. Granville Bantock MD, registrar to the London Surgical Home. Unsurprisingly, he defended the operation and cited a case who had epileptic fits for twelve years and was cured. On the same date, 16 June, 'FRS' wrote suggesting that the clitoris is unimportant with no special nerves and not as important in coital sensation as the vagina – this seems prophetic of future arguments! – '. . . it is of little import whether the clitoris be present or have been removed'. He goes on to say 'The operation for the removal of the clitoris is easily performed, and is devoid of danger – its removal is of little consequence . . .' He refers to the 'harmless operative procedure upon so rudimentary an organ'.

Dr Gage Moore wrote again on 23 June, insisting that 'we have scarcely more right to remove a woman's clitoris than we have to deprive a man of his penis.' (To a modern reader the word 'scarcely' is likely to have particular significance.) That week an anonymous FRCS wrote, 'A relative and patient of mine, not wishing to consult me upon a particular occasion, went to another surgeon. She was told that she had "an ulcer" in the bowel; subsequently, that she had "polypus" and "fissure". Ultimately, she was very strongly urged to have the clitoris removed.' A few weeks later, 14 July, a Dr Pickop from Blackpool wrote that he had watched Baker Brown do clitoridectomies in the London Surgical Home and found the operation 'very unusual, inasmuch as there was no local disease, but a healthy organ made the subject of unnatural use, and thereby, according to Mr Brown's view, a cause of disordered nervous action.'[*] Several doctors pointed out that the operations had been done openly and anyone could go and watch. Others criticised his methods, saying that patients were recorded in his book as being cured yet later proved to need close care for a year or more.

[*] *Lancet*, 1866, ii, 51.

The *BMJ* remained quiet about Baker Brown for much of the summer. This may be because in August the editor, William Orlando Markham, resigned after being appointed a poor-law inspector and his successor, Ernest Abraham Hart, didn't take up his appointment until 22 November. In September a curious announcement was published in the *BMJ* entitled 'Testimonial to Baker Brown Esq., F.R.C.S.'

> The object of this testimonial being to give both the profession and the public generally an opportunity of testifying their opinion and appreciation of the eminent services which Mr. Baker Brown has rendered as a surgeon and operator, it is considered that this will be better shown by the large number of subscribers than by the amount of their individual subscriptions . . .

The editor, or whoever was writing the editorials at the time, commented caustically:

> This notice is followed by a list of subscribers; amongst whom are included several givers of 2s. 6d. and 1s. up to £5.5s. The subscriptions here published seem to amount to about £150.

In November, the new editor instantly showed himself to be even more hostile towards Baker Brown than had been the previous one. Criticism from the surgeons was also gathering momentum. Their letters on the subject became longer and described the opinions of senior surgeons on clitoridectomy. Some of these pronouncements were extremely patriarchal. Dr Charles West, who became the leader in the campaign against Baker Brown had already written prominently in the *Lancet*:

> [I] believe the injurious *physical* effects of masturbation to be the same as those of excessive sexual indulgence, and no others . . . I have not in the whole of my practice seen convulsions, epilepsy, or idiocy *induced* by masturbation in any child of either sex: a statement, I need scarcely add, widely different from the denial that epileptics or idiots may, and not seldom do, masturbate.

Baker Brown replied rather feebly, quoting Maudsley, the distinguished psychiatrist who was to the fore in promoting theories about the inferiority of women; he liked to take the utterances of the great and turn them, seemingly, to support his theories. A few weeks later Maudsley himself wrote dissociating himself from the view that masturbation frequently caused insanity and agreeing with Dr Charles West. Meanwhile, West was preparing a more organised attack. He asked the editor of the *BMJ* to publish a statement, 'in the belief that his former position as a teacher in the largest medical school in London not only justified his doing so but rendered it an act of duty'. He had never, he said, seen epilepsy induced by masturbation. Many were *not* so cured and 'very mischievous' results had followed. He believed that the removal of the clitoris in cases of hysteria, epilepsy, insanity 'and other nervous disease of women' was based on 'erroneous physiology'. He condemned public attempts 'to excite the attention of non-medical persons, and especially of women, to the subject of self-abuse in the female sex [which] are likely to injure society, and to bring discredit on the medical profession.' He thought such attempts were more objectionable when associated with a reference to 'some peculiar mode of treatment and alleged cure practised by one individual'.

> I believe that few members of the medical profession will dissent from the opinion that the removal of the clitoris without the cognisance of the patient and her friends, without full explanation of the nature of the proceeding, and without the concurrence of some other practitioner selected by the patient or her friends, is in the highest degree improper, and calls for the strongest reprobation.

The implication was that, provided these safeguards were observed, it was all right to remove the clitoris. This became the prominent feature in the debate. Among the medical heavyweights there was little questioning of the evils of masturbation or of the operation of clitoridectomy *per se*.

On 3 December there was a meeting of the Obstetrical Society of London at which a paper read by Dr T. Hawkes Tanner on 'Excision of the clitoris as a cure for hysteria, etc.', was followed by a discussion. The *Lancet* reported it a few days later as an 'unusually lively discussion' and commented on 'the remarkable manner in which a peculiarly delicate subject was handled. The current of opinion certainly ran strongly against Baker Brown's operation.

> While we cannot but acknowledge that Mr Brown defended himself with much spirit and no little skill in fencing against the attacks which met him from every part of a crowded room, we are sure that, in a subject which excites such strong prejudice, something much more convincing than general assertions of success after indefinite intervals, or skilful appeals *ad justitiam*, will be required ere the profession will feel disposed to imitate a proceeding which if it be useless is a lamentable mistake, and if it be unnecessary is a cruel outrage.

The following week, 15 December, both the *Lancet* and the *BMJ* gave full accounts of the meeting, which was mostly hostile to Baker

Brown. Later the *BMJ* stated that its proposal for a committee of enquiry was to avoid 'the paper warfare which we saw impending'. Meanwhile, the attack was expanded into another field. On 15 December a paragraph in *The Times* stated that Baker Brown was apparently treating 'women of unsound mind' in the London Surgical Home. On 22 December, the *BMJ* suggested that this was illegal '[u]nless a house be licensed for the reception of persons of unsound mind'. Another doctor wrote that mental disorder begins in the *head* and 'Mr Baker Brown begins his treatment of these cases at the wrong end'. In the same issue Baker Brown himself wrote that 'in deference to many members of my profession, I shall not perform the operation in any case without the sanction of the patient and her friends, nor without consultation with another independent practitioner.'

The *BMJ* continued to be concerned about the 'moral and professional aspects of the charges'. On 19 January 1867 its leading article thundered in rather curious English:

> If terrorism have [sic] been used to frighten patients into submission, where need of operation there was none; if serious operations have been performed upon patients without their knowledge and consent, and without the knowledge and consent of their friends; if one operation have in any case been suggested, in order that another might be performed, the Council, before committing itself to any other inquiry, should make an investigation into these circumstances ... The Obstetrical Society owes a duty to 'science'; it owes another duty to professional honour and public morality.

It is noteworthy that four doctors wrote that the report of the meeting of the Obstetrical Society in the *BMJ* 'differed MATERIALLY from that which they had heard delivered at the Society'. A Dr Greenhalgh admitted he had written it from memory and corrected errors of fact. On 22 December, the *Lancet* said it was a pity that the Obstetrical Society could not express an 'authoritative collective opinion'. It referred in more detail to the original laudatory paragraph in *The Times*, which described Baker Brown as having successfully brought insanity within the scope of surgical treatment. The *Lancet* commented that, the 'question of the causation of epilepsy . . . is not to be solved by excising the clitoris' and added that not only was Brown's operation new, 'but his views of medical ethics are also new'.

The lunacy commissioners followed up the question of the illegal treatment of women of unsound mind and asked the *BMJ* to publish the whole correspondence between them and the London Surgical Home, which it did. The house surgeon of the home had 'substantially admitted the reception into the Home of females of unsound mind'. On January 1867 the commissioners wrote to Baker Brown asking:

> . . . Whether there is any mistake in the paragraph, or on the part of the House Surgeon, as to the objects of the Home; and, if any mistake has arisen, whether you have taken . . . any and what steps to disabuse the public mind upon the subject of this apparent violation of the Lunacy law.

Baker Brown replied immediately. There *had* been a mistake, he said, and added:

> I was very much vexed by the mistake therein, and instantly took steps to ensure correction as I thought would be sufficient. I have been daily waiting to see my hope realised, and am now most willing to take any steps the Commissioners may advise to disabuse the public mind upon the subject of the violation of the Lunacy Law.

The commissioners then demanded from him as senior surgeon to the home, 'a plain and direct contradiction of its being open for the reception of females of unsound mind' and added:

> the Commissioners doubt not that, in possession of such an authoritative contradiction, they will be able themselves to procure for it that necessary publicity which you have failed hitherto to get.

Baker Brown gave them this undertaking. The *BMJ*, still on the attack, twisted his words with irony:

> The profession will take note of Mr. Brown's announcement, that no patient of unsound mind has been cured of that disorder by clitoridectomy, in the Surgical Home. It was understood that such cures were the striking proofs of the efficacy of that procedure.

Two weeks later, on 2 February 1867, the editor returned to the attack.

> In the painful and disgusting case of Hancock *v*. Peaty, the advocate, Dr. Spinks, stated that the unfortunate lunatic had been placed under the care of Mr. Baker Brown, who, unknown to her husband, had performed a most cruel, he might say barbarous, operation upon her.
> As this is one of the great experiments for the cure of mental diseases by surgical operation, to which *The Times*, on unknown authority, alluded, and which Mr. Baker Brown so promptly confused his house surgeon by repudiating . . . when interrogated by the Lunacy Commissioners, the statement of Dr. Spinks is not without importance . . . We have the best authority for stating that the above statements have engaged the attention of the Lunacy Commissioners.

A week later the editor seems to have had an afterthought. It seems that he had only just read Baker Brown's book. In a sub-leader entitled 'Surgery for Lunatics' he quotes Baker Brown's assurance to the lunacy commissioners that the home was not open for the reception of females of unsound mind and never had been. Then he points out that the title of Baker Brown's book was *On the Curability of Certain Forms of Insanity, Etc.*, and that most of the cases described came from the London Surgical Home. He then describes some details from five cases taken from the book, all of whom had undergone Baker Brown's surgery:

> Case 47. Acute hysterical mania.
> Case 43. Incipient suicidal mania.
> Case 42. Epileptic fits with complete idiocy.
> Case 41. Epileptic fits with dementia.
> Case 39. Epilepsy with dementia.

The editor concluded:

> If Mr. Brown has so soon forgotten his reported cases, probably it has also slipped his memory that only last year the papers were sounding a great note of triumph, blown to the benefit of the Surgical Home, and to the tune that Mr. Brown had at that institution discovered or perfected a new cure for insanity in some of its shapes.

The following week there was another sub-leader.

> The Council of the Obstetrical Society
> The Council of the Obstetrical Society are summoned to a special meeting this evening 'to consider two letters from Mr. Baker Brown.' Mr. Brown had addressed a letter to the Council, offering to submit twenty cases of clitoridectomy to investigation. This he announced freely in the press at the time. He has since, we are informed, withdrawn the offer. The proceedings of the Council will be watched with considerable interest.

Clearly, and probably for reasons that were not then apparent, Baker Brown was getting into a muddle of self-contradiction. Reading the accounts gives the impression that he was not in control, had no idea what to do, was trying to placate whoever attacked him in the hope that the row would die down and leave him to practise as before, and that he lacked the judgment to see that this was not going to happen. During the next few weeks he brought even more trouble on to himself. On 9 February, the secretary of the London Surgical Home wrote to the *BMJ*,

> Sir,
> I am directed by the two Senior Surgeons, Mr. Baker Brown and

Mr. Philip Harper, to state that, *solely* in deference to the opinion of the medical press on clitoridectomy, they have determined not to perform the operation in that institution, pending professional inquiry into its validity as a scientific and justifiable operation. An early insertion of this note into your *Journal* will oblige.

Yours etc.,
Woollaston Pym,
Secretary

London Surgical Home,
Stanley Terrace, Notting Hill, W.*

In view of the hostility against him, it may seem extraordinary that he did not keep his word, but the fact is that he did not. On 16 March the *BMJ* printed the following:

*Mr. Baker Brown*

*The following letter has been forwarded to us for publication.*

To the Board of Governors of
the London Surgical Home
17 Connaught Square,
March 12th., 1867.

Gentlemen,

On the 9th. and 13th. of February, there appeared in the medical journals a letter from your Secretary, to the effect that he was directed by Mr. Baker Brown and Mr. Harper to state that the operation of clitoridectomy would not again be performed at the London Surgical Home, pending professional inquiry, etc.

On the 21st of February, a patient in Room No. 11 at the Home was placed under chloroform and the said operation practically carried out by Mr. Baker Brown, although not performed in his usual manner.† I am not aware that any consultation took place to decide on operating in this case; nor do I think that any member of the staff was aware of Mr. Brown's intention to operate.

Considering this act as a decided breach of faith with the profession (all the members of the staff being more or less implicated but having no control in the matter), I came to a decision on the instant that, at the earliest proper opportunity, I must resign my appointment as one of the visiting surgeons; and I now beg leave most respectfully to tender my resignation.

I remain, gentlemen,
Your most obedient servant,
John Locking, MD.

---

* *British Medical Journal*, 9 February 1867, i, p. 154.
† Brown removed the clitoris by cautery instead of by his usual method of scissors.

Two weeks earlier, on 27 February, the honorary secretaries of the Obstetrical Society had written to Baker Brown enclosing a copy of a resolution which informed him that, at two 'Special Meetings of the Council, it had been decided ... that ... the published matters in relation to the performance of clitoridectomy by Mr. I Baker Brown, justify the Council in recommending the Society to put in force against him Law IV, Section II, which provides for the expulsion of a Fellow.'

The *BMJ* informed its readers on 23 March 1867 that the Obstetrical Society had issued to fellows the 'extracts from the published matter' on which they based their recommendation that Baker Brown be removed from the Society. The extracts were 'selected especially which bear upon professional conduct, rather than those which have a surgical bearing'. The council of the Society was not complaining about Baker Brown doing clitoridectomies on all these women but only about the manner in which he went about it. The *BMJ* told its readers, 'the voting will be by papers at a large table' and added,

> The President will, we trust, be supported by all the Fellows in preserving order on this painful occasion, and in restraining injudicious ebullitions of feeling on either side.

Clearly the editor was anxious that Baker Brown should be dispatched with propriety for on 30 March he tackled the subject again,

### The Obstetrical Society

> ... We trust that the discussion will be conducted with prudence and dignity, and that the honour of the Society and the highest interests of the profession at large will be secured by the final result – whatever it may be.*

The meeting of the Obstetrical Society to consider the expulsion of Isaac Baker Brown for unprofessional behaviour was held on 3 April 1867. One member described the occasion as 'one of the most solemn which have ever occurred in the history of the profession'.

The meeting was due to begin at eight o'clock, but members started to arrive soon after seven. Although a specially large room had been booked, it soon filled and, long before the meeting began, there was no room to sit or stand. As well as the London group, about fifty gynaecologists from all over the country had come 'to hear, to judge, and to vote upon the issue presented to them'. If two-thirds of the members voted for Baker Brown's expulsion, this would be carried out. Injudiciously in his defence, Baker Brown was to accuse the council of packing the meeting.

* *British Medical Journal*, 30 March, 1867, i, p. 361.

The account of the meeting was fully reported in fifteen pages of the *BMJ* and the overwhelming impression it gives is hostility. The word 'quackery' was used liberally. The proposer of the resolution announced, 'clitoridectomy is quackery'. The 'disgraceful mutilation' was described. But although there was disapproval of the operation it seems that Baker Brown's crimes, in the eyes of his colleagues, were not that he did the operation but that he did it too often, without gaining the consent of the patient or even of her husband, and often by trickery and threats that failure to undergo it would result in insanity. Cheating the patient was the real professional misconduct. Had he not done that, and had he behaved less flamboyantly, Baker Brown might have retained his professional status and dignity, as well as his clitoridectomy practice.

He tried to justify himself, deploring 'the neglect of the Council in investigating the subject of clitoridectomy as scientific men' and pointing out that he had always been open about what he did, which was true.

> If I did the thing in secret, if I had practised quackery, why should I invite all the profession to come and see me? Why should they come without an invitation?

It was to no avail. The atmosphere of the meeting was very much against him and, according to a participant, 'all were fully impressed by its gravity':

> There was much heat and a strong tinge of personal feeling in some parts of the debate; but this was provoked chiefly by the reprehensible line of defence which Mr. Brown pursued . . . He pronounced his own condemnation.

When the vote was taken the result were:

|  | Votes |
|---|---|
| For the removal of Mr. Brown | 194 |
| Against the removal | 38 |
| Non-voters | 5 |
|  | 237 |

Baker Brown was expelled from the Obstetrical Society and also resigned from the Medical Society of London. His resignation was accepted unanimously. Immediately the *Lancet*, which for some time had refrained from commenting on the case, published a perspicacious leading article.

> For it must be remembered that the verdict which was pronounced on

Wednesday evening bore no direct relation to the utility or uselessness of a particular operation. That is a question which may or may not one day receive its final solution. The point . . . at issue was whether [Baker Brown] was proved to have so far departed from the rules of professional honour as to render his retention in the Society an outrage upon the feelings of the Fellows, and a discredit to the profession . . .

The *Lancet* suggested that the medical profession:

> . . . protests indignantly against the performance of a dreadful operation upon married women *without the consent of their husbands*, and upon married and unmarried women *without their own knowledge of the nature of the operation*. It denounces the behaviour of a surgeon who deliberately insults and compromises a fellow-practitioner by performing in his presence a mutilation as to which his sanction is unasked. [My italics.]

No one seems to have suggested that clitoridectomy was wrong in itself or that it was wrong to do it if suitable permission had been obtained and explanations made. The original reports from which I have quoted extensively reveal much about the beliefs and practice of gynaecologists of the time and their attitudes towards women in relation to surgery. It is interesting to note that the General Medical Council did nothing, although one of its main duties was to deal with just such cases. According to one investigator, J.B. Fleming, the Council's minutes of the period did not even mention Baker Brown.

No sooner was the row over than members of the profession began to conceal the disreputable episode in its history by minimising or ignoring it. In the same year, 1867, a distinguished American gynaecologist, T.G. Thomas, wrote in his book *A Practical Treatise on the Diseases of Women*:

> The excision of the normal organ for the cure of masturbation, nymphomania, or general neurosis, which many years ago was introduced by Baker Brown of London, has long fallen into disuse.

But this was simply not true. Clitoridectomy was discredited in England and doubtless those who continued to practise it did so with caution and circumspection. However, Isaac Baker Brown went to America and found more sympathetic colleagues. The operation was part of standard treatment for many years and was done openly and with an air of respectability. At a meeting of the American Obstetrical Society as late as 1901, Dr W. Gill Wylie said he had not removed a clitoris for years and did not see many cases in private practice where the operation was justified. He then proceeded to report several cases.

One was a nurse with 'severe eczema' of the vulva. The woman was nearly forty years old, so Dr Wylie 'felt no compunctions in regard to this measure and took off the labia freely . . . The patient recovered completely.' Another young woman had refused to speak for two years. She showed 'positive evidences of masturbation', so she was treated accordingly. 'The uterus was dilated and curetted, a drainage tube introduced, and later the clitoris was amputated. She gradually improved in health and was not caught masturbating, for a time at any rate . . . but she would not speak.' Yet another patient impressed Dr Wylie as 'not being one who had become degraded through masturbating but had many fears'. Dr Wylie 'removed the hymen and the little lateral protuberance above the vulva' and 'she quieted down nicely'.

There was an increasing vogue for the operation, along with cauterisation of the spine and genitals. These operations all appeared in standard American textbooks till 1925. Even after 1925, surgery was still sometimes recommended for dealing with masturbation. Holt's *Diseases of Infancy and Childhood* continued till 1936 to be 'not averse to circumcision in girls or cauterisation of the clitoris'.

In America, this kind of surgery only came into particular disrepute through being promoted by a strange medical society which seems to have glorified it and produced the *Journal of Orificial Surgery*, from 1890 to 1925, in Chicago. It is difficult to obtain information about the Society or to see its journal. The profession is not proud of this murky backwater and seldom, if ever, mentions it.

The 'orificial' doctrine of the Society was, like Baker Brown's, a sort of panacea, especially for 'epilepsy'. The treatment was circumcision, clitoridectomy and 'other procedures'. Their activities eventually led to a protest in the *New York Medical Journal* by Meagher, a Brooklyn neurologist. Meagher made a study of the 'cult', he said, 'because nervous and mental patients are particularly likely to be victims of this form of quackery' whose practitioners he regarded as 'especially dangerous to the health of women patients'. He cited a case of 'dementia praecox' – nowadays called chronic schizophrenia – who was 'so badly deteriorated that she looked and acted more like an animal than a human', on whose clitoris one of the 'so-called doctors' wanted to operate for $150. Another patient, a nurse with a headache, submitted to rectal dilatation 'to get the poison out of my system' and then committed suicide. An epileptic girl had a clitoridectomy and went insane shortly afterwards. The 'operator' wrote a 'pseudo-religious' card to her 'whose inner self is noble, sweet and large . . .

freed from the earthtime temple ... no longer bound by material
fetters.' Meagher comments on these practitioners, 'Their audacity
transcends that of all other quacks'. He covers pages with descriptions
of their misdeeds, which seem to have been carried out almost
exclusively for money, together with, perhaps, a perverse excitement
about the 'orifices' on which they operated. Meagher believed this for
he wrote: 'That many of them have certain paranoid trends, and are
also actively sadistic, I believe to be true.' They do not seem to have
had special theories about women, though it appears that most,
though certainly not all, their patients were women. Meagher, writing
in 1923, also makes a point which is important for the theme of this
book.

> Their ridiculous claims are hardly worthy of any serious study. Yet you
> would be surprised at the number of educated people who consult
> them.

This is the essence of unproven medical theories and treatments.
If they are attractive to some people, they will become popular,
regardless of their efficacy. And it may be that middle-class women,
with more time on their hands and free from the drive to earn a living,
were, and are, particularly gullible.

Eventually the members of the Society were run out of town.

Isaac Baker Brown, like most other doctors of the time, may have been
quick to collect his fees, but there is little doubt that he passionately
believed in what he was doing. He maintained this right to the end and
even justified having operated again after promising not to by
saying that the case was so urgent that he felt he had to. He pleaded, 'I
believe that masturbation causes insanity', and the indication is that he
did believe, as did many others of his time, including many doctors.
The picture that comes down to us of him is of a highly intelligent man
with an original mind and plenty of courage and drive, who somehow
went off the rails. During the attacks on him, he seems not to have fully
comprehended what was happening or what he had done. He
continued to make matters worse for himself. He made no attempt to
collect his wits and create a proper defence for himself. In 1888, more
than twenty years after his expulsion, Lawson Tait, in his paper on
masturbation, wrote:

> Mr Baker Brown was not a very accurate observer, nor a logical
> reasoner. He found that a number of semi-demented epileptics were
> habitual masturbators, and that the masturbation was, in women,

chiefly effected by excitement of the mucous membrane on or around the clitoris. Jumping over two grave omissions in the syllogism, and putting the cart before the horse, he arrived at the conclusion that removal of the clitoris would stop the pernicious habit and cure the epilepsy.*

It may seem odd that someone as intelligent and active as Brown could become so obsessed with a theory so patently absurd and stick to it on only anecdotal evidence against such powerful opposition. What happened to him after the case may help to explain it.

Three weeks after his expulsion he was presented with a 'testimonial', a silver dessert service costing three hundred guineas, with his crest engraved on the base. It was from 'several of the nobility, gentry, and members of the medical profession, both in this country and abroad, in token of their appreciation of his marked surgical skill and singular success in the treatment of female diseases.' It quoted a passage from Tacitus which may explain why it is so difficult to find material about the past mistakes of medicine:

> *Precipuum munus annalium reor ne virtutes sileantur, utque pravis dictis factisque, et posteritate et infamia metus sit.*
> The primary function of history is, I believe, that virtues should not be passed over in silence, and that vicious words and deeds should be opposed for fear of future infamy.

Baker Brown resigned from the London Surgical Home and eventually it was closed down. His private practice declined and he was reduced to penury. Early in 1872 his condition was desperate and he was suffering 'from an attack of apparently incurable paralysis'. An appeal was made to members of the medical profession which raised 'the handsome sum' of £404. 10s. 6d. out of which the trustee paid his debts and allowed him two guineas (£2. 2s.) per week. After a few weeks it was thought desirable for him to leave London for the country and he went to a 'hydropathic establishment' which entailed an expenditure of three guineas per week. It seemed that 'considering the acute character of his cerebral illness, his life could not be of long duration.'

A few days later, on the morning of 3 February 1873, Baker Brown died, leaving a widow, three young children and a crippled daughter by a former marriage. 'The Baker Brown Fund agreed to pay £2. 2s. weekly to the widow' for the support of herself and her children.

Lawson Tait did a post-mortem examination on Baker Brown's

---

* 'Masturbation a Clinical Lecture', *Medical News*, 1888, 53, p. 2.

body. He found extensive softening and degeneration of the brain. In 1888 Tait wrote in *Medical News* that Baker Brown had 'carried his efforts to a most injudicious extent, due to the fact that he was suffering from very extensive cerebral softening, and was really incapable of forming a sound judgement.'

This of course explains Baker Brown. It does not explain the beliefs that, in his dementia, he held so strongly and which he shared not only with other doctors but also with many patients and their husbands, so much so that they were prepared to sacrifice so much on his advice.

The rise and fall of interest in and practice of clitoridectomy can be roughly charted through the articles listed in the Index of the Surgeon-General of the United States. In the First Series (1882) 'clitoris' occupies a whole page and in the Second Series rather less. It returns to a whole page in the Third Series (1922) then declines again for the Fourth (1938) where it refers mostly to 'savage tribes'. In the Sixth Series (1961) there is no mention at all and the subjects pass straight from 'clinics' to 'cloaca'.

# XI

# CRITICS AND WOMEN DOCTORS

Advances and improvements in medicine need critical appraisal but instead are often the victims of enthusiasms and power struggles. In the stories of Baker Brown, McDowell and Sims we have already seen the sorts of struggles that went on in the medical world of the nineteenth century, the part played by learned journals and professional meetings, and what patients thought about their treatment. We now need to bring together all these forms of criticism, analyse their importance and assess the effects of their existence or absence.

Browsing through many histories of medicine one could easily think there had been neither criticism nor need for it. Most histories describe the progress of gynaecology, like that of every other branch of medicine, as a steady march of progress for the benefit of patients and humanity. This is achieved by omitting to mention anything dubious in its history, such as the increase in mutilating operations, the imprecise extension of accepted indications for performing many other operations so that they conformed to the surgeon's personal inclinations, and 'orificial surgery'. Likewise, Munro Kerr's substantial *Historical Review of British Obstetrics and Gynaecology*, written by eminent gynaecologists, describes and discusses only what its authors regard as good and progressive. There is no hint of criticism or even appraisal. Harvey Graham in his histories of surgery and midwifery mentions a few slip-ups that occurred in gynaecology, such as the excessive performance of ovariotomy, but overall he is uncritical. Until recently most medical historical writing on the subject was hagiography and much of it still is. The medical establishment does not tolerate much criticism of either its present or its past. Even when a medical institution commissions a professional and established historian to write its history, it usually expects only praise and glory. Historians who attempt even honest appraisal can find themselves in trouble.

Evidence of undesirable aspects of the medical past are often difficult to find and read, but it is impossible to eradicate or delete them from the records altogether. During the nineteenth century there was a huge increase in medical journals, including many specialist journals and most of these are still freely available in medical libraries. Some seem to have vanished, totally or virtually. For example the *Journal of Orificial Surgery* described in the last chapter is difficult to obtain. No copy exists in any library in Britain and there are only two in the United States. But most journals and textbooks remain to bear witness to past triumphs, follies and iniquities. There are also modern appraisals, written with the advantage of hindsight and with modern views and experience of social history.

As we have seen, there was a long tradition of criticism, much of it from doctors, who regarded medicine as little more than 'ineffectual speculation'* or as 'lucrative homicide'.†

During the early years of surgical excitement, after the introduction of anaesthesia and, later, antisepsis, there were many attempts at critical appraisal, some by distinguished members of the profession. There was also hostile criticism, from both members of the profession and others. Criticism is usually more difficult to find in a medical library than are the glories of the profession because, unlike the glories, it is not usually specially collected, has sometimes been cast out by diligent librarians and is less likely to be listed in the catalogue. Many libraries contain no section on criticism or failure. The library of the Royal Society of Medicine in London has a section called 'Criticism in Medicine', but this turns out to be only a tiny section listing a few obscure references and omitting those that might evaluate a treatment or a situation or encourage criticism. Nevertheless, evidence does exist for those prepared to seek it out.

In 1886 a pathologist, Henry Coe, complained in the *American Journal of Obstetrics* that gynaecologists were allowing their enthusiasm for surgery to influence their idea of ovarian pathology. In 1891 Spencer Wells attacked the 'gynaecological proletarians' who, he claimed, were extirpating women's ovaries like the 'aboriginal spayers of New Zealand'. He said that the 'network of reasons' why the operation should be done were now 'so closely woven that few cases of a perplexing nature, that can anyhow be connected with the generative organs or functions, have a chance of escaping laparotomy or something more'. He goes on, 'But would anyone strip off the penis for

---

* Jacob Bigelow: 'On Self Limited Diseases', p. 99.
† Thomas Beddoes, quoted by Roy Porter in a paper read at a seminar at the Wellcome Institute for the History of Medicine, London, 6 February 1990.

a stricture or a gonorrhoea, or castrate a man because he has a hydrocoele or was a moral delinquent?'. He imagines the sexual situation reversed with 'a coterie of Marthas' promulgating 'the doctrine that the most unmanageable maladies of men were to be traced to some morbid change in their genitals, founding societies for the discussion of them and hospitals for the cure of them, one of them sitting in her consultation chair, with her little stove by her side and her irons all hot, searing every man as he passed before her; another gravely proposing to bring on the millenium by snuffing out all the reproductive powers of all fools, lunatics, and criminals . . . ignorant boys being castrated almost impromptu, hundreds of emasculated beings moping about.'

Another surgeon, Alan Hamilton in *The New York Medical Journal*, 1893, said that in the few cases where improvement was noted, it was due to 'the profound impression upon the mind of the subject rather than upon the removal of the ovaries' and cautioned regarding legal implications. 'What the medico-legal complications are that may arise in the future from the wholesale unsexing of women that has gone on in recent years it is difficult to predict.'

Towards the end of the first 'golden period' or 'wild adolescence' of gynaecology, in 1895, the physician Sir William Priestley, MD, LL D decided to publicise his views of the developments he had seen during his forty years of practice. In 1895 he addressed the British Medical Association and chose as his subject 'On Overoperating in Gynaecology'.

He began by praising the great advances in midwifery, particularly in hygiene, where the application of antisepsis was 'marvellous', not only in the saving of lives but also by 'enhancing the esteem' of the medical profession 'in which it must be held as a benefactor of the species'. Self-esteem and self-congratulation seem never to have been far from the minds of the medical establishment. He then praises the improved design of the obstetric forceps and, more sinister, 'modifications of instruments used for 'craniotomy'. In modern times craniotomy, the deliberate destruction of the baby during labour, has become obsolete, being unnecessary where modern standards of obstetric care are even moderately observed. The operation of craniotomy is not in the repertoire of the modern obstetrician, a fact which gives some indication of how much obstetric practice has improved.

Then Priestley turns to gynaecology, where 'in later days the greatest activity is to be noted' and which had brought about 'a revolution in the treatment of the surgical diseases of women, and greatly multiplied the number of possible operations'. He looks back to a time when a woman with an ovarian cyst containing fluid had a life expectancy 'from an actuarial point of view' of five years and 'a great surgeon expressed the opinion that he who attempted the entire removal of an ovarian tumour ought to be indicted for manslaughter!' Ovariotomy had had a 'success in many hands which evokes unqualified admiration' and this, along with other successes, 'seems to have been enough to persuade some persons that the millenium in this field of operations has arrived, and that henceforth there need be no limits prescribed to exploits in abdominal surgery.' Here he introduces caution:

> I have lived long enough to have seen the evil of rushing in too impetuously, and in watching the progress of gynaecology during long periods of time, have witnessed the wax and wane of many enthusiasms which have had their day, and have had a share in bringing something like discredit on a department of practice which, rightly exercised, is productive of great good, but, exercised unwisely, is capable of producing infinite harm.

He then mentions 'a craze for inflammation and ulceration of the os and cervix uteri', during which some said that every woman of a household was apt to be regarded as suffering from these affections, and was locally treated accordingly. Then came 'a brief and not very creditable period when "clitoridectomy" was strongly advocated as a remedy for numerous ills. This was . . . speedily abandoned' and was followed by displacement of the uterus, 'and every backache, every pelvic discomfort, every general neurosis was attributed to mechanical causes, and must needs be treated by uterine pessaries.' Then came oöphorectomy or castration of women not only for restraining bleeding in fibroids but 'also as a remedy for certain forms of neurosis even when the ovaries were healthy and not seriously diseased'. It was soon discovered that this, 'besides unsexing the woman, was frequently followed by more severe nervous penalties than those for which it was being used as a remedy'. Then came ardour for 'stitching up the cervix uteri following childbirth, rents which were described as producing many hitherto unknown evils' and frequently leading to cancer. He cites a doctor who did the operation 300 to 400 times in 900 cases. Lastly there was an 'epidemic' of operations for 'excision of the uterine appendages' and he cites an American writer who:

> . . . characterised the ardour for operations as akin to the excitement of fox hunting and has implored his colleagues in treating diseases of women to recollect that their patients have other organs than those of the pelvis.

In most or all the modes of treatment which I have indicated there is probably some utility, if properly limited and applied in well-selected cases, but the germ of truth has been so obscured by inappropriate use that each one in turn has been pushed aside by fresh innovations . . .

. . . I believe we should get greater credit with other sections of our profession if laudable zeal . . . were tempered by discretion and we were to proceed so cautiously that there should be less need to draw back and limit or even abandon methods which at one time were so popular. It seems to me just now that the tendency is to impart a too large surgical element into the treatment of diseases of women and comparatively to neglect their medical side . . . [A]lthough a just equilibrium will no doubt be attained so far as operations are concerned, by the usual process of evolution, a too reckless attempt at progress not only impairs the reputation of gynaecology but the experience and recognition of faults must be gained at the expense of much suffering to many patients . . .

Here he becomes lyrical in the Victorian manner about the patients and displays his view of women by referring to:

. . . patients of the gentler sex, on whom no man with a spark of chivalrous feeling would desire to inflict unnecessary pain. They are absolutely at the mercy of the medical man, and submit in blind faith to what he recommends.

His tone resembles the way in which feelings about animals are sometimes expressed today.

Priestley proceeds to give common-sense advice, warning against a sort of surgical 'gambling' with 'the lives and liberties of human beings', pointing out that gynaecology is 'an excellent field for the charlatan, who may pretend to cure incurable complaints or persuade helpless patients to submit to unnecessary operations, all for large fees.' He reminds his audience that 'the profession exists for the good of the public, not the public for the profession'. He cautions against demanding patients:

. . . nor should the urgent wishes of the patient be allowed to outweigh the counsels of prudence against it. Caution in this respect is the more necessary because there are always discontented women who magnify their sufferings, and some neurotic women will submit to any martyrdom for the sake of evoking sympathy. They much prefer an active and energetic doctor, however unwise, to one who knows his pathology, and in that knowledge is content quietly to wait. As an extreme example of what neurotic women will endure or even crave for in the way of operation I may mention the case of a woman who suffered successive amputations, beginning with the finger and ending with the removal of the shoulder joint, for injuries which were self-inflicted.

It may be laid down as an axiom that serious and dangerous ailments justify serious remedies, and that even grave incapacitating complaints like fistula etc., may claim the intervention of the surgeon.

He goes on to say that it is 'absolutely unjustifiable' to operate for symptomless fibroids, to open the abdomen for uterine displacements 'attended only by discomfort', or to remove the ovaries for 'indefinite nerve pains or other subjective symptoms'. He cites 'the celebrated Verneuil' who railed against women being 'the victims of carnage' and 'sanguinary debauch'.

The truth is that a mere skilful pair of hands, unless dominated by intellectual capacity and a high sense of responsibility, may become potential of more harm than good.

There is no record of the discussion that followed this paper but it is improbable that he was alone among those in the inner sanctum of the profession to be aware of the dangers inherent in the rapid development of gynaecology. Eleven years earlier, in 1884, Dr T.C. Allbutt, Professor of Physic in the University of Cambridge, had warned that women could become 'entangled in the net of the gynaecologist'. 'Arraign the uterus,' he said, 'and you fix in the woman the arrow of hypochondria, it may be for ever.'

Among the small number of doctors who criticised the medical profession as a whole and the way in which medicine was practised was Johann Peter Frank who called the nineteenth century, 'the poisoning century'. Another, Jacob Bigelow, argued that certain diseases, left to themselves, completed their course without outside intervention. He acknowledged that it was difficult for doctors to stand by and do nothing, but pointed out that attempts to intervene too often left physicians unsure, 'whether the patient is really indebted to us for good or evil'. But this kind of philosophy led to inactivity and retarded progress in knowledge and skill. As scientific knowledge advanced and surgical techniques improved, patients and their families tended to demand more activity. This pressure increased the tendency to treat the symptoms of disease actively, visibly and sometimes heroically, by bleeding, blistering, purging, cutting and so on. Surgery was encouraged by great men like Benjamin Rush, who believed that all disease came from hypertension of the blood vessels. 'There is but one disease in the world . . . morbid excitement induced by capillary tension.' The key was the lancet, or surgical knife. 'Do homage to the lancet . . . I say venerate the Lancet, Gentlemen.' The lancet became the symbol of modern medicine.

Much criticism was directed at gynaecology, probably partly because in its current form it was new and advancing so rapidly. Ovariotomy, or oöpherectomy, attracted particular criticism. We have seen some of this in the debates in the *Lancet*, the *British Medical Journal* and elsewhere concerning Battey and Baker Brown. There are many more, too numerous to quote.

In 1897 *Arena* published a symposium entitled 'A Court of Medicine and Surgery' which concluded that criticism was ineffective because 'the public knew little of the evils which the proposed "court" should abolish'. A few months later *Unnecessary Operations: the Opprobrium of Modern Surgery* was published. The author, G.H. Balleray, wrote that operations were done which were 'unnecessary and unjustifiable' and that this was 'especially true of abdominal and pelvic surgery'. Discussing Battey's operation, he said he believed that 'no greater outrage could be perpetrated upon a confiding woman' and he was convinced that too many ovaries were still removed for small cysts. 'If she did not have pain in her pelvis she would have it some where else.' But 'the uterine adnexae are not the only organs subject to atrocious assault; the uterus itself comes in for more than its fair share. To say nothing about the injury so often inflicted on it by the ignorant, through bungling attempts at dilatation and curettage, or maladroit trachelorrhaphy, the organ is often extirpated for no apparent reason, except the undying fondness of some man for notoriety or money . . . The overzealous gynaecologist seems to be constantly in search of an opportunity to extirpate the uterus.' In the same year an American writer, J.W. Kennedy, gave his article in the *New York Medical Journal* the title 'Frenzied Surgery of the Abdomen', pointing out 'One may be a brilliant operator but a dangerous one'. After this an increasing number of articles counselled conservatism and caution in surgery. During these years greater knowledge of hormones made people realise that many past operations, done in endocrine ignorance, had been foolish, damaging and dangerous. Emil Nowak wrote of 'the irrational and mutilating measures of former days' compared with 'the saner and more conservative methods of the modern gynaecologist'. He said the change was forced on him 'by realization of the futility of the irrational . . . as well as by the awakening of the surgical world to the fact that it is only rarely in accordance with the principles of true surgery to remove tissue that is not the seat of disease, especially when that tissue can be shown to possess a definite and useful function.'

In America increasing consciousness of the poor training received by many surgeons led to other protests. Some were very critical of standards, pointing out that the public had no means of knowing who was well-trained and competent and who was not and that potential doctors found it difficult to distinguish good from bad medical schools. The Carnegie Foundation Report upon Medical Education in the United States was particularly critical. Dr Henry B. Luhn of Spokane, Washington, read a paper called 'Conservatism in Surgery' before the Associations of the Pacific North-west (Section on Surgery) in July 1909, saying that twenty years before few had taken up surgery but since it was safe most now wanted to:

> . . . flaunting themselves upon the public as surgeons without special preparation, and with very limited personal or practical experience.
> . . . much harm is being done to surgery, as they realize that they can operate with very little danger to the patient's life, and they operate with little idea of what they intend doing; and, further, their experience is so limited that they are not really capable of recognizing a pathologic condition when they see it. This class of men will, without an intelligent idea of indication and a diagnosis made only for the patient, attempt operations that have come into prominence through able operators and men of wide experience. The patient will survive, the operation may be noted as a success, though probably no benefit has resulted and oftentimes the patient is worse.

Another paper, read to the thirty-fifth Annual Meeting of the Mississippi Valley Medical Association in October 1909, by Dr Henry H. Cordier of Kansas City, Missouri, referred to 'the many disasters in surgery that are a daily occurrence'.

> Operations are begun that, if completed, are attended by a high rate of mortality; if they are not completed, the case is pronounced an inoperable one, and the patient goes from bad to worse, and either dies or seeks a surgeon who completes the operation with much difficulty and an increased mortality, caused by the previous failure and delay. Organs are sacrificed and functions are destroyed by untimely delay and bad surgery.

One critic wrote that young medical graduates acquire 'their real education at the cost of human life'.

> The young graduate . . . His ostensible mission in life is to heal the sick; but having had little or no actual training in therapeutics, and less in surgery, he naturally finds himself nonplussed . . . Perhaps for years if his preliminary education has been faulty or insufficient, he is forced to cultivate a pompous, overbearing demeanour, the better to hide his ignorance and cloak his oft-recurring blunders . . . If his nature is not robust enough to withstand such corrupting influences, his whole

character may be undermined . . . A system for which he is by no means responsible, forces him to practice [sic] chicanery and deceit . . .

The same critic goes on to say that there were two kinds of dirty or careless surgeons, those who qualified before antisepsis was taught and those who knew but did nothing about it. He cites a Dr M, who used to boast: 'You wash your hands before operating, but I wash mine afterwards.' Apparently he used to put his hands in his pockets or scratch his head in the middle of operations.

Much, but not all the criticism appeared in obscure regional journals. In 1909, the *Journal of the American Medical Association* published an outspoken contribution to the discussion from James E. Moore, the Professor of Surgery in Minnesota.

> Our tolerant attitude is no longer tenable, because these evils are growing, and unless we are outspoken in denouncing them, the whole profession will be condemned for the sins of the few. When the laity wakes up, as they will in the near future, they are likely to have drastic laws enacted which will overshoot the mark and be a serious handicap to legitimate surgery. It behoves the profession, therefore, to give these grave matters careful consideration, and to map out a definite course for their suppression.

A contemporary, Dr Maurice H. Richardson wrote:

> There is in my mind no doubt whatever that surgery is being practised by those who are incompetent to practise it . . . They are unable to make correct deductions from histories; to predict probable events; to perform operating skilfully, or to manage after-treatment.

The difficulties experienced by patients in trying to judge the situation was outlined by the same writer, who described the case of Mrs G, 'a lady of wealth and high social position' who had 'several attacks of appendicitis'. A Dr R recommended and carried out an instant operation, from which she made an uneventful recovery. Mrs G was delighted and recommended the surgeon to all her friends. Then she had another attack of her 'appendicitis', although her appendix had been removed a year before. She tried Dr R again but he was unavailable so she went to Dr S who happened to be a competent surgeon. Dr R was invited to watch the operation and attended. Horrified, he watched Dr S remove the appendix, at which point he cried out, 'My God! What did I take out?' The narrator comments: 'There are many so-called surgeons who could not tell an appendix from an ovary.'

Incompetence was sometimes combined with charlatanry. The same writer describes 'reputable charlatans who advise an operation, then just incise – and show appendix in bottle. This is a highly profitable and tolerably safe form of surgical charlatanry, and it is probably employed to a far greater extent than most medical men are aware of.' He goes on to tell a horrible story of a case of metrorrhagia (excessive bleeding from the uterus). Instead of treating it conservatively the young surgeon tried to do a vaginal hysterectomy (removal of the womb through the vagina) immediately. He cut into the bladder, then felt obliged to open the abdomen in order to repair it. He then removed the uterus by the abdominal route. The patient died. The narrator was convinced that, 'it was the deliberate act of a human fiend whose sole desire was to get all the difficult operations possible, regardless of results, in order to perfect himself as a surgeon.'

We are told of cases in which a 'tumour' that was excised turned out to be a pregnancy and of one in which, during an apparently routine ovariotomy operation, the leg of a foetus suddenly appeared. Another case was of a young woman about to be married who had unspecified symptoms. Her doctor thought her ovaries were diseased. They weren't, but he took them out all the same so that they would give no trouble in the future. Then he removed her perfectly normal appendix. He didn't tell her what he had done but after the marriage he told the husband. In another case an ovariotomy was done for back pain which turned out to be due to flatfoot. An account of the time reported that:

> Some years back, after the advent of gynaecology as a specialty, and when men wholly untrained in the pathology of the female sexual organs removed those organs for symptoms frequently neurasthenic, one might see in almost any hospital numbers of normal organs sacrificed . . . So rabid were the gynaecologists to do surgery that there was nearly a wholesale wiping out of gynaecological therapeutics.

It seems that incompetence, greed and misplaced motives were common in the background to surgical improvement and advance. It is noteworthy that on the whole we find evidence of these practices through contemporary observers rather than through official histories.

Some of the criticism of surgery was of anaesthetists and their methods of working. Although there were now professional anaesthetists specialising in the subject, the intricacies and dangers of anaesthesia were not fully realised and most practising doctors regarded themselves or their colleagues as competent to practise it. Surgeons sometimes administered their own anaesthetics and were not always as careful as they should have been. Some perceptive practitioners were beginning to realise the dangers of this situation. For example Dr J.M. Baldey in his president's address to the American Gynaecological Society, Philadelphia in May, 1908, said:

> The general administration of anaesthetics as performed today is the shame of modern surgery, is a disgrace to the learned profession . . .

A Dr J.T. Gwathmey wrote, 'Anyone and everyone thinks he can give an anaesthetic, and yet there is nothing that requires such constant practice in order to attain perfection.' In another paper read before the American Medical Association, the same doctor emphasised the importance of anaesthetists being 'FULL-TIME'. This paper and the discussion that followed created quite a sensation. Dr R.C. Myles of New York regretted that statistics of fatalities were not available. He remarked ironically that surgeons who lose patients do not give statistics for publication.

An editorial in the *Medical Times* in February 1907 said:

> This subject is of primary importance, though we would hardly think so from the haphazard and incompetent manner in which narcotism is induced. The patient is then really on the borderland between life and death, and much too frequently has this line been crossed in the most ghastly manner when the exhibition of adequate skill and the observance of essential precautions would have obviated any such fatality.

Another story is of a 'young incompetent' who had a nasty experience when his patient swallowed his false teeth. The young anaesthetist was administering chloroform and vowing to himself never to give another anaesthetic when 'the patient passed quickly away on the operating table'. There were also stories about hospital patients being anaesthetised and the surgeon then being late or drunk, or both. 'The patient was removed from the table to his bed still alive, and therefore the operation was accounted a success.' These stories were all published in *Surgery, Gynecology and Obstetrics*, May 1909.

> The giving of the anaesthetic is really the most serious part of every surgical operation . . . Yet how recklessly do we use, or permit the use of, this dangerous adjunct to surgery! . . . the anaesthetizer, rejoicing in what he deems the conclusion of a perhaps tedious task, takes his eyes off the patient and tells the waiting surgeon – . . . 'Go ahead! I've got him under.' Too often has such action got the patient under – the sod.

When one contemplates the highly technical and specialised subject of modern anaesthesia, these accounts of the casual way in which it was practised such a relatively short time ago, are awesome.

The protests about anaesthesia came mostly from the medical profession for few people other than doctors had sufficient technical knowledge to appraise or criticise it. Even among doctors, few realised the supreme importance of the anaesthetist in the practice of surgery. But surgery itself, including gynaecology, was more visible and to a small extent the laity did protest. Some criticism came from those who believed that male medical practice was misogyny translated into medical treatment. In the 1880s, when ovaries began to be removed not only for the cure of cysts and tumours but also for 'ovarian prolapse' and exploratory operations for suspected ovarian disease also began to be performed, some patients were wary and some cases are recorded of women who refused to undergo ovariotomy. Some women protested not so much specifically at gynaecology as at the male attitude towards women. Catherine Esther Beecher crusaded against local treatment. In *Letters to the People on Health and Happiness* Beecher describes the ineffectuality of the string of 'talented, highly-educated and celebrated' doctors who had tried to cure her own severe nervous ailments. She took sulphur and iron and let one doctor sever the 'wounded nerves from their centres', she let another cover her spine with 'tartar emetic pustules', she had animal magnetism, the water cure, but all without success.

She says nothing of her personal experiences of local treatment but says it was roughly equivalent to rape because the surgeon seldom allowed a lady to keep her 'honour'. The treatment was 'performed', 'with bolted doors and windows, and with no one present but patient and operator' by doctors who have all too often 'freely advocated the doctrine that there was no true marriage but the union of persons who were in love'. Beecher was cured by a timely tip from a woman doctor, Elizabeth Blackwell. A generation later Beecher's talented grand-niece, Charlotte Perkins Gilman, in her novel, *The Yellow Wallpaper*, protested against Weir Mitchell's rest cure. Gilman's heroine knows that the true cure is work and intellectual stimulation.

There was criticism also from the midwives, who disliked the way in which male doctors had usurped their traditional role.

One wrote that 'pregnancy has too generally been considered as a state of indisposition or disease: this is a fatal error and the source of almost all the evils to which women in childbearing are liable.'* In America a strong-minded woman called Lydia Pinkham built up a thriving business selling 'Lydia E. Pinkham's Vegetable Compound', but regarded herself as part of the reform movement. The product was

---

* M. Mears: *The Pupil of Nature of Candid Advice to the Fair Sex*, 1797.

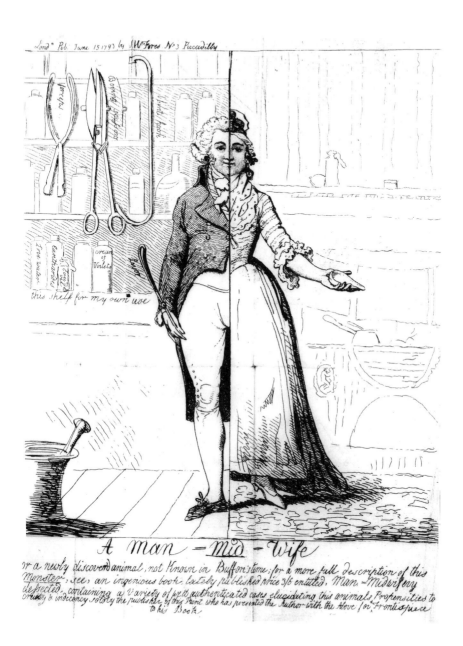

A Man — Mid — Wife

or a newly discovered animal, not known in Buffon's time; for a more full description of this Monster; see an ingenious book lately published price 3/6 entitled, Man = Midwifery defected, containing a variety of well authenticated cases elucidating this animals Propensities to cruelty & indecency to lay the publisher of this Print who has presented the Author with the Above for, Frontispiece to his Book.

**GRADUALLY THE MAN-MIDWIFE WITH HIS INSTRUMENTS OF SCIENCE OVERCAME THE COSY, DOMESTIC WOMAN MIDWIFE**

launched in 1875 and she believed it to be more effective and less dangerous than the medical profession. In a banner headline, she proclaimed herself 'Saviour of her Sex'. Like most vendors of patent medicines, she liked to publicise unsolicited testimonials, such as:

> Dear Mrs Pinkham,
> I have been afflicted with a malady that my physician tells me he has never met before and I write to ask you the cause and what the cure is.

Pinkham always diagnosed poisoning by the doctors and recommends her own product. 'Take the Compound according to directions and let Doctors alone.'

Patent medicines and their vendors flourished in this era but direct criticism of the medical profession, whether it came from within the profession or from outside, was largely ignored and occasionally rejected by the powerful body of what we would now call established thought. In America there was little supervision and discipline was largely unorganised. In Britain, institutions that might have been thought to protect patients, such as the General Medical Council, the British Medical Association and the Royal Colleges, were much more concerned with the prestige of the profession and the advancement of those who dominated it.

We have seen that criticism came from those with medical and surgical knowledge as well as from the laity. A particularly sinister form of criticism was that surgeons, or some of them, were sadists. This was expressed forcibly in 1910 by Barnesby in a chapter entitled 'The Gynaecological Pervert'. He discusses the human tendency to 'kill, injure or destroy', whose commonest expression is the infliction of pain, injury or mutilation upon other living beings and says that 'in medicine and surgery, particularly the latter . . . there has grown up a spirit of cruelty and heartless indifference to human suffering that makes one wonder if we are yet a civilized people.' He says that where the desire to injure and cause suffering exists in 'a man of intelligence and refinement' – there is a pervert.

> Perversion plays a part in surgery, and especially gynecology, never before suspected, finding therein a license and security possible in no other legalized profession or occupation.

He advises that women should not read the textbooks of perversion but 'they should know of its existence and of the danger to which they are exposed if their medical adviser should be one of this depraved class.' An educated man searching for gratification of this sort may well become a gynaecologist. 'Soon he has gained the confidence of a host of feeble-minded or ignorant women, some of whom are ill, many of whom are simply hypochondriacs – and one and all of whom he had absolute license to operate just as much or as little as he chooses.' He cites surgeons who replace healthy bits of ovary in old women but rip the whole lot out in young women as well as a surgeon in Chicago, an 'expert gynecologist' who, when operating on young women for any reason, 'he often cuts off the two labia minora [the small folds or lips lying just within the labia majora]. Why does he do this? When asked for his reason for so remarkable an act his reply is rather vague, and at best unconvincing.' Barnesby goes on to say:

> Let us suppose the case of a young man, intellectual, talented and perhaps, with great aptitude in surgery, but nevertheless at heart a sexual pervert. He begins practice and soon acquires a reputation as a skilful surgeon. But he feels, stirring within him, sadistic tendencies which he cannot or will not repress. He looks about him for a means of gratification that will be well within the law, and his search is soon rewarded. He becomes a gynecologist ... never so happy as when cutting out ovaries.

Some people thought that the way to temper the unpleasant treatments devised by male surgeons and the unpleasant motives of some who carried them out was to encourage women doctors. Women, it was agreed, were purer in heart and motive than men: they were gentle and good and would be a civilising influence on men and on the medical profession. This was one of the arguments used to further them.

We must now look at the part played by women doctors in the struggles for power and the expansion of surgical practice that took place in the second half of the nineteenth century, particularly in gynaecology. How far did these women influence and modify the trend, so noticeable in many of their male colleagues, towards ever more gynaecological interference? Did they go along with the idea that women were easily, or even inherently, sick? Or that a woman's place was solely in the home? Or that study would damage the female brain? Were they a restraining and 'civilising' influence on the subject? Were they anxious to wield the scalpel themselves? Did they object to what was happening and if so how much and in what way? Did they identify with the women patients or with the men who seemed so eager to cut them up? Did they support the innovators or the critics?

Some historians, such as for example, Ann Wood (Douglas), (1974), Hurd-Mead (1938), Lovejoy (1957) and Doyle (1934) have all tried to show that women took up medicine with the primary aim, often unconscious, of freeing women from the tyranny of men, whether professional or domestic, and also of treating women's diseases, which they thought were the result of women's traditional submission. The theory is that they furthered science because their mistrust of the male doctor made them reject aspects of medical practice that were not scientific. It led them to distrust drugs and to believe in hygiene and good sanitation. Sometimes they were hostile to science, regarding it as an invasion of privacy, for example in gynaecological surgery. Their real goal was advancement of their sex. For example, Harriot Hunt, in her *Glimpses* (1856) describes her stunned realisation of the profound ignorance of male doctors treating female diseases. Her sister had a course of remedies similar to those given to Beecher and she and Harriot came away having 'lost all confidence in medicine'. She thought the doctor was deliberately making women sick and that the professional exploitation was a mask for a deeper, sexual exploitation. Like Beecher, she was loudly against local examinations by finger or by speculum. They were 'too often unnecessary' and their moral effects were terrible. She believed that many medical men were sceptics who 'lived sensually' and contaminated their patients. She described local examination as a violation, with the doctor taking advantage.

Ideas such as these seem to have been held by some women doctors, but were certainly not common to all. Women doctors were not a homogeneous group and they had few common beliefs. They were a number of different individuals who wished, from a variety of motives, to be doctors. There were such wide differences between them that it is impossible to generalise except to say that, in taking up a profession, they went against the customs and beliefs of the time concerning how women should behave. This does not mean that they all had the same idea, were all rebels or necessarily acted against the norms and expectations of their own circle. Many, like Elizabeth Garrett Anderson, had strong support from their relatives and friends.

The motives of the early women doctors were manifold. Some seriously sought control over their own lives and wanted satisfying outlets for their energy. Others had experience of sickness which influenced their choices. For example, there were those who had been sickly as children and had become interested in their own problems. Some had nursed relatives through serious illnesses. Many confessed to simply being ambitious, whether or not they were active in the women's rights movement or even believed in its aims. Some wanted to convince men that they could do as well. Some sought social status or a means of earning money that was more lucrative and interesting than traditional female occupations such as teaching or being a governess. Some, like Elizabeth Blackwell, sought to escape from romantic yearning and to 'place a strong barrier between me and all ordinary marriage'.* Some felt divinely inspired or were strongly moralistic and many shared the idea that women were morally superior to men. Others, such as Elizabeth Garrett Anderson and Mary Putnam Jacobi, were fascinated by science, by surgery and by medical skills, and worked hard to develop them.

There were women doctors who, like Elizabeth Garrett Anderson, trained as surgeons and practised gynaecological surgery, despite the fact that it was very difficult for a woman to learn. It is noteworthy that in 1888 the first panhysterectomy in America was done by a woman surgeon, Dr Mary A. Dixon Jones. But the strong objection of some women doctors to what was going on sometimes reached the extent of protesting against *all* surgical treatment. Women tended to practise in 'gentler' fields. In medical school, Elizabeth Blackwell was shocked at the 'horrible exposure of women to male physicians and local treatment'. She became one of those women doctors who tended to oppose medical intervention, scientific experiment and vivisection wherever they met it. On 27 November 1854 Blackwell wrote to her sister Emily, who was studying medicine in Europe:

> A lady called on me today three weeks returned [from Paris] . . . This lady had had the red hot iron applied to the uterus by Jobert, for ulceration, [so she said] and felt so much better that she thinks there is nothing like it, and means to advise all her friends to be scorched – she came to me hoping that I would apply it to a sister-in-law! So Milly you must be prepared to cut and burn, and practice [sic] every conceivable abomination, for it is perfectly evident to me that the more unnatural the application, the more the women like it. This lady was frizzled twice, the smoke filled the room and she is desirous now to find someone who will practice as Jobert did.

Elizabeth Blackwell crusaded against ovariotomy and called it 'the castration of women'. She wrote: 'The great increase in ovariotomy, and its extension to the insane is a notable result of this *prurigo secandi* (itch to cut). She estimated that in Europe one woman in 250 had been 'castrated' and she collected newspaper clippings which supported her belief that young doctors were doing the operation only

* *Pioneer Work*, p. 28.

in order to obtain professional expertise. For Blackwell, ovariotomies simply dramatised the anti-woman bias of much contemporary science. She eschewed all drugs and vaccinations etc. This distrust of science has been interpreted as a distrust of masculinity. In America Dr Marie Zakrzewska lamented the fact that women were coming to her Boston Hospital insisting that their ovaries be removed for birth control. Writing to Dr Elizabeth Blackwell on 21 March 1891, she noted that women came to the New England Hospital begging for operations 'on the slightest cause'. Married women 'between 28 & 40 years' came in asking for ovariotomies 'because causing [sic] dismenorrhea & children were not desired'. When surgeons were thus tempted, she mused, 'do you wonder . . . [that they] go the whole length of disregard for Nature?'

Throughout the period the women doctors and would-be doctors were themselves struggling to gain enough power to storm the citadel of the male medical establishment and to gain a foothold within it. The resistance from men was strong, particularly amongst the obstetricians and gynaecologists, who formed the group most in competition with the women. Sophia Jex-Blake, writing in 1887, said that opposition to women doctors was fading away but remained strongest among obstetricians and gynaecologists.

One of the objections to women entering the medical profession was that they would not be strong enough to do the work. This argument was strengthened by the prevailing beliefs that they were dominated by their sexual organs and incapacitated by menstruation. In a specific attack on women becoming professional rivals rather than patients, an obstetrician addressing the London Obstetrical Society in January 1874 said 'women are unfitted to bear the physical fatigues and mental anxieties of obstetrical practice, at menstrual periods, during pregnancy and puerperality . . .'

Despite her concessions to current, and almost universal, prejudices, Elizabeth Garrett Anderson believed that the doctors were wrong and was pleased when results come from Massachusetts Labor Bureau, which made the first report on the health of American college women and found that their health actually *improved* during college education. In 1886 John Dewey analysed the figures and concluded that worry over personal matters damaged health more than did over-study.

Much of the demand for women doctors came because of the apparently vast amount of gynaecological disease and because of problems of modesty in intimate examinations. The advance of science demanded direct observation and examination but custom did not and many women patients and male doctors were worried by this. Hostility to local examinations was common but by no means universal. Most patients who consulted women doctors were women and many women doctors worked largely or exclusively with 'women's problems', children and preventive medicine. Many of them planned to concern themselves only with these.

Many women doctors were also convinced of the need for treatment that was not confined to one area or organ of the body and was gentler and non-invasive. Unlike other professions, medicine has a tradition of female healers. In March 1905 an article by Ella Flagg Young in the *New York Times* stated, 'every woman is born a doctor. Men have to study to become one.' Indeed, women were the traditional healers of the people, or rather, they had been before the arrival of regulations that necessitated education, study and quali- fications from which women were automatically excluded.

The story has been told many times of the long struggle of men to exclude women from their traditional role as healers and the long struggle of women to maintain and improve it. Especially from the eighteenth century onwards, the increasing need for specific and technical education and training enabled men to demand specific training for medical practice and to exclude women from it by denying their eligibility for that training. Against this, women put up a long struggle to be included.* For example, physicians had to be graduates of the universities of Oxford or Cambridge – from which women were excluded. The Royal Colleges and the Society of Apothecaries extended their power over medical education – but were all-male preserves. The leaders of the medical profession wanted it to stay that way and realised that as long as they excluded women from education and reinforced the idea that they were incapable of it, they were safe from having to accept them as colleagues. In 1856 a woman, Jessie Merlton White, successfully petitioned the University of London to allow her to matriculate. The influential medical journal the *Lancet* opposed her on the grounds of decency and chronicled much of the opposition. Permission must be an oversight on the part of the senate. No one would want to marry such women, for they would be impure. *Real* ladies like their position as guardian angels of the home and so on. In January 1859 the newspapers announced that Elizabeth Blackwell, the Englishwoman who had qualified in medicine in America, was visiting England. The Press varied from casual contempt to insulting hostility. A typical comment was, 'It is impossible that a

---

* The story is told clearly in Jean Donnison's *Midwives and Medical Men*.

woman whose hands reek with gore can be possessed of the same nature of feelings as the generality of women.' At the same time the medical profession excluded many of the 'traditional' female traits — caring, succouring, watching, waiting. Increasingly, the emphasis was on discovery and control, power and acquisition, whereas women also had a tradition of quietness, gentleness and non-violence. While attempting to obtain a medical education, Elizabeth Garrett Anderson experienced innumerable frustrations due to men using her gender as an excuse for excluding her from what she was trying to do and from examinations and qualifications.*

Few women doctors in the nineteenth century criticised male colleagues but many believed that they themselves had a special sympathy for women and children and could treat them, and do preventive medicine, better. A typical observation, by Anna Longshore-Potts, was that the attitudes of male doctors were 'cut and dried' and if women had pursued medicine earlier, 'today women would have had more healthy bodies'.† Female health educators spoke constantly of women's humanising effect on medical practice. One woman, Eliza Mosher, wrote in 1916: 'Educated medical women touch humanity in a manner different from men; by virtue of their womanhood, their interest in girls and young women, both moral and otherwise; in homes and in society.' Others argued that medicine was a natural extension of women's sphere and peculiarly suited to the female character which was self-sacrificing, empathetic and altruistic. Many women doctors saw themselves as the professional allies of mothers.

There has been a tendency to believe that treatment tended to be polarised according to sex, with men using instruments and women being caring and natural. This is not so. One study found men more callous towards patients and more eager to use forceps and other forms of intervention, yet a comparison between the records of two Boston hospitals, one staffed by men, the other by women, revealed no unanimity. Many male doctors were hostile towards 'meddlesome midwifery' and many women doctors revealed 'male' values. The only difference they found between men and women in their management of childbirth was in the administration of drugs. Men gave more than women. The authors concluded that what drew women together was not a 'party line' about how to manage illness but a belief that women had a right to good health, that their own role was to facilitate that

* This is well described in Jo Manton's *Elizabeth Garrett Anderson*, 1965.
† Anna Longshore-Potts: *Discourses to Women on Medical Subjects*, San Diego, 1897.

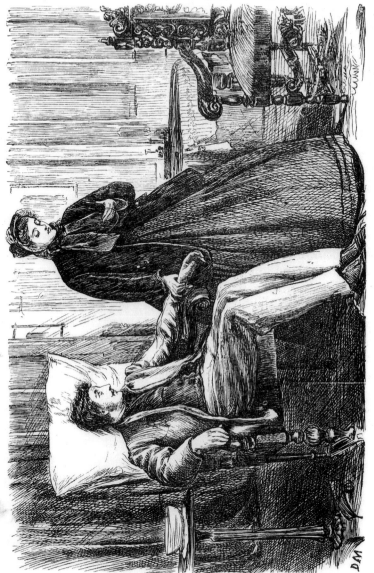

LADY-PHYSICIANS.

Who is this Interesting Invalid? It is young Reginald de Braces, who has succeeded in Catching a Bad Cold, in order that he might Send for that rising Practitioner, Dr. Arabella Bolus!

*PUNCH* WAS SCEPTICAL ABOUT WHY WOMEN DOCTORS WERE CALLED IN . . .

right and that better health among them was possible in the future. Few women doctors believed that women had to suffer illness because of the way they were made. Even if they advised caution, for example in menstruation, they tended to look for the abnormalities rather than regard the whole feminine state as responsible. The authors of this study read the MD theses produced in the Women's Medical College of Pennsylvania during the 1850s to 1870s and found that the predominant idea was that pregnancy was a normal state, with gradually increasing popularity of interference. These historians came to the conclusion that it was impossible to uncover a uniform approach among these women on how to treat, diagnose or prevent illness. Women internalised many 'male' values, just as men were sometimes advocates of 'female' positions. The conclusion seems to be that, although certain trends can be discerned as part of this history of the nineteenth century, it is impossible to generalise.

Although women doctors, like everyone else, were products of their age and conditioned by it, they all rebelled against their traditional role while still being part of it. They were profoundly influenced by the attitudes of society, which conditioned them from birth to regard themselves as adjuncts to men and as patients rather than doctors. Many things that seem certain to us or which we take for granted, were sources of doubt and difficulty to them. In looking at their history and their varied relationships with the Victorian age, with the medical profession in general and with the new surgical expertise, one cannot but be struck by the variety of their attitudes and responses and by the relentless determination with which they tried to understand their situation and to further their cause.

# XII
# MODERN TIMES

Enthusiasm for surgery increased still more as the twentieth century approached, and it was rapidly becoming more popular, diverse and ambitious. In the 1890s the interest of many surgeons moved to appendicitis and there were lengthy battles about whether and when the appendix should be removed or conserved. Gynaecology, running parallel with general surgery and sometimes struggling for a separate existence, was established and flourishing on both sides of the Atlantic, though there were many doubts and warnings. In 1896 the preface to Allbutt and Playfair's distinguished textbook suggested that advances in gynaecology had been 'perhaps more remarkable than in any other field of medicine' but that 'adventurousness' and 'unbalanced zeal has had its inevitable result of injudicious practice, which is to be regretted.' But surgeons, increasingly confident, were certain they could now do even major operations with adequate skill and safety, and many had become routine procedures. In 1905, a medical editorial on *The Future of Gynecology* in the American journal *Surgery, Gynecology and Obstetrics* even claimed that 'the specialty is so far advanced that there is not very much more progress to be made in it'. This was part of a widespread belief that surgery was now 'safe', although not everyone agreed. In July 1912, Dr James Barr, in his presidential address to the British Medical Association, criticised the profession's tendency to uphold self-constituted moralists, denounced the falling birth-rate and called for quantity rather than quality.*

The new surgery had spread to many parts of the body, particularly within the abdomen, but the majority of patients were still women. In line with the thinking behind the 'retroversion' and

* James Barr, *British Medical Journal*, 27 July 1912.

'displacement' arguments, other organs were now diagnosed as being displaced or were thought to have 'dropped' in a condition called 'ptosis'. The stimulus for this concept seems to have come from X-rays, which came into use from 1889. People were usually X-rayed standing up, which meant that, under the influence of gravity, the position of their internal organs was lower than in the corpses and patients undergoing operation to which surgeons were accustomed. No one seems to have looked at 'normal' people to see whether their organs were also 'dropped'. They concluded that the symptoms of which the patients complained, such as dragging back pain, constipation, foul breath, nausea, vomiting, menstrual disorders and so on were due to this 'abnormal' position of the organs, which they then corrected by developing a number of operations. There were five to seven times more women than men among these patients and the justification for operating on them depended not only on a disregard of the effects of gravity, but also on current ideas about 'neurasthenia'. Surgeons busily stitched abdominal organs into the position where they believed they should be. The operations became popular even though the rationale for doing them was illogical. Their popularity lasted for about forty years. An operation might be repeated several times or several operations were done to 'cure' one condition. For example, for a condition of 'simple dilatation of the stomach, and of gastroptosis' the stomach was sewn to the upper abdominal wall, and the author concluded that operations on the stomach alone would probably not be sufficient, but should be assisted by an operation to fix the kidney as well. '[In] women similar supporting operations will be necessary upon the genital organs as well.'* The invention of ptosis enabled surgeons to devise new operations to 'correct' it, in whatever organ it was believed to have occurred. In 1910 several papers gave favourable evaluations of operations for the relief of neurasthenia and associated visceral ptosis. A review of fifty-one female patients noted that twenty-nine per cent were completely relieved of neurasthenia after surgery and the remainder equally divided between those improved and those unchanged.

But some surgeons were sceptical and regarded it as a new craze that did not help the patients. Robert Morris led a public battle from 1908, when, at the American Medical Association's Section of Surgery and Anatomy, he spoke against the temptation of 'the technique that inspires a feeling of security' and 'surgical art for art's sake'. He urged that surgeons look at their death- and recovery-rates and compare

---

* Curtis, 1900.

them with those of other surgeons and also with spontaneous recoveries in cases where nothing was done. There was a feeling that the techniques of surgery should be re-united with the art of medicine. In 1910, at the height of the ptosis craze, Richardson, a Boston surgeon, stated that after several operations neurasthenic symptoms reappeared 'as soon as the glamour of the operation was lost and the patient returned to the humdrum of home from the professional atmosphere of the operating-room and clinic, in which great interest was shown in her case and in which she herself felt a stimulated interest.'

The craze for the 'disease' of ptosis was joined by other such crazes, for example those for gastrointestinal symptoms caused by 'putrefaction' or 'auto-intoxication', thought to be due to an abnormally long large bowel and too much digestive movement. At the same time an elaborate theory developed that chronic appendicitis was due to local conditions which interfered with the movements of the gut. The more one reads the original accounts of these operations, the more one realises that they were fantasies of their inventors. One of the most ardent of these inventors was the London surgeon Arbuthnot Lane whose surgery for constipation became extremely popular. Lane's ideas about bowels exactly suited the growing fantasies of the age about the dangers of constipation and its alleged accompaniment, 'auto-intoxication'. The operation to which Lane gave his name consisted of cutting imaginary 'adhesions' attached to the bowel, excising a large part of the colon, including a part known as 'Lane's kink' (now known to be a normal part of everyone's anatomy), and joining the two cut ends. The theory was that this cured 'chronic intestinal stasis'. Other surgeons invented variations and additions to Lane's operation.

Outside the abdomen operations such as removal of the thyroid were recommended for mental disturbance or dementia praecox. A curious theory arose in which a force named the 'kinetic drive' was thought to exist in conditions as far apart as epilepsy, neurasthenia, hypertension, hyperthyroidism, and many others. Surgeons invented operations for 'dekineticisation', which usually involved cutting sympathetic nerves or removing endocrine glands. Since little was known about these glands, the onward march of surgery was not impeded by knowledge or understanding. These are only a few of the many bizarre operations that were popular in the early part of the century. One must however remember that they developed alongside many that saved life, including operations to relieve internal disasters such as haemorrhage and obstruction, or which relieved chronic discomfort or pain – for example operations for hernia, fistula and so on. Many people were restored to health who, only a few years before, would have died or been doomed to miserable or painful lives.

What happened to all the operations as the twentieth century advanced? Some declined in popularity, revealed as useless or dangerous and not useful to the increasingly dignified profession of surgery; some proved their value, improved conception and technique and so multiplied or were superseded by improved procedures; new operations were invented and either flourished and developed or declined into oblivion. Some have attracted criticism, even ferocious criticism, especially from the new women's movement that has existed since the 1960s.

Operations for 'retroversion' and 'displacement' continued far into the century and even those performed without immediate local cause of symptoms or discomfort are still occasionally done today, especially in the private sector. The idea that retroversion caused symptoms and required operations became part of the institutional truth of gynaecology. No amount of criticism affected it. As late as 1940 the Chicago Gynaecological Society heard that 'retroversion of the uterus will probably always be one of the more common gynaeco-logical conditions requiring treatment and surgical intervention for the cure of symptoms in some cases.' In 1947 Atlee protested against the so-called 'acceptable indications' for the treatment of retroversion of the uterus' and referred to 'the really atrocious numbers of useless suspensions at present being done'. Gradually there was a complete reversal of opinion about the value of these operations but the fashion for doing them had lasted for several generations, largely because it was taken up by the highest and most influential doctors on both sides of the Atlantic and became part of gynaecology's received wisdom. Despite the fact that many of the operations were mechanical failures and did not do what they set out to do, leading gynaecologists were reluctant to abandon them, especially as many patients lost their symptoms, at least temporarily. But gradually it was realised that many 'successful' operations did not cure the patient and were not as safe as had been thought. A small but consistent number of patients died from the operation or had serious post-operative complications, especially during pregnancy. Also, gradually, there was greater understanding of female physiology and the techniques of surgery, and also of low back pain, the condition for which the operation was frequently performed. Improved understanding of the causes of prolapse, improved care during childbirth and the arrival of anti-biotics greatly reduced the number of women suffering from prolapse.

Even the most die-hard resister of new ideas came to realise that a retroverted uterus was a variation of the normal and existed in a substantial proportion of women, both healthy and sick. All this led to a decline in interest and today gynaecological textbooks barely mention the subject. Today we have returned to the belief prevalent in pre-anaesthetic days and articulated by Colombat d'Isère in 1838: 'Those inclinations that take place in the non-gravid womb require no special treatment.' *Plus ça change . . .*

Doctors gradually came to understand something of the 'placebo effect', which is the improvement that occurs simply as a result of *having* treatment rather than the result of the treatment itself. It includes the effect of the doctor as a person and the fact that, during the treatment, the patient is an object of attention. The placebo effect has been responsible for an enormous amount of medical treatment being accepted because the patients were apparently 'cured' or improved when really coloured water or chalk pills, given with professional authority and ritual, would have had the same effect. It required the development of both psychology and of statistical methods for this to be understood.

Another operation that has become increasingly popular during the twentieth century is Caesarean section, the removal of the baby through the mother's abdominal wall. This procedure performed on living women became a serious possibility only after anaesthetics were introduced. The operation has saved the lives of countless women and even more babies, but it has also been done with increasing frequency, sometimes on flimsy grounds. Ever since it became part of the routine repertoire of obstetricians it has been performed proportionately twice as frequently in the United States as in Britain and there have also been marked differences between European countries and, within the same country, between different districts and surgeons. The proportionate number of women having the operation increased enormously on both sides of the Atlantic during the post-war years and the operation became a battle ground between the obstetricians who wanted to control childbirth and women who demanded more control over their own bodies. It came to be done, or was influenced by, such factors as the doctor's convenience and working hours, the times the laboratory was open and the increasing danger of being sued for negligence if it was not performed.

Caesarean sections and the rate at which they were performed were the subject of particular controversy in 1986, in the discussions and arguments about the obstetrician Wendy Savage. She was suspended from her consultant post in a London teaching hospital largely because she did fewer Caesareans than her colleagues, the implication being that she was not safe. An enquiry found that her record of maternal health and infant survival was at least as good as that of her colleagues and she was cleared. The case highlighted the differences in attitude that existed between many modern women and the doctors who cared for them in pregnancy and childbirth. These women were, and still are, convinced that many gynaecologists are arrogant, sexist and controlling and that these attitudes profoundly influence the way they treat their patients. The women accuse the doctors of managing childbirth for their own convenience rather than for their patients', of creating pathological conditions which they then proceed to cure and of using their patients as pawns in their games of power. Today many women, while acknowledging that gynaecologists may save their lives or health and, increasingly, can enable the infertile to have children, complain bitterly about them.

A gynaecological subject that again attracted interest and criticism in Britain in recent years was mutilating genital operations, which most people thought had been abandoned in Britain during the nineteenth century. With the exception of ovariotomy, (the word now discarded and the operation discredited or restricted to well-defined indications), and certain types of hysterectomy, mutilating operations on females (in contrast to circumcision on males) have never been done on a large scale in western countries. Mutilation incurs disapproval, even though it has certainly been done on many occasions without good reason. It incurs even more disapproval if the indications for which it is done are not part of the accepted belief or practice of the time. A few years ago there was unease in the British medical profession about the ethics of British gynaecologists in private practice who were performing operations such as clitoridectomy, infibulation and female circumcision on young Arab girls, operations that are still the custom in parts of the Middle East and Africa. The argument put forward by these surgeons was that the operations were going to be done anyway and so it was better that they should be done in a British hospital by a British surgeon than under unsterile conditions in the patients' own countries. Here is a personal description of such an operation written by a woman who later became a doctor. She had the operation when she was six years old. One can only speculate on the difference it would have made to her had it been done in a British hospital with full aseptic techniques.

I was six years old that night when I lay in my bed, warm and peaceful in that pleasurable state which lies halfway between wakefulness and sleep ... I felt something move under the blankets, something like a huge hand, cold and rough, fumbling over my body, as though looking for something. Almost simultaneously another hand, as cold and as rough and as big as the first one, was clapped over my mouth, to prevent me from screaming.

They carried me to the bathroom. I do not know how many of them there were, nor do I remember their faces, or whether they were men or women. The world to me seemed enveloped in a dark fog which prevented me from seeing ... I was frightened ... something like an iron grasp caught hold of my hand and my arms and my thighs, so that I became unable to resist or even to move. I also remember the icy touch of the bathroom tiles under my naked body, and unknown voices and humming sounds interrupted now and then by a rasping metallic sound which reminded me of the butcher when he used to sharpen his knife before slaughtering a sheep for the *Eid*.*

She thought that thieves had broken into the house and were going to cut her throat 'which was always what happened with disobedient girls like myself in the stories that my old rural grandmother was so fond of telling me.'

She continues, 'I strained my ears for the rasp of the metallic sound. The moment it ceased, it was as though my heart stopped beating with it ... I imagined the thing that was making the rasping sound coming closer and closer to me. Somehow it was not approaching my neck as I had expected but another part of my body. Somewhere below my belly, as though seeking something buried between my thighs. At that very moment I realized that my thighs had been pulled apart.' Her legs were held wide apart, 'gripped by steel fingers that never relinquished their pressure. She thought the knife was about to be plunged down her throat but 'suddenly the sharp metallic edge seemed to drop between my thighs and there cut off a piece of flesh from my body.'

In spite of the 'tight hand' held over her mouth, she screamed with pain, 'for the pain was not just a pain, it was like a searing flame that went through my whole body'. Soon afterwards she 'saw a pool of blood around my hips'. She did not know what they had cut off her body and she did not try to find out. She just wept and called out for her mother. Then she received the 'worst shock of all'. Her mother was standing by her side. 'Yes, it was her, I could not be mistaken, in flesh and blood, right in the midst of these strangers, talking to them and smiling at them ...'

* A Festival of Sacrifice.

She was put back to bed and then saw them catch hold of her sister, two years younger. 'The look we exchanged seemed to say: "Now we know what it is. Now we know where lies our tragedy." '

When she returned to school, she found that all her classmates, from all walks of life, had been through the same experience.*

A scrupulous surgeon is likely to refuse to perform an operation solely on the grounds that if he does not do it, someone else will, even with the knowledge that the other is likely to be more dangerous. When the operation is unacceptable in his own culture, he is even less likely to perform it. But some surgeons do. A well-known gynaeco-logist told a colleague that he would perform 'any operation the patient asks for, provided it is safe', and there are others who follow this policy without saying so. Some surgeons are willing to perform clitoridectomy on English women if they or their husbands request it. Many major, unnecessary operations have been done, and still are, simply because the patient, usually, though not always, a woman, wants to have it. Disturbed people sometimes fix their problems on to some part of their anatomy, often the nose, eyebrows, womb, or their children's tonsils, and demand that these be re-shaped or removed when there is no recognised indication for so doing. Some of these requests are overtly sexual, for instance asking to have their clitorises moved forwards for greater sexual enjoyment (the reverse of Victorian operations, which were done to destroy sexual feeling), or their vaginas re-shaped to fit their husbands' penises. Such stories may be myths. There are people, again most of them women, whose mental balance has come to depend on having an operation every so often. Only then can they bear the burdens and tensions in their lives. Surgery makes them feel important for a while and gains them the attention they feel unable to achieve otherwise. This boosts their flagging self-esteem and means they can avoid, for a while, doing things they dislike while gaining other advantages. Sometimes their husbands recognise the situation consciously or unconsciously and support it, knowing that life will be easier until the next operation. These patients are a burden to doctors who do not believe that it is their duty to comply. The woman determined to have a hysterectomy is known to every gynaecologist and, if she persists, she is likely to get one. Rarer, but in the same category is the woman who demands a Caesarean section to avoid the pain and uncertainties of labour. Some surgeons avoid the problem by entering into the patient's delusion and persuading themselves that an operation is necessary, or maybe at least harmless.

* Nawal El Saadawi, *The Hidden Faces of Eve*, 1980.

The persistent patient is likely to end up in the operating theatre either training a young surgeon or enriching an older one. There is as yet little serious debate on the ethical problems involved in questions such as, 'Should a woman be able to demand a Caesarean or any other operation?' or 'How much trouble should doctors take in explaining complicated medical situations to patients in a way that enables them to make an informed judgment?' But women are beginning to ask these questions and doubtless eventually the gynaecologists will follow.

In the last decades the interests of gynaecologists have changed, as has what they feel needs to be done and discovered. In their meetings and conferences, in journals and books designed to keep the profession up to date there has been less emphasis on operations and more on matters of direct concern to large numbers of women. A series of volumes entitled *Progress in Obstetrics and Gynaecology** is 'a forum for postgraduate debate and education'. Each volume contains essays by different specialists on subjects of special current interest to obstetricians and gynaecologists. Volume 3 (1983) refers to the 'schism between British and American practice' as 'an incomprehensible embarrassment' and discusses the difference in attitudes to interference in labour. The argument for and against induction of labour 'swings like a pendulum' and this is part of discussions on Caesarean section and mid-cavity forceps. There is a chapter on the sequelae of hysterectomy and the 'post-hysterectomy syndrome'. The author regarded the subject as particularly important because more and more hysterectomies were being done. There is comment on the high incidence of pre-existing psychiatric problems in women who undergo hysterectomy and discussion on the possible association between psychological and gynaecological disease reflecting hormonal associations between the ovaries and the brain or perhaps indicating that some women with psychiatric problems have difficulty coming to terms with their menstruation or may present psychological distress in the form of physical complaints, thus reflecting prevalent unsympathetic attitudes to emotional illness in the community. It was thought that there was little danger that the operations would *cause* new psychological problems, though new cases seemed to emerge. The authors emphasise the importance of 'determining whether

* Edited by John Studd.

hysterectomy is indeed the correct therapy', what the women's emotional and physical responses are likely to be, as well as adequate preparation of patient and partner, and arranging prompt psychiatric treatment where necessary.* There is also discussion about intra-uterine devices, a subject of much controversy and anger at the time of writing, with great emphasis on safety. 'IUD users have a mortality rate of 3–5 deaths per million women annually, mainly due to infection.' On the subject of the traditional major gynaecological operations there is concern about vesico-vaginal fistula in the Third World and the revelation that in some countries the chief cause is still 'pressure necrosis associated with obstructed labour', just as it was in the time of Marion Sims. It notes that there were still 350 cases per year in England and Wales but does not specify the cause. It may well have been cancer, though some of the patients may have come from the Third World.

In the same review there is also concern about male infertility, a subject that appeared increasingly in the gynaecological literature of the 1980s. Perhaps it was the many rumours that some gynaecologists were submitting infertile women to invasive surgery before even asking for a specimen of their partners' sperm that prompted the declaration, 'It is essential to investigate both partners of an infertile marriage fully, as there is no simple test for infertility'. The following year (1984) five out of eight gynaecological articles were directly concerned with infertility, the other three being 'Doubtful Gender at Birth', 'Pre-menstrual Syndrome' and 'Sexually Transmitted Disease of the Vulva'.

The review also now contained a general section with two papers, 'Factors Affecting the Relationship between Gynaecologist and Patient', and 'Medico-Legal Aspects of Obstetrics and Gynaecology'. Of the former the editor writes, 'To the best of my knowledge, there is almost no literature on the subject and no specific research has been done on it.' The subject had been discussed at two international congresses (the World Congress on Psychosomatic Obstetrics and Gynaecology in Berlin in 1980 and the World Congress in Dublin in 1983). There is also increasing awareness of the influence of psycho-logical attitudes on medical practice. One article discusses 'androgyny' and points out that the relationship between a male gynaecologist and a female patient will to a great extent be determined by his attitude to women: 'If the doctor sees a woman as someone whose main function is to serve and reproduce, his feeling of

* Lorraine Dennerstein & Margaret Ryan: 'The Post-hysterectomy Syndrome', in Studd (ed): op. cit., vol. 3, 1983.

superiority – already present in any doctor-patient relationship – will be intensified.' Also, 'a masculinist view of society can have a direct influence on the interpretation of gynaecological complaints and the choice of treatment for them.' An example of this is provided by the attitudes of gynaecologists (in the past) towards undesired pregnancy, the surgical treatment of vaginism, and spasm of the vaginal muscles on penetration. These attitudes are only slowly disappearing, amid the rapid and increasing frequency of hysterectomy as a solution for such disparate complaints as abdominal pain, dyspareunia (pain during sexual intercourse) and menstrual disorders. The author advises male gynaecologists to develop their feminine sides – solidarity, identification and empathy rather than authority, ascendancy and sympathy, and also points out that a female gynaecologist may feel envy, often unconscious, towards the women on account of what she has renounced or delayed in order to reach her present position. He also acknowledges the existence of sexuality (without implying a sexual relationship) in the doctor-patient relationship. Slowly, slowly, it seems, gynaecology was moving with the times, though it has to be remembered that these are probably the words of the more enlightened members of the specialty.

Of the twelve gynaecological articles in the 1986 volume (Volume 5), only three concerned surgery and the rest included 'Puberty', 'Intersex' and 'Psychosexual Counselling', contraception and the menopause. Clearly the gynaecologists were trying to become expert in psychological and sexual aspects of life. They continued to be interested in infertility, including male infertility, and helping infertile couples with dramatic treatments such as IVF has become a gynaecological subject of high public profile. Like other surgeons, gynaecologists were also moving towards less traumatic invasions of the body through the increasing use of ultrasound (in which sound-waves are bounced off organs to make images) and endoscopy (the examination and treatment of internal organs through tiny tubes, often with the ability to operate). Endoscopy, pelviscopy, colposcopy, hysteroscopy are all coming into their own and are emphasised in the 1989 edition (Volume 7), which also contains articles on contraception and 'The Sex Ratio; and ways of manipulating it'. Again, there are only three articles on 'conventional' gynaecological subjects – one on prolapse of the womb and two on cancer.

Probably the operation that has caused most controversy during the twentieth century is hysterectomy, the surgical removal of the womb.

It is performed for cancer, excessive bleeding and a host of other reasons, many of them disputed. Like Caesarean section, it is an ancient operation, though it had virtually never been successful until anaesthetics were established. It had also been done mainly on the dead, for practice. Surgeons had thought about the possibility of performing such an operation and in 1787 it had been suggested by H.A. Wrisburg, Professor of Obstetrics at Göttingen as a treatment of cancer. The suggestion was repeated in 1814. Neither of these surgeons attempted to perform the operation. There were too many impediments, particularly the dangers of shock and haemorrhage which were far greater than in ovariotomy, and infection, which was a problem with all operations. Another difficulty was to distinguish between different conditions, particularly fibroids (benign tumours of the muscle of the uterine wall) from cancer. Until the time of William Hunter in the mid-eighteenth century, fibroids were confused with malignant growths and the whole subject was confused by ignorance and old wives' tales. Both had been called *scleroma* by Galen and for many generations the term 'mole' was used for any strange intra-uterine growth. An 1817 textbook said:

> The housewives believed that moles not only take the form of certain animals, but that they even walk, run, fly, try to hide themselves even to re-enter the womb from which they came; indeed, if no obstacle be offered they will kill the woman just delivered of them.*

The first attempt at removal of a uterus through the wall of the abdomen was performed in 1825 by Langenbeck, but the operation proved too difficult. He abandoned it and the patient died several hours later. In the same year Lizars described a case on whom hysterectomy had been performed. He said it was 'one of the most cruel and unfeasible operations that ever was projected or executed by the head or hand of man.' This was echoed by James Johnson, editor of the *London Medico-Chirurgical Review*, who wrote:

> We consider extirpation of the uterus, not previously protruded or inverted, one of the most cruel and unfeasible operations that ever was projected or executed by the head or hand of man. We are very far from discouraging bold or untried operations, but there is a limit beyond which it may not be prudent to go, even should a solitary instance or two of success rise up as precedents to bear out the operation.†

By the middle of the century this view was still held. In 1848 the authoritative Professor Meigs wrote about operations on fibroids:

* Joseph Capurin: *Traité des Maladies des Femmes*, 1817.
† *London Medico-Chirurgical Review*, 1825, 3, N.S., p. 264.

As to doing anything about those [fibroids] that grow outwardly towards the peritoneum, I look upon it as hopeless. I detest all abdominal surgery, save that which is clearly warranted by the otherwise imminent death of the patient.

In 1844 Ashwell showed the distinction between fibroids and cancer, but there was still uncertainty as to whether or not fibroids were liable to become malignant and only much later was it realised that they did not. The earlier laporotomies (operations for opening the abdomen) undertaken for removal of ovarian cysts often revealed large fibroid masses which the surgeons were too scared to remove as well. Ovariotomy was seen as dangerous, but uterine surgery as impossible. The commonest cause of death in ovariotomy was peritonitis (inflammation or infection of the membrane covering the abdominal organs), but with uterine surgery, shock and haemorrhage were also extremely likely to occur. It seems that seven-eighths of the attempts to remove a fibroid uterus before 1863 were either abandoned or ended fatally and Ricci says that 'the voice of the profession rose in unison against this phase of surgery'.

Even as late as 1863, Sir James Simpson said in his *Clinical Lectures on Diseases of Women*:

Judging of it *a priori*, we should regard the operation as unjustifiable, and experience serves only to confirm this judgment ... I have no hesitation in saying that it should even then be rejected, as an utterly unjustifiable operation in surgery.*

The first completed operation of hysterectomy was done in 1845 by A. M. Heath of Manchester. This patient, who had fibroids, also died, probably from shock and haemorrhage. The next completed operation was done by Charles Clay on a woman whose large fibroid uterus weighed twenty-four pounds and who also had a cystic ovarian mass weighing eight pounds. Clay removed both. The patient recovered, but was dropped by a nurse on the thirteenth day and died. This may or may not be a reflection on the quality of nursing in those pre-Nightingale days but it certainly reminds us of the long period in which patients stayed in bed and were incapacitated. Even a generation later, in London's Chelsea Hospital for Women, patients stayed in hospital for an average of seven weeks. An operation usually led to many weeks or even months of weakness and illness. There were, of course, no blood transfusions and no antibiotics. The woman who lost much blood or who became infected (as most did) had to replace her own blood, fight the infection – and often both together – on her own.

* See p. 65.

The first deliberate abdominal hysterectomy for a fibroid uterus that was correctly diagnosed was done by the American surgeon John Bellinger in 1846. This patient also died. The operation's prospects did not look good.

The first successful removal of a fibroid uterus in America was in June 1853 by Walter Burnham of Lowell, Massachusetts, who did it by mistake. He thought he was removing an ovarian cyst. The tumour fell out through the incision and, unable to replace it, he had to remove it. Although the patient survived, it was still thought that the operation was too dangerous to be recommended. Later, this surgeon did fifteen cases with three recoveries. At one stage, in each of eight consecutive operations, the patient died. In another series, eighteen patients out of twenty-four died and in another ten died in eleven operations. During the years 1881 to 1885, the leading surgeons in the field operated 400 times with a death-rate of fifty per cent. The enthusiasm of these surgeons and the persistence with which they continued to operate despite such appalling results is difficult to understand. Did some people regard women, or some women, as expendable?

Gradually techniques improved and, during the twentieth century, hysterectomy became enormously popular. It became safer, increased in popularity and replaced ovariotomy as a common operation that could be done even when the problem was vague or psychiatric. Increasing knowledge of endocrine function and female physiology made it increasingly difficult to justify wholesale ovariotomy. As its popularity grew and it became relatively safe, some gynaecologists sought to extend the indications for doing it, for instance finding reasons for removing the uteri of women who 'wouldn't need them any more'. If this could become established practice it would provide an unlimited opportunity for young surgeons to learn their art and for their elders to enrich themselves. Hysterectomy became a substitute for ovariotomy for those with beliefs and desires that urged them to operate on women's internal organs and by the middle of the twentieth century hysterectomy was becoming the most commonly performed operation in the West. It was but a short step to extending it almost universally. In 1969, Wright advocated routine removal of the uterus after the last planned pregnancy on the grounds that it was potentially cancer-bearing. He writes, 'The uterus has but one function: reproduction. After the last planned pregnancy, the uterus becomes a useless, bleeding, symptom-producing, potentially cancer-bearing organ and therefore should be removed.' It may be significant that this was the year when the new women's movement was gathering strength and was beginning to affect the lives and consciousness of countless women. Many of these feminists had other views about their organs, even when they were beyond the age of childbearing. Nevertheless, pressure from gynaecologists for approval of wholesale excision of the womb continued. One textbook, by Nowak, describes the uterus of a woman who has completed her family as 'a rather worthless organ'. In 1973 a gynaecologist, J.B. Skelton, addressed the American College of Obstetricians and Gynaecologists and advocated 'prophylactic elective total hysterectomy and bilateral salpingo-oöphorectomy after completion of childbirth as proper preventive medicine.' He argued that it eliminates the risk of cancer developing, ensures sterility, reduces the need for later, often multiple gynaecological operations, 'relieves the women of unpleasant and uncomfortable monthly bleedings', 'allows smooth maintenance therapy with feminizing hormones, eliminating bothersome cyclic variations, tensions and emotionally altered states which affect the woman's world', and 'decreases the frequency of unpleasant, humiliating pelvic exams and tests and allows better utilization of available health personnel, facilities and time. And all this can be achieved with one single operation. Seldom in life do we risk so little to gain so much.'

This, at the height of the new women's movement, went to the heart of the modern controversy. Opposition to the medical argument grew. In 1976 it was shown that if prophylactic hysterectomies were done on 1,000,000 women, the average lifespan would be increased by just two months – 'or about the time it takes to go through the operation and convalescence'.* But by this time, although the operation was much safer, it was being performed on so many women that, at least in the United States, there were now more deaths from hysterectomy than from cancer of the womb. A 1975 study by Cornell University Medical College indicated that 787,000 hysterectomies were performed in the US in 1975, resulting in 1,700 deaths. Surgery was regarded as unnecessary in twenty-eight per cent of cases and in this group there were 374 deaths.†

Hysterectomy was also being advocated and performed as a sterilising procedure, an alternative to cutting the Fallopian tubes. At one centre twenty per cent of all hysterectomies were done for sterilisation. At another, the number of elective hysterectomy operations done for purposes of sterilisation increased by 742 per cent in three years. Yet several studies showed that hysterectomy was much

* P. Brown & E Druckman: 'Elective Hysterectomy: Pro and Con', *New England Journal of Medicine*, p. 264–68.
† *New York Times*, 1 Feb 1976.

more dangerous than simple cutting of the tubes and that it led to many more complications and discomforts.* Other studies began to reveal some bad psychological effects of hysterectomy. One found that two and a half times more women were referred to psychiatrists after hysterectomy than after cholecystectomy (removal of the gall bladder), the ratio being much greater when those women who had previously been referred to psychiatrists were eliminated from the count.

There had long been concern about the number of hysterectomies performed, especially in the United States, where proportionately twice as many are done as in Britain. In 1946 a prediction was made that 'a tragedy, painful and far-reaching in its implications' would arise from the discovery that a third of the pathology reports from a series of hysterectomies in ten US hospitals revealed no evidence of disease.

Another survey concluded:

> What is clear is that in many instances there is little evidence of informed consent by the patient and that these operations have been 'sold' to the public by surgeons in a manner not unlike many other deceptive marketing practices.†

Interestingly, in 1984 a New York jury found no malpractice on the part of a gynaecologist who had performed a hysterectomy but awarded damages to the patient because he had failed to obtain her consent.§ This goes back in American law to 1914 when it was judged that 'a surgeon who performs an operation without his patient's consent commits an assault for which he is liable in damages'.‡

In 1977, the Congressional Commerce Oversight Committee investigated unnecessary surgery. Critics within the medical profession testified that perhaps as many as forty per cent of the hysterectomies performed were 'questionable'. They cited cases where the doctor removed the uterus for 'hysterical' symptoms – obsessive fear of pregnancy or cancerphobia. Of the 725,000 hysterectomies

---

* William Ledger & Margaret Child: 'The Hospital Care of Patients undergoing Hysterectomy: An Analysis of 12,026 Patients from the Professional Activity Study', *American Journal of Obstetrics and Gynaecology*, 1973, 117; Russell K. Laros & Bruce Work: 'Female Sterilisation', *American Journal of Obstetrics and Gynaecology*, 1975, 122; Hibbard: 1982.

† Bernard Rosenfeld, Sidney Wolfe, & Robert McGarrah: *Study of Surgical Sterilisation: Present Abuses and Proposed Regulations*, Washington, DC, Health Research Group, October 1973, p. 2.

§ *New York Times*, 22 February 1984.

‡ *Schoendorf v. Society of New York Hospitals.*

performed in 1975, only twenty per cent could be justified as treatment for cancer or other life-threatening disorders. There has been widespread concern about unnecessary surgery, especially, though not exclusively, in the United States. In 1974, a senate investigation reported 2.4 million unnecessary operations causing 11,900 deaths and costing about $3.9 billion. More deaths are caused annually by surgery in the US than the annual number of deaths during the wars in Korea and Vietnam.* We know that many more women than men undergo surgery. In the United States, and probably elsewhere in the western world, of the commonest ten operations, five are women's operations – dilatation and curettage, Caesarean section, hysterectomy, bilateral destruction or occlusion of Fallopian tubes, and oöphorectomy and salpingo-oöphorectomy.

Much of such criticism applies more to America than to Europe, but disquiet also exists in Britain. In 1988 the results of a survey carried out by workers in Oxford were published as *Do British Women Undergo Too Many or Too Few Hysterectomies?* This discusses the processes involved in hysterectomy from the moment when the woman decides she requires a medical consultation. The survey revealed an increase in the demand for hysterectomy so that it was now one of the most commonly performed surgical operations in England and Wales and was being done (in 1985) at the rate of more than 66,000 women (twenty-eight per 10,000) per year. Even though this was far less than the United States, it was still more than twice the rate in Norway and more than some other countries. There were also enormous differences between different districts whose women appeared to have similar social conditions and health. The authors pointed out that differing rates might mean that some women were being deprived of operations they needed rather than that unnecessary operations were being performed. Many women are highly satisfied with the results of their hysterectomies, even where the indications for doing them would be regarded by some surgeons as dubious. The authors of this survey argued for a thorough evaluation of the impact of hysterectomy on the quality of life and a more thorough consideration of what is meant by and involved in 'patient demand', so often the reason or excuse for operating.

Feminists struggle for individual rights, patient rights. They believe that every competent adult should be the final judge of whether or not an operation should be done. They also try to 'raise consciousness' about this so that people become more involved and

* M. Weitz: *Health Shock*, Englewood Cliffs, NJ, Prentice Hall, 1982.

better able to think along such lines. There is increasing questioning of gynaecological processes and the necessity to perform them, and of the motives of some gynaecologists. Gynaecology has become part of the dispute between women and the medical profession. Many women have become suspicious, some after unfortunate personal experiences. One example is a woman I met recently who had started to bleed heavily immediately after her male gynaecologist had fitted her with an intra-uterine contraceptive device. On a number of occasions she asked him to remove it but each time he refused, saying that the bleeding had nothing to do with the device and that she needed a hysterectomy. Finally she went to another gynaecologist, a woman, who said there was nothing wrong with her womb and removed the device. 'The bleeding stopped within ten minutes,' she said, and added vehemently, 'I'll never, *ever* go to a male gynaecologist again.'

Increasingly, individual women, especially the growing number of feminists, criticise gynaecologists and object to the arrogance and authoritarian attitudes of some. This account of one woman's gynaecological experience is fictional but it has the ring of personal experience.

> I've a high failure rate in gynaecologists. The first one I saw was a misogynist and an extortionist, the second a lecher. The third one might have been all right, I can't positively say he wasn't but we moved house before I had a chance to find out. The fourth one, Mr Gamble, I haven't met yet. He's been recommended by my doctor and by several people I know who variously say he's sympathetic, attractive, dishy. A surgeon's wife I share the school run with told me Mr G is the envy of his colleagues, who've had to watch him sweep the gynaecological board, not just of the county's childbearers, but of the menopausal. They seek him out, according to her, for hysterectomies, for removal of ovarian cysts and ovaries, and for Hormone Replacement Therapy. This is enough to put me off him, but I'm telling myself to keep an open mind.*

Arrogance and conceit have existed among some gynaecologists ever since the specialty emerged. In 1900, Englemann, the president of the American Gynaecological Society, said in his presidential address:

> We seem to have attained the apex of surgical achievement but there are peaks beyond and new fields to conquer . . . The task before us now is that we reduce morbidity as we have mortality; now that we can with impunity remove organs, we must endeavour to restore healthy functional activity.

* Georgina Hammick: 'A few problems in the day case unit', in *People for Lunch*, London, Sphere Books, 1988.

More recently, Russell G. Scott pontificated:

> If like all human beings, he [the gynaecologist] is made in the image of the Almighty, and if he is kind, then his kindness and concern for his patient may provide her with a glimpse of God's image.*

The tendency of many to concentrate on their own handiwork rather than on the patient is shown in an interview with a young resident gynaecologist.

> The thing with surgery is that you have something to show. You have a headache and I give you an aspirin and it goes away, fine. If you have postpartum bleeding and you need a hysterectomy and I take your uterus out and everything is fine, you can say 'look at that fine piece of surgery I did.'†

Another source of anger among women has been the gynaecologists' preoccupation with surgery, which affects comparatively few women, and their lack of interest in subjects which affect nearly all women at some time in their lives, particularly abortion and birth control.

Both these subjects are largely outside the scope of this book and so have not been discussed in any depth. In 1967 the Abortion Act contained a 'social clause' which made abortion lawful if the continuation of pregnancy threatens the well-being of the mother's existing children. The British Medical Association and Royal College of Obstetricians and Gynaecologists objected strongly to this clause. One critic, Andrew Malleson, said in 1973 that the doctors 'pick facts to support their prejudices'. He demonstrated how they twisted facts and misquoted other people's results and conclusions. The authors, he said, have 'erroneously convinced themselves that abortion is a dangerous operation, then excluded social affliction as a legitimate indication for abortion.' The report said that for girls under the age of sixteen it would encourage promiscuity, and then that the legal right to perform abortions should be restricted to consultant gynaecologists in the National Health Service. This, said Malleson, was closed-shop tactics. He then went on to discuss how few women (less than ten per cent) had had professional help with contraception – yet the College had never concerned itself with this.

The Royal College of Obstetricians and Gynaecologists was founded in 1929 to encourage the study and improve the practice of

---

* Russell C. Scott: *The World of a Gynaecologist*, London, Oliver & Boyd, 1968, p. 25.
† Diana Scully: *Men Who Control Women's Health*, p. 104.

obstetrics and gynaecology. All its officers and executives were men. In 1949, it elected its first and only woman president, Dame Hilda Lloyd. The adulatory biographer of the College saw this as 'a revolutionary step' which evoked doubts in some male fellows but, he says 'there was no need to fear'. On the whole members of the College were opposed to contraception or else ignored it. It formed no part of the training of doctors and most contraceptive clinics (or 'Family Planning Clinics' as they were called) had to be held outside health service premises and away from hospitals. It was only in 1950 that the first contraceptive clinic was opened in a teaching hospital and it was years before others followed. It was not until 1970 that the College asked the first question about contraception in its diploma examination. Malleson comments, 'It does not appear that the College has been unduly concerned that young doctors should have a knowledge of contraceptive techniques' and found that the archives of the Family Planning Association revealed no support for contraceptive education from the Royal College of Obstetricians and Gynaecologists, 'who are meant to be improving the practice of obstetrics and gynaecology'.

In 1959, the Family Planning Association wished to advertise its services in *Family Doctor*, the British Medical Association's magazine for the general public, but because some doctors disapproved the council for the BMA withdrew the advertisements. A row followed. Even *The Times* disapproved of the BMA's actions. In a leader on 12 December it criticised the BMA for its timidity. The BMA retaliated by commenting that during World War II *The Times* had refused to advertise the slogan 'Wash your hands after going to the W.C.'

The Family Planning Association's advertisements did not appear in *Family Doctor*. Malleson commented, 'It is not surprising that sometimes people get misogynists and gynaecologists mixed up' and suggested that if gynaecologists did not want to do abortions, midwives should be allowed to do them. The medical profession has always been inclined to adopt a dog-in-the-manger attitude, insisting on power over an area of human life which it intended to ignore. Abortion is a typical subject for such treatment. It has become increasingly clear to feminists and others that the attitudes of the medical profession towards abortion are highly moralistic and are often not related to what women perceive as their needs.

Many complaints against gynaecologists formulated by modern feminists are made in terms of power, control and self-determination. They may attack the medical profession's tendency to diagnose women's illness as psychosomatic. The present troubles in the maternity services are often focused on the question of who has control of the mother. The cases of Wendy Savage and her colleague Pauline Bousquet and the 'radical midwives', and their 'persecution' by the medical establishment, have all added to this, often in conflict with that part of the nursing establishment that identifies itself with male dominance. It has become increasingly obvious that there is a tendency on the part of the medical establishment to attack women practitioners who 'step out of line'.

New techniques and treatments are embraced eagerly by gynaecologists. Many advances are still based on ignorance. Experimentation is an attempt to conquer this ignorance. Gynaecologists in training are urged to do research, to find new 'facts' and devise new procedures, but without rocking the boat or deviating too far from the party line. The implication is that medicine is based on the male body and women are considered only when they differ from men. Technology supports authoritarianism and mechanistic medicine is concerned not with health but with curing disease. Intervention is social intervention and control.

The National Health Service did not change power relationships or the bias of gender and class in medicine. In practice, it reinforced it. The part played by politics in medicine is closely linked to medicine in politics. Women often feel lost in this predominantly male world. Many of them, as part of their conditioning as women, have internalised masculine expectations of themselves, especially in health matters where the line between medical and social judgment has become thin and confused.

Many more women are now aware of these matters and have become articulate about them. Many have turned to alternative medicine as being better suited to their needs. Women's health groups have sprung up. These are informal gatherings of up to about eight or nine women which attempt to study women in the context of their lives – home, work, community. Patients in our society are expected to be passive and so are women. These groups aim to make what knowledge they have generally available to all and to restore to women control over their bodies, establishing confidence through understanding.

# CONCLUSION

It is easy to take a single viewpoint of the story told in this book, perhaps that it charts advances in science and medical progress, or describes exploitation of women by men. Each view is both true and false, and neither fully explains what happened.

The theory and practice of medicine essentially concerns healing so it is easy to ignore or forget the influence of other motives on its development and practice, yet these are often more powerful. If we are to understand the attitudes of past or present surgeons towards women, we have to try to understand the men themselves – their ambitions, greed, love of discovery, problem-solving or scoring off others. Many motives can be detected in reading the accounts of the first generation of surgeons that was able to progress rapidly in skill and knowledge. To achieve this they had to experiment, as happens in most advances in medical techniques. Inevitably, those who experimented most were those who enjoyed doing so. Surgeons with imagination and sometimes grandiose ideas became prominent. They needed patients on whom to operate. They sought them among both the poor in the public hospitals and among those who could pay for their services. The latter were often ailing middle-class women who lacked interesting occupations and were caught up in the prevalent myths about women being inherently ill and dominated by their reproductive organs. These women were a gift to the surgeons. By offering themselves and believing that surgery might cure them of their discontents, they encouraged the doctors to extend the possible areas in which surgery might be practised and to rationalise the possible benefits. The surgeons became excited and persuaded themselves that they were doing the right thing. They communicated their excitement to their patients, who trusted them and believed them. So the surgeons (or ovariotomists) were able to increase the professional empire they had built through operating on the huge ovarian cysts which had given them their new skills. Moreover, like other men of their time and class, they were all imbued with Victorian ideas about women, as indeed were the women themselves. They achieved much, but at what cost?

The history of surgery is not just a thing of the past. Many of these battles are still with us.

# GLOSSARY

ABDOMEN The cavity of the body, lying in front of the spine and below the chest, from which it is separated by a partition of muscle, the diaphragm. The cavity continues downwards into the pelvis. It is the largest body cavity and contains the organs of digestion – stomach, intestines, liver, etc, – and also the organs of excretion – kidneys, bladder, etc, – and the female reproductive organs – womb, ovaries, tubes, etc. It is lined by the peritoneum, a membrane which also covers the organs and enables them to slide smoothly over one another.

ABSCESS A localised collection of pus formed after invasion by pyogenic organisms and separated by a wall of inflammation and damaged tissue.

ACUTE In lay terms, used to mean 'severe'. In medical terms, it refers to a condition of rapid onset, severe symptoms and rapid resolution. Compare with Chronic.

ALBUMINURIA The presence of the protein albumen in the urine. Since the molecule of albumen is the smallest of the proteins of the blood, it is the first to appear through a stressed or damaged kidney. Albuminuria is common in fevers, diseases of the kidney or heart, and in pregnant women as an early sign of toxaemia of pregnancy.

AMAUROSIS Blindness, partial or total.

ANAEMIA A condition in which the haemoglobin of the blood is reduced so that it can carry less oxygen.

ANALGESIC Drug that reduces pain.

ANDROLOGY Term once suggested for the special study of diseases of the male sex. The idea of this specialty did not appeal to the medical profession and did not develop.

ANIMAL MAGNETISM A doctrine of medical treatment developed by Franz Anton Mesmer, based on the idea that electricity and magnetism could cure disease.

ANOREXIA NERVOSA A psychological illness, mostly of young women, which has been described as 'the relentless pursuit of thinness'. There is refusal or inability to eat, and loss of weight and starvation may be so great as to be fatal if not properly treated. It was described in the nineteenth century but thought to be very rare until, in the second half of the twentieth century, many other 'diseases' (for example, many cases of 'debility', Simmonds' disease, 'anaemia', 'neurasthenia') were found to be anorexia nervosa. This coincided with an 'epidemic' of the condition comparable to the prevalence of chlorosis in the nineteenth century.

ANTIBIOTICS Substances or drugs, originally produced from microorganisms, which inhibit the growth of other microorganisms and so help the body to fight infection, or invasion by those organisms.

ANTIPHLOGISTIC An outdated medical term, much used before the days of aseptic surgery and antibiotics. Literally, 'against burning or roasting', but used to describe the regimen which included 'all the rules, prohibitions and observances which are prescribed in cases of fever, inflammation and diseases of excitement'. It included bloodletting, purging, clean air, exclusion of sunlight, regulation of diet and drink. Also 'no talking in the room' and the muffling of noise outside by laying down straw in the street. It seems to have been essentially a middle-class regimen.

ANTISEPSIS System devised by Lister to prevent infection in surgical wounds. Since it was believed that infection was carried in the air, operations were done under a spray of carbolic acid in order to kill the germs. This was damaging to both patients and surgeons. The system was replaced by asepsis.

ASCITES, ASCITIC FLUID Fluid that has collected in the peritoneal (abdominal) cavity. It is an abnormal condition caused by many diseases, including tuberculosis, heart failure, liver damage and cancer.

ASEPSIS The complete absence of bacteria and other microorganisms that can cause infection. It is the aim in every surgical operation that it be performed under aseptic conditions. Asepsis as a concept replaced Lister's antisepsis in the late nineteenth century. Its basis is scrupulous cleanliness with sterilisation of all instruments, dressings etc, and as far as possible a no-touch technique during operation and afterwards.

ATOM The smallest particle of a chemical element.

AUSCULTATION Examination of the body by listening, usually with a stethoscope, to movements of muscle (including heart muscle), gas or liquid inside the body. It is often used to listen to the movement of air in the lungs and of gas and liquid in the abdomen. Occasionally it is used to listen to joints and other parts of the body.

BACTERIA Microorganisms of a particular and widespread group. Some are harmful to man or animals, others are harmless or beneficial. They play an important part in breaking down foodstuffs and organic matter both inside and outside the body.

BATTEY'S OPERATION See Oöphorectomy.

BLISTERING A former treatment by applying irritant substances such as mustard, hartshorn or cantharides (Spanish flies) to the skin. It was used in many conditions, especially diseases of the lungs and joints.

BLOOD-LETTING This, the very opposite of most treatment today, was a popular treatment for many centuries. It was used in fevers, fits, asthma, and even in haemorrhage. It was also done regularly on some people with the idea that it kept them healthy.

BMA British Medical Association. An organisation comparable to a trade union for doctors.

BMJ *British Medical Journal*, the weekly journal of the British Medical Association.

BRITISH MEDICAL ASSOCIATION See BMA.

BRITISH MEDICAL JOURNAL See *BMJ*.

CAESAR, CAESAREAN SECTION A surgical operation for delivering a baby through an incision in the abdominal wall. The operation became practicable on living women only after the introduction of anaesthetics and became reasonably safe only after the introduction of asepsis.

CANCER A malignant condition arising from the abnormal division of cells that tend to invade or destroy surrounding tissues and may travel to distant parts of the body and form secondary 'tumours'.

CANCEROUS Pertaining to Cancer.

CATALEPSY Episodes of abnormal posture in which the limbs are held in weird positions, often for long periods of time. A condition associated with psychosis and hysteria and much less common nowadays than it was in the nineteenth century.

CATALEPTIC FITS See Catalepsy.

CAUTERISATION Use of the cautery.

CAUTERY An instrument which is heated to burn tissues. It can be used to check bleeding during surgery, to remove small warts or other growths, or to 'clean up' infected tissue.

CELL Basic unit of all living organisms. All bodies are made up of collections of different types of cells.

CERVIX The narrow lower part or 'neck' of the uterus (womb) whose mouth (os) opens into the vagina.

CHLOROSIS The nineteenth-century 'green sickness' of young women that is now no longer seen. It was probably a mixture of iron-deficiency anaemia and lack of fresh air.

CHOLECYSTECTOMY Surgical operation for removal of the gall bladder.

CHRONIC In lay terms, often used to mean 'severe' but as a medical term it is the opposite of acute and refers to a disease of slow onset and long duration, regardless of severity. Sometimes a condition may start with an acute attack, and then proceed to become chronic. Sometimes a chronic disease may have acute phases, known as acute-on-chronic.

CHRONIC SCHIZOPHRENIA A form of schizophrenia that is usually of slow onset (though it may start with an acute attack) and which eventually 'burns itself out', leaving the sufferer impaired to a greater or lesser degree.

CLITORIDECTOMY Surgical operation for removal of the clitoris.

CLITORIS The female genital organ, situated in the anterior part of the vulva, that is most sensitive and which corresponds, anatomically speaking, to the male penis.

COLPOSCOPE, VAGINOSCOPE Instrument that displays the vagina.

COLPOSCOPY Examination of the vagina with a colposcope.

CONVULSIONS Involuntary multiple and repeated contraction of muscles leading to temporary contortion of body and limbs. They occur in epilepsy, and also sometimes in brain damage, fevers and in infancy.

CRANIOMETRY Measuring the skull. This was popular in nineteenth-century anthropology, often as a means of asserting the superiority of the Anglo-Saxon male.

CRANIOTOMY Obstetric operation in which the skull of the foetus is perforated during labour so that the head collapses and can then be delivered. Improved obstetrics have led to the disappearance of this operation. The word is also used to refer to the surgical removal of a piece of skull in order to operate on the brain or meninges.

CUPPING A procedure in which vacuum glasses (often hot glasses or glasses in which paper or spirits were burned) were applied to any part of the body with the idea of drawing blood and fluid to that part. It was sometimes used in preparation for blood-letting, but 'dry cupping', (without blood-letting) was regarded as useful in many general disorders. Now obsolete.

CURETTAGE Surgical operation of scraping the lining of the uterus (womb) or another organ with a curette. It is a method of performing abortion or is done to diagnose or treat disease. See also Dilatation and Curettage.

CURETTE A small, sharp, spoon-shaped instrument used for scraping the inside of the uterus (womb) or other organs.

CYST An abnormal hollow or space in the body and filled with liquid or semi-liquid contents.

CYSTIC Referring to a cyst.

D & C see Dilatation and Curettage.

DEMENTIA PRAECOX Nineteenth-century term for schizophrenia.

DILATATION AND CURETTAGE Obstetric operation of dilating the cervix (neck of the womb) in order to perform curettage.

DIURETIC Substance that increases the volume of urine.

DROPSY See Oedema.

DYSPAREUNIA Painful or difficult sexual intercourse, usually referring to the woman.

ECLAMPSIA A dangerous condition affecting women in pregnancy or childbirth. Raised blood pressure is followed by chemical changes, swelling of the body (oedema), convulsions, coma and often death. In the nineteenth century the condition was comparatively common but twentieth century antenatal care has made it extremely rare.

ECTOPIC PREGNANCY Pregnancy which occurs outside the uterus (womb), usually in a Fallopian tube. The growth of the foetus causes the tube to split and bleed into the abdominal cavity, an acute emergency. The condition is extremely dangerous and, before the introduction of anaesthetics and the development of abdominal surgery, was usually fatal.

EMETIC A substance or drug that induces vomiting.

ENDOCARDITIS Inflammation of the lining of the heart.

ENDOCRINE GLAND A gland that discharges its product straight into the blood stream. The secretion is called a hormone.

ENDOSCOPE An instrument that is passed into the interior of the body in order to view it.

ENDOSCOPY The process of using an endoscope.

EPILEPSY A group of brain disorders in which there are fits or convulsions.

EPILEPTOID Related or similar to epilepsy.

EPITHELIUM The tissue that covers the external surfaces of the body and also the hollow structures inside.

EVOLUTION The process by which species of organisms develop.

EXCORIATION The soreness and inflammation that results from destruction or removal of the skin or mucous membrane.

EXCRESCENCE An abnormal growth on the surface of the body or a part of the body, such as a wart.

EXTIRPATION Complete surgical removal. A word used much more during the nineteenth century than today.

FALLOPIAN TUBE The tube leading from an ovary to the uterus (womb) down which the ova (eggs) pass.

FEVER, PYREXIA A rise in body temperature above the 'normal', usually taken to be 98.4° Fahrenheit or 37° Celsius.

FIBROID Tumour consisting of muscular and fibrous tissue which grows in the wall of the uterus (womb). Often several fibroids grow at the same time.

FISSURE A split or cleft. In anatomy this is a normal structure. In pathology it is abnormal, a defect caused by disease, eg anal fissure.

FISTULA An abnormal passage between two hollow organs, eg bladder and vagina (vesico-vaginal), rectum and vagina (recto-vaginal). Sometimes used to describe an abnormal passage between a hollow organ and the exterior, though this is strictly a sinus, eg anal fistula, fistula-in-ano.

FISTULA-IN-ANO An abnormal passage or sinus between the anus and the exterior. If it is higher than the controlling sphincter or muscles, there is incontinence of faeces.

FITS Sometimes used loosely for 'temper', 'anger', 'scene' or 'hysteria', but for technical meaning see Convulsions.

FORCEPS Surgical instrument with two opposing blades designed to compress or grasp an object. Examples include Spencer-Wells forceps, designed to compress blood vessels and so stop bleeding, and obstetric forceps, designed to pull out the foetus.

FORCEPS, MID-CAVITY The process of applying obstetric forceps before the baby's head is at the pelvic outlet.

GALL BLADDER An oblong sac lying under the liver. It stores bile, the juice from the liver.

GANGRENE Death or decay of part of the body due to deficiency or absence of the blood supply. A constant supply of blood is needed to keep most tissues alive. See also Necrosis.

GASTROPTOSIS A downward displacement of the stomach. It is now mostly regarded as a normal variation but, in the early days of extensive surgery and X-rays, it was thought to be the cause of many complaints.

GASTROTOMY Surgical operation in which the stomach is opened.

GENERAL PARALYSIS OF THE INSANE (GPI) An advanced form of syphilis affecting the brain.

GLAND An organ or group of cells that produce a substance which the body uses. Glands are either exocrine, discharging their products through a duct where they are needed, or endocrine, discharging them into the blood stream which then carries them elsewhere.

GLOSSECTOMY Surgical operation for removal of the tongue, or part of it.

GLOSSODECTOMY See Glossectomy.

GONORRHOEA A venereal disease affecting the genitals of either sex.

GPI See General Paralysis of the Insane.

GRANULATION TISSUE The tissue formed when a wound or infection is healing.

GREEN SICKNESS See Chlorosis.

GYNAECOLOGY The study or specialty of diseases of women, chiefly those of the reproductive organs. The term was invented in the mid-nineteenth century. Before then these diseases were classified under obstetrics.

HAEMOGLOBIN Substance that makes blood red. It is carried by the red cells of the blood and carries oxygen round the body.

HAEMOLYTIC STREPTOCOCCUS Bacterium that can destroy red blood cells and is responsible for many diseases, including tonsillitis, scarlet fever and acute nephritis. During the nineteenth century, the organism was virulent and dangerous but for reasons unknown it lost much of the virulence spontaneously, shortly before the introduction of antibiotics.

HAEMOSTASIS The arrest of bleeding.

HAEMOSTATIC Refers to an instrument or substance that stops bleeding.

HEMIPLEGIA Paralysis or part-paralysis of one side of the body.

HERNIA Protrusion of an organ or tissue out of the body cavity or structure in which it normally lies (rather as the inner tube of a car wheel may bulge through the outer tubes). See also Strangulated Hernia.

HERNIAL SAC The space or potential space into which the hernia protrudes.

HORMONE Secretion from an endocrine gland.

HORMONE REPLACEMENT THERAPY (HRT) Controversial modern procedure for replacing hormones no longer secreted after the menopause, with the aim of keeping the body young.

HOSPITAL FEVER Infection of wounds leading to septicaemia once thought to be an inevitable accompaniment of surgery. After the introduction of antisepsis and asepsis, it diminished and disappeared.

HRT see Hormone Replacement Therapy.

HYDROCOELE Accumulation of fluid in the scrotum or sac that

surrounds the testis. Most cases are benign and are treated by drainage or by surgical removal of the lining of the sac.

HYPEREMESIS Severe vomiting.

HYPEREMESIS GRAVIDARUM Condition of excessive vomiting in pregnancy. Untreated it may lead to death.

HYSTERECTOMY Surgical operation for removal of the uterus (womb). It may be done via the vagina or through an incision in the abdominal wall. It may or may not be accompanied by removal of other organs such as Fallopian tubes and ovaries. The operation is a cause of much controversy at the present time.

HYSTERIA Nervous condition of varied and sometimes confused terminology. Characteristics are overreaction (with a purpose) and the tendency to convert psychological symptoms into physical ones, eg paralysis, 'fits', or 'lump in the throat'. Typically associated with young women, but by no means confined to them.

HYSTERICAL FITS Sometimes there are 'fits' in hysteria which used to be confused with epilepsy.

HYSTERO-EPILEPSY Term much used in the nineteenth century for 'fits' thought to be due to hysteria.

HYSTEROSCOPY Surgical procedure of passing a hysteroscope or uteroscope into the uterus (womb) in order to gain a direct view of its interior.

IN VITRO FERTILISATION (IVF) Fertilisation of an ovum outside the body. A controversial procedure at the present time.

INFIBULATION Operation on the female external genitals in which the labia are bound together.

INFLAMMATION Reaction of living tissue to injury, infection or irritation. Characterised by pain, redness, swelling and loss of function of the affected part.

INGUINAL CANAL Passage in the groin through which various structures pass from the abdomen. A common site for hernia, especially in males.

INTERSEX Possession of both male and female anatomical characteristics.

LABIUM (LABIA, PL) A lip-shaped structure, one of two pairs of skin-folds, that enclose the vulva. The larger, outer pair are called the labia majora and the smaller, inner pair are called the labia minora.

LANCET Small knife used for bleeding, opening abscesses and other minor surgery. Became a symbol of the medical profession.

LANCET, THE Independent medical weekly of high prestige. Founded in 1823 by Thomas Wakley.

LAPAROTOMY Surgical operation of incision into the abdominal cavity.

LAUDANUM Preparation of opium and alcohol widely used in the nineteenth century as a narcotic and analgesic. Still obtainable today.

LEECHES A kind of worm, *Herudo medicinalis*, for many centuries applied to the human body to suck blood, pus or other fluid.

LEUCORRHOEA Whitish or yellowish discharge from vagina, not necessarily abnormal.

LITHOTOMY The surgical removal of stone from the bladder.

LITHOTOMY POSITION Surgical position of the patient lying on his or her back with legs in the air, suspended in stirrups.

MALIGNANT Cancerous. Invading the surrounding tissues and/or spreading to distant parts of the body. See Cancer.

MANIA Abnormal mental state with excitement, restlessness, insomnia, excessive energy, unrealistic ideas and objectives, followed by depression. The word is also often used to describe an obsession with something or someone.

MANUAL REMOVAL Refers to the procedure carried out if the placenta is not born soon after the baby or if part of it is left behind. See Retained Placenta.

MEDICINE, MEDICAL These terms may relate to the diagnosis, treatment and prevention of disease, or to disease or procedures that do not concern surgery and surgeons but are dealt with by physicians.

MENINGES Membranes covering the brain.

METRORRHAGIA Non-menstrual or excessive bleeding from the uterus (womb).

MICROORGANISMS (MICROBES) Organisms too small to be seen with the naked eye. They include bacteria, viruses, rickettsiae and some fungi.

MOLE Used to describe either an abnormal growth in the skin or defective form of pregnancy forming a tumour in the uterus, with no foetus and no placenta. Formerly any tumour of the uterus.

MOLECULE A small unit of a chemical substance, consisting of linked atoms.

MOLIMEN A strange word used by nineteenth-century gynaecologists to describe a woman's 'striving' menstruation.

MONOGENIC THEORY Anthropological theory of the nineteenth century that all human beings are descended from one race. This is now the prevalent theory. See Polygenic Theory.

MUCOUS MEMBRANE The moist membrane lining many tubes and cavities of the body, including the mouth, nasal passages, gastrointestinal tract, bronchial passages and bladder.

NARCOTIC Substance that induces sleep. Misnamed in America's 'war against drugs' to include drugs which alert and waken. A complex and misleading invention of the twentieth century.

NARCOTISM Refers to either a condition of being anaesthetised or to dependence on a narcotic drug.

NECROSIS Death of cells or tissues as a result of disease, injury, poisoning or loss of blood supply.

NEURASTHENIA, NEURASTHENIC Nineteenth-century term for a set of psychological symptoms including weakness, fatigue, inability to withstand stress, headache, anxiety, dizziness and so on. Now classified with the neuroses and related to hysteria.

NEUROSIS, NEUROSES Psychological condition in which contact with reality is maintained but in which anxiety leads to irrational ways of thinking and reacting.

NO-TOUCH TECHNIQUE Part of the system of asepsis involving the manipulation of surgical instruments, dressings, dissection, etc without touching them directly.

NULLIPARA A woman who has not been pregnant.

NYMPHOMANIA Extreme degree of sexual promiscuity in a woman. During the nineteenth century many doctors and others were seriously concerned about it and used it as a justification for performing mutilating operations.

OBSTETRICS The branch of medicine concerned with pregnancy and childbirth. Until the middle of the nineteenth century the term also covered diseases of women.

OEDEMA Excessive accumulation of fluid in the body tissues. Popularly known as dropsy.

OÖPHORECTOMY Surgical operation for removal of an ovary or both ovaries. During the nineteenth century, the term was sometimes confined to the operation for removing ovaries that showed no signs of disease (Battey's Operation), while extirpation or ovariotomy was used when referring to removal of diseased ovaries.

OÖPHORO-ELILEPSY A nineteenth-century term dating from the days when all women's problems were thought to be due to their reproductive organs. Fits and hysteria were thought to originate in the ovary and to be caused by a disorder there.

OPIUM The juice of the poppy *Papaver somniferum*, used throughout history to soothe, calm, allay anxiety, ease pain and aid sleep.

ORGANS Aggregations of tissues built up into a specific structure in the body, with a specific function or functions.

OS CERVIX The mouth of the cervix, which points into the vagina.

OS UTERI see Os Cervix.

OVARIAN CYST Tumour or growth of the Ovary.

OVARIAN DROPSY old term for Ovarian Cyst.

OVARIOTOMY Old term for surgical operation to remove an ovary or both ovaries because of disease. A more accurate term is oöphorectomy.

OVARY Organ in the female pelvis responsible for forming the ova or eggs. See Ovariotomy.

OVULATION The production of an egg which usually occurs halfway through the menstrual cycle.

OVUM (OVA PL) The female germ cells which develop in the ovary and pass down the Fallopian tube to reach the uterus.

OXYGEN Gas present in the air which is necessary to the life of all living creatures, tissues and cells.

PALPATION Examination of a patient by touch and direct feeling with the hands and fingers.

PANHYSTERECTOMY Surgical operation for removal of the uterus (womb), ovaries, tubes and surrounding glands and tissue. Usually done for cancer.

PARACENTESIS Tapping. The process of drawing off abnormal fluid from the abdomen, ovary or elsewhere through a hollow needle or tube.

PARAPLEGIA Paralysis or partial paralysis of both legs.

PATHOLOGIST Doctor who specialises in the study of disease processes and the examination of abnormal tissues and cells.

PATHOLOGY Study of disease processes and tissues.

PATIENT DEMAND Pressure put on doctors by patients to treat certain symptoms or to give a certain kind of treatment.

PEDICLE, PEDUNCLE The stump left after excision of an organ, eg the ovary.

PELVIC Concerning the pelvis.

PELVIS The pelvic bones (the large, flat bones that connect the legs with the spine) and that part of the abdomen that lies within them.

PELVISCOPY Direct examination of the female internal organs through an instrument.

PERCUSSION Examination of the body by tapping it and listening to the effect.

PERINEUM, PERINAEUM The floor of the pelvis. Important in midwifery (obstetrics).

PERIPHERAL EXCITEMENT (IRRITATION, STIMULATION) Nineteenth-century term used by doctors and scientists researching into the behaviour and function of nerves, but also used as a euphemism for masturbation.

PERITONEAL Refers to the peritoneum.

PERITONEUM The membrane that lines the abdominal cavity and covers many of its organs.

PERITONITIS Inflammation or infection of the peritoneum.

PESSARY A plastic, metal or ceramic object, specially designed to be inserted into the vagina, usually to prop up a descending uterus (womb). See Prolapse. Also a drug or tablet inserted into the vagina for the treatment of disease.

PHLEBITIS Inflammation in a vein.

PHYSICAL SIGNS What the doctor can see, hear, feel, or otherwise elicit as abnormalities or signs of disease. Contrasted with symptoms, which are what the patient complains of. They may sometimes be the same, for example a patient may complain of cough (symptom) and the doctor may observe him coughing (sign).

PHYSICIAN A general term for 'medical practitioner', especially in America, or describes a doctor learned in internal disease (often called 'internist') who treats patients other than by surgery.

PLACEBO An inert, ineffective substance given to a patient because he has faith in it. New drugs are tested against placebos to eliminate the 'placebo effect'. Placebos are one of the great inventions of twentieth-century medicine.

PLACENTA The thick, plate-like structure attached to the wall of the pregnant uterus (womb) which feeds the foetus and provides it with oxygen.

PLACENTA PRAEVIA A dangerous condition in pregnancy in which the placenta lies in front of the baby. If not treated, when labour starts the placenta separates from the wall of the uterus and the baby usually dies. Because the wall is still distended by the foetus inside, there is excessive, potentially fatal, bleeding. Nowadays placenta praevia is diagnosed during antenatal care and treated by caesarian section.

POLYGENIC THEORY Anthropological theory of the nineteenth century that different races of humans have different descents. The theory was largely promulgated to assert the superiority of the Anglo-Saxon races over all others. It gradually fell into disrepute.

POLYP, POLYPUS A growth, usually benign, growing from mucous membrane. Polyps are common in the nose, bowel and vagina.

PROCIDENTIA, TOTAL PROCIDENTIA Descent (prolapse) of the uterus (womb) so that it lies wholly outside the body.

PROLAPSE Descent of the womb into the vagina.

PROTEIN Group of chemicals that are the basis of life.

PSYCHOSEXUAL The area of thought and feeling that concerns sexuality in any of its forms.

PSYCHOSEXUAL COUNSELLING Professional help (talking) with sexual problems.

PTOSIS Dropping of an organ or part of the body. In the late nineteenth century and early in the present century it was fashionable diagnosis in relation to abdominal organs, now known to be normal variations.

PUBERTY The onset of sexual maturity and the beginning of menstruation, wet dreams and secondary sexual characteristics.

PUBIS The area in front of the pubic part of the pelvic bones. In adults it is covered with pubic hair and in women it is called the mons veneris.

PUS A thick yellowish liquid that forms where there is bacterial infection. It consists mostly of white blood cells, dead bacteria and fragments of dead tissue.

RADICAL In surgery, refers to an extensive operation removing everything that might cause trouble later, eg radical mastectomy for cancer of breast, in which the surrounding tissues and glands are also removed.

RETAINED PLACENTA Condition in which the birth of the placenta is delayed. It is a potentially dangerous source of bleeding or infection. It is removed under anaesthetic but in past times it was sometimes a life-and-death matter to remove it without anaesthetic to save the life of the mother, who often then died from shock.

RETENTION Usually refers to the inability to pass urine due to nervous disease or to obstruction.

RETROFLEXION Condition in which the uterus (womb) is bent backwards instead of, as is more common, forwards. Distinguish from retroversion, in which it is *pointing* backwards.

RETROVERSION Condition in which the uterus (womb) is pointing backwards instead of, as is more common, forwards. Distinguish from retroflexion, in which it is *bent* backwards.

RICKETS Condition in which the bones become soft due to lack of Vitamin D – often due to lack of sunlight.

RUPTURE Can refer to breaking, eg rupture of a cyst, or to hernia, especially inguinal hernia.

SAC A chamber or bag in the body, either normal or abnormal.

SACRUM The lowest part of the spine, where, in humans, five vertebrae are fused into a plate-like bone, attached to the vestigial tail or coccyx.

SALPINGO-OÖPHORECTOMY Surgical operation to remove the ovaries and Fallopian tubes.

SCARLET FEVER Infectious illness caused by the haemolytic streptococcus. Until the 1930s when the organism underwent spontaneous change and became less virulent, it was a dangerous disease of childhood.

SCHIRROUS, SCIRROUS, SCIRRHUS Means hard. Usually refers to cancers, especially of the breast.

SCHIZOPHRENIA Serious mental disorder which may be acute or chronic. See Acute and Chronic.

scleroma A hardened patch of tissue consisting of Granulation Tissue.

SEPSIS Invasion with pus-forming bacteria.

SEPTICAEMIA Invasion of the blood by bacteria, leading to fever and illness.

SHOCK Physical shock is a condition of lowered blood pressure and circulatory collapse, often due to haemorrhage or to severe allergy. Insufficient blood circulates to the tissues and the patient is cold, clammy and seriously ill.

Psychological shock can occur as the result of any personal tragedy or sudden, overwhelming psychological stress. The blood pressure is normal and the condition, though unpleasant, is not potentially fatal.

SIGNS see Physical Signs.

SINUS Passage between a hollow organ and the exterior of the body. See also Fistula.

SLOUGH, SLOUGHING The separation of dead tissue from healthy tissue. See Gangrene and Necrosis.

SOFT TISSUES All the tissues of the body except bone and cartilage.

SPASM Sustained involuntary contraction of muscle which can be painful.

SPENCER–WELLS FORCEPS Forceps designed to stop bleeding.

SPERMATAZOA Male germ cells.

STAPHYLOCOCCUS Bacteria responsible for most local infections of skin, boils, etc and sometimes for more serious conditions such as pneumonia.

STRANGULATED HERNIA Condition in which the blood supply to a hernia is cut off leading to gangrene or necrosis. The term usually refers to abdominal herniae such as inguinal or femoral herniae (named from the region in which they protrude). A strangulated hernia is usually an acute surgical emergency.

STRICTURE Narrowing of a tube in the body, eg the intestine or urethra.

SURGICAL Refers to surgery and to conditions treated, or which may be treated, by surgery.

SYMPTOMS What the patient complains of, in contrast to signs, which the doctor elicits for himself.

SYNDROME A collection of symptoms and signs that are recognised as being often associated.

SYPHILIS A serious chronic infectious disease transmitted sexually and so classified as a venereal disease.

TESTES Male organs that produce spermatazoa.

THERAPEUTICS Branch of medicine concerned with treatment, particularly by drugs.

THERAPY Word applied, often somewhat indiscriminately, to different attempts and methods designed to alleviate disease and suffering.

TISSUES Collections of cells specialised to perform a particular function. Aggregates of tissues constitute Organs.

TOXAEMIA A condition of poisoning in the blood, usually from bacteria.

TOXAEMIA OF PREGNANCY Condition of raised blood pressure, albuminuria and oedema which can precede eclampsia in pregnancy. Much antenatal care is devoted to preventing and treating this potentially dangerous condition.

TRICHOMONAS Infection, usually of the vagina, with the parasite trichomonas.

TUBERCULOSIS Chronic infection due to the tubercle bacillus. Now largely conquered where there are adequate medical services.

TUMOUR An abnormal swelling or growth.

ULCER A break in the skin or mucous membrane that fails to heal.

ULTRASOUND (ULTRASONIC WAVES) Modern alternative to X-rays for producing images of structures inside the body by using extremely high frequency waves which 'bounce off' whatever they encounter.

URETHRA The tube connecting the bladder with the exterior.

URINARY RETENTION Inability to pass urine, usually due to paralysis or obstruction.

VAGINA The passage connecting the exterior with the mouth of the uterus (womb).

VAGINISM, VAGINISMUS Condition of spasm of the muscles of the vagina making sexual intercourse difficult or impossible.

VAGINOTOMY Surgical operation involving cutting into the vagina.

VENEREAL Transmitted by sexual intercourse.

VESICO-VAGINAL FISTULA Abnormal passage between the bladder and the vagina, leading to incontinence of urine. Usually due to obstructed and mishandled childbirth. Nowadays very rare.

VIRUS A minute microorganism that can reproduce only in a living cell. Viruses are responsible for many diseases.

VULVA The external genitalia of the female.

VULVECTOMY Surgical operation of removing the vulva.

# BIBLIOGRAPHY

ALAYA, Flavia, 'Victorian Science and the "Genius" of Woman', *J. Hist. Ideas*, 38, April-June, 1977, pp. 261–80.

ALEXANDER, William, *Women Physiologically Considered*, 1839.

ALLBUTT, H. Arthur, *The Wife's Handbook: How a woman should order herself during pregnancy . . . with hints . . . on other matters of importance necessary to be known by married women*, 2nd edn., London, 1886.

ALLBUTT, H. Arthur, *Artificial Checks to Population: Is the popular teaching of them infamous? A history of medical persecution*, 14th edn., London, 1909.

ALLBUTT, Thomas Clifford, & ROLLESTON, Humphry Davy (eds.), *A System of Medicine*, 9 vols., London and New York, Macmillan, 1898.

ALLBUTT, Sir Thomas Clifford, 'Medicine in the 19th Century', *Bull. of the Johns Hopkins University*, 1898, 9, pp. 277–85, reprinted with explanatory note by A.M. Chesney in *J. Med. Educ.*, 1956, 31, pp. 460–68.

ALLBUTT, T.C., & PLAYFAIR, W.S. (eds.), *A System of Gynaecology*, London, 1896, especially article by Handfield-Jones.

ASHWELL, Samuel, *A Practical Treatise on the Diseases Peculiar to Women*, 3rd edn., London, 1848.

ASTRUC, J.A., *Treatise on all the Diseases Incident to Women*, London, Cooper, 1743.

ATLAY, J.B., *Sir Henry Wentworth Acland, Bart, KCB, FRS: a memoir*, London, Smith, Elder & Co, 1903.

AUSTIN, G.L., *Perils of American Women; or, A Doctor's Talk with Maiden, Wife and Mother*, Boston, 1883, 198, pp.158–60.

AUSTOKER, Joan, 'The Treatment of Choice: Breast cancer surgery 1860–1985', *Soc. Soc. His. of Med. Bull.*, December, 1985, pp. 100–107.

AVELING, J.H., 'British Gynaecology, Past and Present', *Brit. Gyn. J.*, 1885–6, 1, pp. 72–95.

BALLINGALL, G., *Outlines of Military Surgery*, London, 1833.

BALLS-HEADLEY, W., *The Evolution of the Diseases of Women*, London, Smith, Elder & Co, 1894.

BANDLER, S.W., *Medical Gynaecology*, 3rd edn., Philadelphia, W.B. Saunders & Co, 1914.

BANNISTER, Robert C., *Social Darwinism: Science and myth in anglo-American social thought*, Philadelphia Temple University Press, 1979.

BANTOCK, G.G., 'Table of 238 Cases of Ovariotomy (163 to 400 inclusive) with remarks', *Brit. Gyn. J.*, 5, (1889–90), pp 373–76, 430–37.

BARBER, B., & HIRSCH, W. (eds.), Collier Macmillan *The Sociology of Science*, New York, The Free Press and London, 1962.

BARKER-BENFIELD, Ben, 'Sexual Surgery in Late Nineteenth Century America', *Int. J. Health Serv.*, 1975, 5, pp. 279–98.

BARKER-BENFIELD, Ben, 'The Spermatic Economy: A nineteenth century view of sexuality', *Feminist Studies* 1*11, Summer, 1972. Also in GORDON, Michael (ed.), *The American Family in Social-Historical Persepctive*, New York, St. Martin's Press, 1973.

BARKER-BENFIELD, G.J., *The Horrors of the Half-Known Life: Male attitudes toward women and sexuality in nineteenth century America*, New York, Harper & Row, 1976.

BARNES, B., & SHAPIN, S., *Natural Order: Historical studies of scientific culture*, London, Russell Sage, 1979.

BARNES, Benjamin J., 'Discarded Operations: Surgical Innovation by Trial and Error' in BUNKER, John P. et al. (eds.), *Cost, Risks and Benefits of Surgery*, New York, Oxford University Press, 1977, pp. 109–123.

BARNES, Robert, 'Lectures on the Diseases of Women', *Lancet*, 1880,

1, pp. 4–6, 155–7; 2, 121–3, 923–25.

BARNES, Robert, *On the Relations between Medicine, Surgery, and Obstetrics in London*, New York, W. Wood & Co., 1884.

BARNES, R., & BARNES, R.S.F., *A System of Obstetric Medicine and Surgery*, 2 vols., London, Smith, Elder & Co., 1884

BARNES, Robert, 'On Vicarious Menstruation', *Brit. Gyn. J.*,1886-7, 2, pp. 151–83.

BARNES, Robert, 'Women, Diseases of,' in R. Quain (ed.), *A Dictionary of Medicine: including general pathology, general therapeutics, hygiene, and the diseases peculiar to women and children*, 2 vols., London, Longmans Green, 1882, ii, 1987.

BARNES, Robert, 'The Foundation of the British Gynaecological Society,' *Brit. Gyn. J.*, 1885–6, 1, pp. 233–8.

BARNES, Robert, 'Obstetric Physician to St Thomas's Hospital Lumleian lectures, 1873', *Lancet*, 1873, 1, 513, 549, 585, 619. – Subject: The convulsive diseases of women. Also in *BMJ*, 1873, pp. 391–4, 421–5, 453–5, 483–5.

BARNES, Robert, 'On the Correlations of the Sexual Functions and Mental Disorders of Women,' *Brit. Gyn. J.*, 1890–91, 6, 390–413, 416–30.

BARNES, Robert, 'An Address on Obstetric Medicine and its Position in Medical Education', *Obstetrical Journal of Great Britain and Ireland*, 1875–76, 3, pp. 289–99.

BARNESBY, Norman, *Medical Chaos and Crime*, Mitchell Kennerly, New York, 1910.

BARRETT, C.R.B., *The History of the Society of Apothecaries of London*, E. Stock, London, 1905, pp. 40, 50.

BARROW, M., *Women 1870–1928: A select guide to printed and archival sources in the United Kingdom*, London, Mansell, 1981.

BELL, John, *The Principles of Surgery*, Edinburgh, 1801.

BELLERS, John, *An Essay towards the Improvement of Physick*, London, 1714.

BENNET, J.H., *A Practical Treatise on Inflammation of the Uterus, its Cervix and Appendages, and on its Connection with other Uterine*

*Diseases*, Churchill, London. See also review of 4th edn., *BMJ*, Nov 2, 1861.

BENNET, J.H., *A Practical Treatise on the Chronic Inflammation of the Uterus, its Cervix and Appendages and on its Connection with other Uterine Diseases*, Philadelphia, 1864, p. 237. See also his letters to the *Lancet*, 1864.

BERNARD, Claude, *Introduction to the Study of Experimental Medicine*, translated by H.C. Greene, Macmillan, New York, 1927.

BIDDIS, Michael, 'The Politics of Anatomy: Dr Robert Knox and Victorian racism', *Proc. Roy. Sec. Med.*, 1976, 69, pp. 245–50.

BIDDIS, Michael, *Father of Racist Ideology: The social and political thought of count Gobineau, New York*, 1970, London, Weidenfeld, 1975.

BIGELOW, Jacob, 'On Self Limited Diseases,' presented before the Massachusetts Medical Society, May 27, 1835, reprinted in BRIEGER, Gert H., *Medical America in the Nineteenth Century*, Baltimore, The John Hopkins Press, 1972, p. 99.

BLACKWELL, Elizabeth, *Pioneer Work in Opening the Medical Profession to Women*, New York, 1895, (pp. 257–59 re midwifery lectures), and New York, E.P. Dutton. 1914.

BLACKWELL, E., *Essays in Medical Sociology*, New York, Arno Press, 1920. and the *New York Times*, 1972.

BOLT, C., *Victorian Attitudes to Race*, London, and Toronto, University of Toronto Press, 1971, especially pp. 1–28.

BOOTH, Charles, *Life and Labour of the People of London*, London, Macmillan, 1902.

BRANCA, Patricia, *Silent Sisterhood: Middle class women in the Victorian home*, London, Croom Helm, 1975.

BRANCA, Patricia, 'Image and Reality: The myth of the idle, Victorian woman', in Hartmann & Banner, *Clio's Consciousness Raised*, 1974.

BRETT, S. (ed.), *The Faber Book of Diaries*, London, Faber, 1987.

BRIEGER, Gert H., *Medical America in the Nineteenth Century*, Baltimore, John Hopkins Press, 1972.

BRIFFAULT, Robert, *The Mothers: A study in the origins of sentiments and institutions*, 3 vols., London and New York, 1927.

BROCA, Paul, 'On Anthropology', *Anthrop Rev.*, 1868, 6, p. 50. Fee's 1979 paper gives a good account.

BROCKBANK, W., & KENWORTHY, F., *Diary of Richard Kay, 1716–51*, Manchester University Press, 1968.

BRODY, H., *Stories of Sickness*, New Haven, Yale University Press, 1987.

BROOKS C. McC., & CRANfiELD, P.F., (eds.), *The Historical Development of Physiological Thought*, New York, 1959.

BROWN, F.K., *Fathers of the Victorians*, Cambridge, 1966.

BROWN, G.H., *Lives of the Fellows of the Royal College of Physicians of London, 1826–1925*. London, Royal College of Physicians, 1955. A continuation of *The Roll of the Royal College of Physicians of London comprising Biographical Sketches of all the Eminent Physicians*, by William Munk, London, The Royal College of Physicians, 1878.

BROWN, Isaac Baker, *On Surgical Diseases of Women*, London, 1854.

BROWN, Isaac Baker, *On the Curability of Certain Forms of Insanity, Epilepsy, Catalepsy and Hysteria in Females* London, R. Hardwicke, 1866.

BROWN, P., & DRUCKMAN, E. (eds.), 'Elective Hysterectomy: Pro and Con', *NEJM*, 1976, 295 (5), pp. 264–268.

BROWNE, W.A.F., 'The Moral Treatment of the Insane', *J. Ment. Sci.*, 1864, 10, pp. 309–37.

BRUMBERG, Joan Jacobs, *Chlorotic Girls, 1870–1920,: A Historical Perspective on Female Adoloscence*, in LEAVITT, Judith Waltzer, *Women and Health in America*, University of Wisconsin Press, 1984.

BUCHAN, William, *Domestic Medicine*, 1st American edn., Philadelphia, 1771, printed for and sold by R. Aitken, at his bookstore.

BUCKLE, H.T. 'The Influence of Women on the Progress of Knowledge', presented to the British Royal Society in 1858 and published in Essays, New York, 1486.

BUCKLEY, T., & GOTTLIEB, Alma, *Blood Magic: The anthropology of menstruation*, London, University of California Press, c.1988.

BUCKNILL, J.C. & TUKE, D.H., *A Manual of Psychological Medicine: containing the history, nosology, description, statistics, diagnosis, pathology, and treatment of insanity*, London, J. Churchill, 1858.

BUER, M.C., *Health, Wealth and Population in the Early Days of the Industrial Revolution*, 1968 (1926).

BULLOUGH, V. & VOGHT, Martha, 'Women, Menstruation, and Nineteenth Century Medicine', *Bulletin of the History of Medicine*, 47, 1973, pp. 66–82. Also in LEAVITT, J.W. (ed.) *Women and Health in America*, University of Wisconsin Press, 1984.

BUNKER, J.P., *Costs, Risks and Benefits of Surgery*, OUP, 1977.

BUTLER, M.W., *The British Practice of Battey's Operation, 1872–1890*, University of Cambridge, 1982.

BUTLER, H. T., *Manual of Gynecology*, 2nd edn., Philadelphia, P. Blakiston, 1897, pp. 180–5.

BURKE, W.L., *The Age of Equipoise*, New York, 1965.

BURSTYN, Joan N., *Victorian Education and the Ideal of Motherhood*, London, Croom, Helm, 1980, bib.

BYFORD, William H., *A Treatise on the Chronic Imflammation and Displacement of the Unimpregnated Uterus*, Philadelphia, 1864, p. 22–41.

BYNUM, W.F., & PORTER, R., *Medical Fringe and Medical Orthodoxy, 1750–1850*, London and New Hampshire, Croom Helm, 1987.

CAMERON, H.C., *Mr Guy's Hospital 1726–1948*, London, Longmans Green, 1954.

CARTER, Robert Brudenell, *On the Pathology and Treatment of Hysteria*, London, John Churchill, 1853, p. 21.

CASTIGLIONE, A., *A History of Medicine*, 2nd edn., Alfred A. Knopf, 1947

'CENSOR' (pseud.), 'Use of the Speculum Vaginae', *Lancet*, 1845, 1. pp. 105, 223.

CHADWICK, 'Obstetric and Gynecological Literature, 1876–1881', *Transactions of the American Medical Association*, 1881, 32, p. 254.

CHAMBERLAIN, Geoffrey, *Contemporary Gynaecology*, London, Butterworths, 1984.

CHAMBERLAIN, Mary, *Old Wives' Tales: their history, remedies and spells*, London, Virago Press, 1981.

'CHELSEA HOSPITAL FOR WOMEN, THE', *Lancet*, 1894, 1, 365, 631–2, 709; 1, 160–1, 200–1, 214, 462–3, 595–7.

CHESLER, Phyllis, *Women and Madness,* New York, Doubleday, 1972 and Harmondsworth, Penguin Books, 1979.

CHURCHILL, Fleetwood, *Observations on the Diseases Incident to Pregnancy and Childbed,* Dublin, Martin Keene, 1840.

CHURCHILL, Fleetwood, *On the Diseases of Women: including those of Pregnancy and Childbed,* 4th edn, Dublin, Fannin & Co, London, Longman and Co, 1857. Said by *BMJ,* 1857, to show well the present state of knowledge and to be very up to date.

CHURCHILL, Fleetwood, *Outlines of the Principle Diseases of Females: chiefly for the use of students,* Dublin, Martin Keene, 1835.

CHURCHILL, Fleetwood, *On the Principle Diseases of Females,* 2nd edn., Dublin, Martin Keene, 1844. Second edition corrects some errors, adds some references and some engravings; third edition, 1850, extensively changed.

CIANFRANI, Theodore, *A Short History of Obstetrics and Gynecology,* Springfield, Charles C. Thomas, 1960.

CLARKE, Edward C., *Sex in Education; or A Fair Chance for Girls,* Osgood, Boston, 1873.

CLAY, Charles, *Peritoneal Section for the Extirpation of Diseased Ovaria,* 1848.

CLAY, Charles, review article on 'Extirpation of Diseased Ovaria', *British and Foreign Medical Review,* 1843, 16, pp. 387–402.

CLOUSTON, T.S., 'Women from a Medical Point of View', *Popular Science Monthly,* 24, 1883, pp. 214–34.

CLOUSTON, T.S., *Clinical Lectures on Mental Disease,* 4th edn., 1896, p. 521. This book was first published in 1883 and had its 6th edn. in 1904.

COBBE, Frances Power, *The Duties of Women: A course of lectures,* 1881, pp. 161–2.

COBBE, Frances Power, 'The Little Health of Ladies', Contemporary Review, 1877, xxxi, 276–96.

COBURN, K. (ed). *The letters of Sara Hutchinson from 1800–1835,* London, Routledge & Kegan Paul, 1954.

COLLIE, Michael, *Henry Maudsley, Victorian Psychiatrist: a bibliographical study,* St. Paul's Bibliographies, 1988.

COLOMBAT D' ISÈRE, *Amer, J. Med. Sci., 1840.*

COLOMBAT D' ISÈRE, *Traité des Maladies des Femmes et de l'Hygiène Spéciale de leur Sexe,* Paris, Librairie Médicale de Labé, 1838. Translated by Charles Meigs, 1845.

COLOMBAT D'ISÈRE, *Hygiene in Females,* 1845.

COMFORT, Alex, *The Anxiety Makers: Some curious preoccupations of the medical profession,* London, Nelson, 1967.

COMINOS, Peter, 'Innocent Femina Sexualis in Unconscious Conflict' in Vicinus', *Suffer and be still,* p. 155–72.

COMINOS, Peter, 'Late-Victorian Sexual Responsibility and the Social System', *Internat. Review of Social History,* 1963, 8, pp. 18–48, pp. 216–50.

CONNELL, R.W., *Gender and Power: Society, the person and sexual politics,* Cambridge, Polity Press, 1987.

CONOLLY, John, *Treatment of the Insane without Mechanical Restraints,* 1856. Reprinted, London, Dawson's, 1973, p. 161.

CONWAY, Jill, *The Female Experience in Eighteenth Century America: A guide to the history of American women,* Princeton, Princeton University Press, 1985.

CONWAY, Jill, 'Stereotype of Femininity in a Theory of Sexual Evolution', *Victorian Studies,* 1970–1, 14, pp. 83–9.

CONWAY, Jill, 'Women Reformers and American Culture 1870–1930', *Journal Society of History,* 1971–2, pp. 164–77.

COOPER, James Fenimore, *Gleanings in Europe,* edited by Robert E. Spiller, New York, 1930.

COOPER, Wendy, *The Fertile Years,* 1978.

CORSI, Pietro & WEINDLING, Paul, *Information Sources in the History of Medicine,* London, Butterworth Scientific, 1983.

CRAWFORD, P., 'Attitudes to Menstruation in Seventeenth-Century England', *Past and Present,* 1981, 91, pp. 47–73.

CROUZET, François, *The Victorian Economy,* translated by A.S. Forster, London, Methuen, 1982.

DALE, W., *Present State of the Medical Profession,* London, 1860.

DALY, Mary, *GYN/Ecology*, Beacon Press, Boston, 1978, and Women's Press, London.

DAVENPORT-HINES, Richard, *Sex, Death and Punishment: Attitudes to sex and sexuality in Britain since the Renaissance*, London, Collins, 1990.

DAVIDOFF, Leonore, *The Best Circles: Women and society in Victorian England*, New Jersey, Totowa, 1973.

DAVIDOFF, Leonore & HALL, Catherine, *Family Fortunes: Men and women of the English middle class, 1780–1850*, Chicago, University of Chicago Press, 1987.

DAVIDSON, M., *Medicine in Oxford*, 1953, p.49.

DAVIES, Celia, 'Making Sense of the Census in Britain and the USA: The changing occupational classification and the position of nurses', *Sociol. Rev.*, N.S., August 1980, 28, 3, 607.

DAVIES, Emily, *Thought on Some Questions Relating to Women*, 1910.
DAVIES, Emily, *The Higher Education of Women*, London, Stahan, 1866.

DAVIES, Margaret Llewellyn, (ed.), *Life as we have known it, by Co-operative Working Women*, Hogarth Press, 1932. Reprinted with an introductory letter by Virginia Woolf and a new introduction by Anna Davin, Virago Press, 1977.

DAVIES, Margaret Llewellyn (ed.), *Maternity: Letters from working women, collected by the Women's Co-operative Guild*, London, G. Bell & Sons Ltd, 1915 and Virago, 1978.

DAVIES, S.E., 'Female Physicians', *The Englishwoman's Journal*, 1861.

DAVIS, J.B., 'Contributions towards Determining the Weight of the Brain in Different Races of Man', *Philosophical Transactions*, 1868, 158, pt. 2, pp. 505–27.

DEGLER, Carl N., 'What Ought To Be and What Was: Women's sexuality in the nineteenth century', in LEAVITT, Judith Waltzer, (ed.), *Women and Health in America*, University of Wisconsin Press, 1984.

DEGLER, Carl N., *At Odds: Women and family in America from the Revolution to the present*, New York, Oxford University Press, 1980.

DELAMONT, Sara, & DUFFIN, Lorna, *The Nineteenth Century Woman: Her cultural and physical worlds*, Croom Helm, 1978.

DELANEY, Janice, et el., *The Curse: A cultural history of menstruation*, New York, 1977.

DE MOULIN, D., 'A Historical-Phenomenological Study of Bodily Pain in Western Medicine', *Bull. His. Med.*, 1974, 48, pp. 540–70.

DENMAN, T., *An Introduction to the Practice of Midwifery*, 2nd edn., London, vol. 1. 1792, p. 179–80.

DENNIS, F. S., *A System of Surgery*, Philadelphia, 1895.

DESMOND, Adrian, *The Politics of Evolution: Morphology, medicine and reform in radical London*, Chicago University, 1990.

DEVITT, N., 'The Statistical Case for Elimination of the Midwife: Fact verses Prejudice, 1890–1935', *Women and Health*, 1979, 4.

DICKINSON, Robert Latou, 'Bicycling for Women from the standpoint of the Gynaecologist', Amer. J. Obst., Jan. 1895, 31, pp. 24–37.

DICTIONARY OF NATIONAL BIOGRAPHY, Oxford University Press, 1882–1986.

DIGBY, Anne, 'Women's Biological Straitjacket', in MENDUS & RENDALL, *Sexuality and Subordination*, Routledge, 1989.

DIRCKX J.H., *The Language of Medicine: Its evolution, structure and dynamics*, New York, Praeger, 1983.

DISTANT, W.L., 'On the Mental Differences between the Sexes', *Journal of the Anthropological Institute*, 1875, 4, p. 87.

DIXON Edward H., *Woman and her Diseases from the Cradle to the Grave*, New York, 1857, 134, 140.

DIXON, Norman, *On the Psychology of Military Incompetence*, London, Cape, 1976.

DONAJGRODZKI, A.P. (ed.), *Social Control in Nineteenth Century Britain*, London, Croom Helm, 1977, pp. 108–37.

DONNISON, Jean, *Midwives and Medical Men: A history of interpersonal rivalries and women's rights*, London and New York, Heinemman Educational, 1977. A powerful account of how men replaced women in the obstetrical services.

DONZELOT, Jacques, *The Policing of Families*, translated by Robert Hurley, New York, Pantheon Books, 1979.

DOYLE, Helen McKnight, *A Child Went Forth*, New York, 1934, especially pp. 15–18.

DYHOUSE, C., 'Social Darwinistic Ideas and the Development of Women's Education in England, 1880–1920', *History of Education*, 1976, 5, p.1.

EARLE, A. Scott, *Surgery in America: from the colonial era to the twentieth century*, Philadelphia, Sanders, 1965

ECKER, Alexander, 'On a Characteristic Peculiarity in the Form of the Female Skull, and its Significance for Comparative Anthropology', *Anthropological Review*, 1868, 6, pp. 350–56.

EDEL, Leon, *The Diary of Alice James*, Harmondsworth, Penguin Books, 1982.

EDES, R., 'Points in the Diagnosis and Treatment of some obscure common Neuroses', *JAMA*, 1896, 27, pp. 1077–82.

EDES, R., 'The Relations of Pelvic and Nervous Diseases', *JAMA*, 1898, 31, pp. 1133–36.

EDGERTON, M., JACOBSON, W., & MEYER, E., 'Surgical/Psychiatric Study of Patients seeking Plastic (Cosmetic) Surgery: 98 consecutive patients with minimal deformity', *Brit J. Plastic Surgery*, 1960, 13, pp. 136–45.

EDIS, A.W., 'On the Relations of Gynaecology to General Therapeutics', *Brit. Gyn. J.*, 1889–90, 4, pp. 7–23.

EDWARDS, Susan M., 'Femina Sexualis: Medico-legal control in Victoriana', *Bull. Society Soc. Hist. Med,.* 1981, 28, pp. 17–20.

EGERTON, George, *Keynotes and Discords*, London, Virago, 1983.

EHRENREICH, Barbara, & ENGLISH, Deirdre, *Complaints and Disorders: The sexual politics of sickness*, Glass Mountain Pamphlet no. 2, Old Westbury, New York, Feminist Press, 1973.

EHRENREICH, Barbara, & EHRENREICH, John, *The American Health Empire: Power, profits and politics*, New York, Vintage Books, 1971.

EHRENREICH, Barbara, & ENGLISH, Deirdre, *For Her Own Good: 150 years of experts' advice to women*, London, Pluto Press, 1979.

EHRENREICH, Barbara, & ENGLISH, Deirdre, *Witches, Midwives and Nurses: A history of women healers*, Glass Mountain Pamphlet no.1, Old Westbury, New York, Feminist Press, 1973 and London, Writers' and Readers' Publishing Co-operative, 1976.

EHRENREICH, J. (ed.), *The Cultural Crisis of Modern Medicine*, New York, Monthly Review Press, 1978. See essay by Zola.

EICHLER, M., *The Double Standard: A feminist critique of feminist social science*, London, Croom Helm, 1980.

ELIADE, Mircea, *The Forge and the Crucible: The origins and structures of alchemy*, 1971.

ELLERMAN, M., *Thinking about Women*, London, Macmillan, 1968.

EL SAADAWI, Nawal, *The Hidden Face of Eve: Women in the Arab World*, translated and edited by Dr Sherif Matata, London, Zed Press, 1980.

ENCYCLOPAEDIA BRITTANICA, Sections on Gynaecology, 11th ed., London, 1910.

FARR, W., *Vital Statistics*, edited by N.A. Humphreys, London, 1885.

FASBENDER, H., *Geschichte Der Geburtshilfe*, Jena, 1906.

FAULDER, Carolyn, *Talking to your Doctor*, 1978.

FAULDER, Carolyn, *Whose Body Is It: The troubling issue of informed consent*, Virago, 1985.

FAWCETT, M.G., *Education of Women of the Middle and Upper Classes*, London, 1868, 17, pp. 511–17.

FEE, Elizabeth and FOX, Daniel, (eds.), *Aids: The burdens of history*, Berkeley, University of California Press, c. 1989.

FEE, Elizabeth, 'Nineteenth Century Craniology: The study of the female skull', *Bull. Hist. Med.*, 1979, 53, pp. 415–433.

FEE, Elizabeth, The Sexual Politics of Victorian Social Anthropology, *Feminist Studies*, 1 (3/4) 1972/3, pp. 23–39, also in Hartman & Banner, *Clio's Consciousness Raised*, 1974.

FEE, Elizabeth, *Science and the Woman Question, 1860–1920: A study of English scientific periodicals*, PhD thesis, Princeton University, 1978.

FEE, Elizabeth, *Women and Health: The politics of sex in medicine*, 1983.

FIGLIO, K., 'Chlorosis and Chronic Disease in Nineteenth Century Britain: The social constitution of somatic illness in a capitalist society', *Social History*, vol. 3, no. 2, 1978, pp. 167–9.

FIGLIO, K., 'Sinister Medicine? A critique of left approaches to medicine', *Radical Science Journal*, 1979, 9, pp. 14–68.

FOUCAULT, Michel, *The Birth of the Clinic: An archaeology of medical perception*, London, Tavistock, 1973.

FOX-GENOVESE, Elizabeth, & GENOVESE, 'Placing Women's History in History', *New Left Review*, 1982, 133. pp. 5–29.

FREIDSON, E., *Profession of Medicine: A Study of the Sociology of applied knowledge*, New York, Dodd, Mead, 1973. (1970). See especially pp. 23, 47, and 71ff.

FREIDSON, E., *Professional Dominance: The social structure of medical care*, New York, Atherton Press, 1970.

FREMANTLE, A., (ed.) *The Wynne Diaries*, 3 vols., London, Oxford University Press.

FRENCH, R.D., *Antivivisection and Medical Science in Victorian Society*, Princeton, 1975.

FROW, John, 'Structuralist Marxism', *Southern Review*, July, 1982, xv, 2, pp. 208–17.

FULLER, Margaret, *Women in the Nineteenth Century*, (1855), New York, W.W. Norton, 1971.

GALLAGHER, Catherine & LAQUER, Thomas, (eds.), *Making of the Modern Body: sex and society in the nineteenth century*, Berkekey, University of California Press, c. 1981.

GALTON, Frances, *Hereditary Genius: an inquiry into its laws and consequences*, London, Macmillan, 1869.

GAMARNIKOW, Eva, 'Sexual Division of Labour: The Case of Nursing' in KUHN, Annette, and WOLPE, Ann Marie (eds.), *Feminism and Materialism: Women and modes of production*, Routledge & Kegan Paul, 1978.

GARRISON, F.H., *A Medical Bibliography: An annotated checklist of texts illustrating the history of medicine*, 4th edn., Aldershot, Grafton. 1983.

GARRISON, F.H., 'Medicine in the Tatler, Spectator and Guardian', *Bull. Hist. Med.*, 2, 1934, pp. 477–503.

GILMAN, Charlotte Perkins, *The Yellow Wallpaper*, (1892), Virago.

GOTHAM, Deborah, *The Victorian Girl and the Feminine Ideal*, Indiana, Bloomington, 1982.

GOULD, Donald, *The Black and White Medicine Show: How doctors serve and fail their customers*, London, Hamish Hamilton, 1985.

GOULD, Stephen Jay, *The Mismeasure of Man*, New York, W.W. Norton, 1981.

GRAHAM, Harvey, *Eternal Eve*, 1st edn. 1950; 2nd edn. 1960, London, Hutchinson.

GRAHAM, Harvey, *Surgeons All*, 2nd edn., Rich & Cowan, 1956.

GRANSHAW, L., & PORTER, R., *The Hospital in History*, London, Routledge, 1989.

GRANSHAW, L., *St Mark's Hospital: A social history of a specialist hospital*, King Edward's Hospital Fund for London, 1985.

GREEN, Thos. H., *Gynecology: The Essentials of Clinical Practice*, Boston, Little, Brown, 1971, p. 436.

HALEY, B., *The Healthy Body and Victorian Culture*, Cambridge, Mass., Harvard University Press, 1978.

HALL, Marshall, *Commentaries on Some of the More Important of the Diseases of the Female*, 3 pts, London.

HAMILTON, A., 'The Abuse of Oöpherectomy in Diseases of the Nervous System', *New York Medical Journal*, 1893, 57, pp. 180–83.

HAMILTON Alexander, *A Treatise on the Management of Female Complaints*, 7th edn., Edinburgh, 1813.

HAMILTON, R., *The Liberation of Women*, London, Allen & Unwin, 1976.

HANDFIELD-JONES, M., 'The Development of Modern Gynaecology', in Allbutt & Playfair, *A System of Gynaecology*, London, 1896.

HANDLIN, Oscar, *Race and Nationality in American Life*, 5th edn., Boston, 1957, pp.139–66.

HARRIS, I., ed., *Family Memorials: Chiefly the memoranda Left by Isabella Harris with Some Extracts from the Journal of Her Mother*, privately printed, n.p., 1869, quoted in Porter's *In Sickness and in Health*.

HARRIS, Seale, *Woman's Surgeon: The life story of J. Marion Sims*, New York, 1950.

HARRISON, Brian, 'Women's Health and the Women's Movement in

Britain: 1840–1940' in WEBSTER, Charles (ed.) *Biology, Medicine and Society*, Cambridge University Press, 1981.

HARRISON, Brian, *Separate Spheres: The opposition to women's suffrage in Britain*, 1978.

HEMLOW, J. (ed.), *The Journals and Letters of Fanny Burney (Madame D'Arblay)*, 12 vols., Oxford, Clarendon Press, 1972–84.

HESELTINE, Michael, *The Early History of the General Medical Council, (1858–1886)*, [London], 1949. Reprinted from the Medical Press, no. 5757, 1949.

HIEBERT, E., *Historical Roots of the Principle of the Conservation of Energy*, Madison, 1962.

HOBBS, A.T., 'Surgical Gynaecology in Insanity', *BMJ*, 1897, 2, pp. 769–70.

HOLLICK, Frederick, *The Diseases of Women, their Cause and Cure Familiarly Explained*, New York, T.W. Strong, 1849.

HOLLIS, P (ed.), *Women in Public: The Women's Movement 1850–1900*, Allen & Unwin, 1979.

HOLLIS, Patricia, *Pressure from Without in Early Victorian England*, London, Edward Arnold, 1974.

HOLLOWAY, F., 'Medical Education in England, 1830–1858', *History*, 1964, 49. pp.299–324.

HOLMES, G., *Augustan England: Professions, state and society, 1680–1730*, London, George Allen & Unwin, 1982.

HOLMES, O.W., 'The Contagiousness of Puerperal Fever', *NEJM*.

HOLMES, O.W., 'Currents and Counter-Currents in Medical Science', in a collection of papers of the same title, 1860.

HOUGHTON, Walter, *Ideas and Beliefs of the Victorians, An historical revaluation of the Victorian age*, New York, Dutton, 1966.

HOUGHTON, Walter, *The Victorian Frame of Mind*, Yale University Press, 1957.

HUIZER, G., & MANNHEIM, B., *The Politics of Anthropology: From Colonialism and sexism toward a view from below*, The Hague, 1979.

HUNT, Harriot K., *Glances and Glimpses, or Fifty Years Social,*

*Including Twenty Years Professional Life*, Boston, 1865 and Source Book Press, 1970.

HUNT, T., (ed)., *The Medical Society of London, 1773–1973*, London, Heinemann, 1972.

HURD-MEAD, Kate Campbel, *A History of Women in Medicine from the Earliest Times to the Beginning of the Nineteenth Century*, Haddam Ct, Haddom Press, 1938.

HURD-MEAD, Kate Campbell, *Medical Women of America: A short history of the pioneer medical women of America and a few of their colleagues in England*, New York, 1933 and London, 1938.

ILCHESTER, The Earl of, ed., *Lady Holland's Journal*, 2 vols., Longmans Green, London, 1908.

JALLAND, Pat & HOOPER, John, *Women from Birth to Death: the female life cycle in Britain, 1830–1914*, Harvester Press, c. 1985.

JAMESON, Edwin M., *Gynecology and Obstetrics*, New York, 1962. May, 1977.

JARDINE, Alice and SMITH, Paul, (eds.), *Men in Feminism*, New York and London, Methuen, 1987.

JONES E.L., *Chlorosis; the Special Anaemia of Young Women*, London, Bailliere, Tyndall and Cox, 1897.

JONES, G.S., *Outcast London: A study of the relationship between classes in Victorian society*, Oxford, 1971.

JONES, Greta, *Social Darwinism and English Thought: The interaction between biological and social theory*, Brighton, Sussex, 1980.

JORDANOVA, L.J., 'Natural Facts: A historical perspective on science and sexuality', in MCCORMACK, C., and STRATHERN, M., *Nature, Culture and Gender*, Cambridge, 1980.

JORDANOVA, Ludmilla, *Sexual Visions: Images of gender in science and medicine between the eighteenth and twentieth centuries*, University of Wisconsin Press, 1989.

JORION, P,. 'The Downfall of the Skull', RAIN, 1982, 48, pp.8–11.

*Journal of Orificial Surgery*, Chicago.

KAISER, Barbara L. & KAISER, Irwin H., 'The Challenge of the Women's Movement to America Gynecology', *Amer. J., Obst. Gyn.*, 1974, 120, pp. 652–665.

KAISER, Irwin H., 'Reappraisals of J. Marion Sims,' *American Journal of Obstsetrics and Gynaecology*, 1978, 132, pp.878–884.

KANNER, S. Barbara, *The Women of England in a Century of Social Change*, 1815–1914, in VICINUS, Martha, *Suffer and be Still*.

KEELE, Kenneth B., *The Evolution of Clinical Medicine*, 1963.

KELLER, E.F., *Reflections on Gender and Science*, New Haven, Conn., 1985.

KELLY, H.A., 'The Ethical Side of the Operation of Oöpherectomy', *American Journal of Obstetrics*, 1898, 27, pp. 208–09.

KELLY, H.A., *Medical Gynaecology*, Philadelphia Saunders, 1909, pp. 67, 72–3.

KELLY, H.A., 'Reminiscences in Development of Gynecology', *Connecticut State Medical Journal*, 1937, p. 463.

KELLY, H.A., *Hysterorrhaphy*, 1887, New York, W.F. Wood & Co.

KEMBLE, F., *Journal of a Residence on a Georgian Plantation in 1838–1839*, 1863. Reprint ed., 1961, with an introduction by John A. Scott, Athens, Georgia.

KENNEDY, David, *Birth Control in America: The career of Margaret Sanger*, New Haven, 1970.

KETT, Jospeh, *The Formation of the American Medical Profession: the role of institutions, 1780–1860*, Yale University Press, 1968.

KITZINGER, Sheila, *The Midwife Challenge*, London, Pandora, 1988,

KITZINGER, Sheila, & DAVIS, John (eds.), *The Place of Birth*, London, 1978.

KITZINGER, Shelia, *Good Birth Guide*, London, 1983.

KLEIN, Rudolf, *Complaints Against Doctors*, London, 1973.

KLEIN, Viola, *The Feminine Character: History of an ideology*, London, Routledge & Kegan Paul, 1946. See also third edition, 1989.

KLEIN, Viola. 'The Emancipation of Women: its motives and achievements', in Houghton, W. *Ideas and Beliefs of the Victorians*, p. 261.

KLINE, P., & COOPER, C., *Rigid Personality and Rigid Thinking, British Journal Educational Psychology*, 1985, 55, pp.24–27.

'LANCET, The Obstetrical and Gynaecological Section of the Royal Society of Medicine', *Lancet*, 1907, 2, pp. 427–41.

LANE, Joan, 'The Role of Apprenticeship in Eighteenth Century Medical Education in England', in BYNUM W.F., and PORTER, R., *William Hunter and the Eighteenth Century Medical World*, Cambridge University Press, 1985.

LANE, Joan, ' "The Doctor Scolds Me": The Diaries and Correspondence of Patients in Eighteenth-Century England', in PORTER, R., (ed.), *Patients and Practitioners*, pp. 207–47.

LANGE Helene, *Higher Education of Women in Europe*, New York, Appleton, 1901.

LARNED, Deborah, 'Caesarian Births: why are they up 100%?,' *Ms Magazine*, October, 1978.

LARSON, M.S., *The Rise of Professionalism: A sociological analysis*. Berkeley, University of California Press, 1977.

LAYCOCK, Thomas, *A Treatise of Nervous Disorders of Women*, 1840. Laycock was Professor of Medicine and Lecturer in Medical Psychology at Edinburgh.

LAYTON, T.B., *Sir William Arbuthnot Lane, Bt: An enquiry into the mind and influence of a surgeon*, Edinburgh and London, E. & S. Livingstone, 1956.

LEAVITT, Judith Walzer (ed.) *Women and Health in America*, University of Wisconsin Press, 1984.

LEONARDO, R.A., *History of Gynaecology*, New York, Froben Press, 1944.

L'ESPÉRANCE, Jeanne, *Doctors and Women in Nineteenth Century Society: Sexuality and role*, in WOODWARD J. &. RICHARDS, D. (eds.) *Health Care and Popular Medicine*, 1977.

LEWIS, Jane, *Women in England, 1870–1950: Sexual divisions and social change*, Bloomington, University of Indiana Press, 1984.

LEWIS, Roy & MAUDE, Angus, *The English Middle Classes*, London, 1949.

LINDEMANN, E., 'Observations on Psychiatric Sequelae to Surgical Operations in Women', *Amer. J. Psychiatry*, 1941, 98, p. 132. 'Observations of Women after Operations', *Amer. J. Psychiatry*, 1958, 98, p. 132.

LONGO, Lawrence D., The Rise and Fall of Battey's Operation: a fashion in surgery', *Bull. Hist. Med*, 1979, 53, pp.244–67.

LORBER, Judith, *Women Physicians*, New York, Tavistock, 1984.

LOUDON I.S.L., 'The Nature of Provincial Medical Practice in Eighteenth-Century England', *Medical History*, 1985, 29, pp.1–32.

LOUDON, I.S.L., 'Deaths in Childbed from the Eighteenth Century to 1935', *Medical History*, 1986, 30, pp.1–41.

LOUDON, I.S.L., 'Chlorosis, Anaemia and Anorexia Nervosa', *Journal of the Royal College of General Practitioners*, 1980, 30, pp.1669–87.

LOUDON, I.S.L., *Medical Care and the General Practitioner, 1750–1850*, Oxford, Clarendon Press, 1986.

LOUDON, I.S.L., 'The Concept of the Family Doctor', *Bull. Hist. of Med.*, 1984, 58, pp. 347–62.

LOUDON, J.B., *Social Anthropology and Medicine*, London and New York, Academic Press, 1976.

LOVEJOY, Esther, *Women Doctors of the World*, New York, Macmillan, 1957.

LUTZKER, Edythe, *The London School of Medicine for Women*, 1972.

LUTZKER, Edythe, *Women Gain a Place in Medicine*, New York, McGraw-Hill, 1969.

MACAULAY, Alexander, *A Dictionary of Medicine, designed for popular use, containing an account of diseases and their treatment*, 10th ed., Edinburgh, Adam and Charles Black, 1849.

MACFARLANE, Alan, *The Family Life of Ralph Josselin*, Cambridge, Cambridge University Press, 1976.

MACFARLANE, Alan, *Orgins of English Individualism*, Oxford, Blackwell, 1978.

MACKENZIE, M., 'Specialism in Medicine', *Fortnightly Review*, 1885, 37, N.S., p.773.

MALLESON, Andrew, *Need Your Doctor be so Uuseless?*, London, Allen & Unwin, 1973.

MANTON, Jo, *Elizabeth Garrett Anderson*, London, Methuen, 1965.

MARCY, H.O., 'The Early History of Abdominal Surgery in America', *Transactions of the Section of Obstetrics and Gynecology of the*

*AMA*, 1909, pp.248–266, and *JAMA*, 1910, Feb. 19, 54, no.8, pp.600–605.

MARGACH, J., *The Anatomy of Power*, W. H. Allen, London, 1979.

MARKOWITZ, G., & ROSNER, D.K., 'Doctors in Crisis: A study of the use of medical education reform to establish modern professional elitism in medicine', *Amer. Quart.*, 1973, 25, p.83.

MARTINEAU, H., *Life in the Sick-Room: Essays by an invalid*, 2nd edn., London, 1854.

MARTINEAU, H., *Autobiography*, 2 vols., London, Virago, 1983. First edition 1877.

MAUDSLEY, Henry, 'Sex in Mind and Education', *Fortnightly Review*, April 1874.

MCDOWELL, E., 'Three Cases of Extirpation of Diseased Ovaria', *Eclect. Repert.*, Philadelphia, 1817, p.242.

MCKEOWN, T., *The Origins of Human Disease*, Oxford, Blackwell, 1988. McKinley, J., 'Epidemiological and Political Determinants of Social Policies Regarding the Public Health', *Soc. Sci. Med.*, 1979, 13A, pp. 541–58.

MEADOWS, A., 'On Certain Obstetric and Gynaecological Operations', *BMJ*, 1886, 2, pp. 356–8.

MEIGS, Charles D., *Females and their Diseases: A series of letters to his class*, Philadelphia, Lea & Blanchard, 1848.

MEIGS, Charles D., *Lecture on some of the Distinctive Characteristics of the Female, Delivered Before the Class of the Jefferson Medical College, January 5, 1847, 5*. Philadelphia, Collins, 1847.

MEIGS, Charles D., *Woman: Her Diseases and Remedies: A series of letters to his class*, 3rd edn., Philadelphia, Blanchard & Lea, 1854.

MELVILLE, L. (ed.), *The Berry Papers: Being the correspondence hitherto unpublished of Mary Agnes Berry, 1763–1852*, London, John Lane, 1914.

MENDUS, Susan, & RENDALL, Jane, *Sexuality and Subordination*, Routledge, 1989.

MEYER, D., *The Postive Thinkers*, Garden City, New York, Doubleday, 1965.

MICHELET, Jules, *La Femme*, translated by J.W. Palmer, MD, New York, 1870. Originally published Paris, 1863.

MICHELET, Jules, *L'Amour*, translated from 4th Paris edn. by J.W. Palmer, MD, New York, Carleton, Publisher, 1868.

MORANTZ, R.M., 'The Perils of Feminist History' in LEAVITT, *Women and Health in America*.

MORANTZ, R.M., & ZSCHOCHE, Sue, 'Professionalism, Feminism and Gender Roles: A comparative study of ninetenth-century medical therapeutics' in LEAVITT, *Women and Health in America*.

MORANTZ, R.M., 'Making Women Modern' in LEAVITT, *Women and Health in America*.

MORGAN, Elaine, *The Descent of Woman*, London, Souvenir Press, 1972.

MORGAN, Elaine (ed.), *Sisterhood is Powerful*, New York, Vintage Books, 1970.

MORGAN, Elizabeth, *The Making of a Woman Surgeon*, 1981.

MORTON, Leslie T., & MOORE, Robert J., *A Bibliography of Medical and Biomedical Biography*, Aldershot, Scolar, 1989.

MOSCUCCI, Ornella, *The Royal College of Obstetricians and Gynaecologists, 1929–1989*, forthcoming.

MOSCUCCI, Ornella, *The Science of Woman: British gynaecology 1849–1890*, DPhil thesis, University of Oxford, 1984.

MOSCUCCI, Ornella, *The Science of Woman: Gynaecology and gender in England, 1800–1920*, Cambridge, Cambridge University Press, 1990.

MOSELEY, William, *Eleven Chapters on Nervous and Moral Complaints*, 1838.

MOSHER, Eliza, 'The Value of Organization; What it has done for women', *Woman's Medical Journal*, June 1916, 26, pp. 1–4.

MURPHY, J., 'The Influence of Surgery on Gynaecology', *Provincial Medical Journal*, 1891, 10, pp. 403–4.

MYRDAL, Alva, & KLEIN, Viola, *Women's Two Roles: Home and Work*, London, Routledge & Kegan Paul, 1956.

NEALE, R.S., *Class and Ideology in the Nineteenth Century*, London, 1972.

NEWMAN, Charles, *The Evolution of Medical Education in the Nineteenth Century*, London, 1957.

NUMBERS, Ronal L. & SCHOEPFLIN, Rennie B., 'Ministries of Healing: Mary Baker Eddy, Ellen G. White, and the religion of health' in LEAVITT, *Women and Health in America.*

OAKLEY, Ann, *The Captured Womb: A history of the medical care of pregnant women*, Oxford, Blackwell, 1984.

OAKLEY, Ann, *Sex, Gender and Society*, London, 1972, and New York, 1973.

OAKLEY, Ann, *Subject Women*, London, Fontana, 1982.

OUTRAM, Dorinda, *The Body in the French Revolution*, Newhaven, Yale University Press, 1989.

'Ovariotomy in the Royal Medical and Chirurgical Society', *BMJ*, 1862, 2, pp. 521–2.

'Ovariotomy', *BMJ*, 1862, 2, p. 494.

OWEN, David, *English Philanthropy 1660–1960*, Cambridge, Mass., Belknap Press, 1965.

PARRY, Noel & Jose, *The Rise of the Medical Profession: A study of collective social mobility*, London, Croom Helm, 1976.

PEASLEE, E.R., *Ovarian Tumours: their pathology, diagnosis and treatment; especially by ovariotomy*, Lewis, London, 1873. Dedicated to the memory of Ephraim McDowell and to Spencer Wells.

PECHEY, John, *A General Treatise of the Diseases of Maids, Bigbellied Women, Child-Bed Women, and Widows*, London, 1696.

PERKIN, Harold, *Origins of English Society, 1780–1880*, London, 1969.

PERNICK, M.S., *A Calculus of Suffering: Pain, professionalism and anesthesia in nineteenth century America*, New York, 1985.

PETERSEN, M. Jeanne, *The Medical Profession in Mid-Victorian London*, University of California Press, 1978.

PHILIPS, Angela & RAKUSEN, Jill (eds.) *Our Bodies, Ourselves: A health book by and for women*, Boston Women's Health Book Collective.

PICK, Daniel, *Faces of Degeneration: A European disorder, c. 1848–1918*, Cambridge University Press, 1990.

PINKER, R., *English Hospital Statistics, 1861–1938*, London, Heinemann, 1966.

PLOSS, H.H., BARTELS, M., & BARTELS, P., *Woman: An historical gynaecological and anthropological compendium*, 3 vols., London, 1935. First published in German, 1885.

POIRIER, Suzanne, 'The Weir Mitchell Rest Cure: doctors and patients', *Women's Studies*, 1983, 10, pp. 15–40.

POOVEY, Mary, ' "Scenes of An Indelicate Nature": The medical "treatment of Victorian women" ', *Representations*, 1986 14, p. 146.

PORTER, R., 'Was There a Medical Enlightenment in Eighteenth-Century England?', *British Journal For Eighteenth-Century Studies*, 1982, 5, pp. 46–63.

PORTER, D., & PORTER R., *Patient's Progress: The Dialectics of Doctoring in Eighteenth Century England*, Cambridge, Polity Press, 1989.

PORTER, R., & WEAR, Andrew, *Problems and Methods in the History of Medicine*, London, Croom Helm, 1987.

PORTER, R. & D., *In Sickness and in Health: The British experience 1650–1850*, Fourth Estate, 1988.

PORTER, R., *Disease, Medicine and Society in England, 1550–1860*, Macmillan Education, 1987.

PORTER, R., *Health For Sale: quackery in England 1660–1850*, Manchester, Manchester University Press, 1989.

PORTER, R. (ed.) *Patients and Practitioners: Lay perception of medicine in Pre-Industrial society*, Cambridge University Press, 1985.

PORTER, R., 'Medicine and the Decline of Magic,' *Soc. Soc. Hist. Med.*, 41, December 1987.

PORTER, Theodore, *The Rise of Statistical Thinking, 1820–1900*, Princeton University Press, 1986.

POYNTER, F.N.L. (ed.) *Science and Medicine in the 1860s*, London, 1966.

POYNTER, F.N.L., 'Medicine and Culture', proceedings of an historical symposium organised jointly by the Wellcome Institute of the History of Medicine, London, and the Wenner-Gren Foundation for Anthropological Research, New York, 1969.

QUAIN, R. (ed.), *A Dictionary of Medicine: including general pathology, general therapeutics, hygiene, and the diseases peculiar to women and children*, 2 vols., London, 1882, ii, 1789. New revised edn., Longmans Green, London, 1894.

REISER, S.J., *Medicine and the Reign of Technology*, Cambridge, Cambridge University Press, 1978.

RICCI, James V., *One Hundred Years of Gynaecology 1800–1900*, Philadelphia, 1945.

RICCI, James V., *The Development of Gynaecological Surgery and Instruments: a comprehensive review of the evolution of surgery and surgical instruments for the treatment of female diseases from the Hippocratic age to the antiseptic period*, Philadelphia, Blakiston Company, 1949.

RICCI, James V., *The Genealogy of Gynaecology: History of the development of gynaecology throughout the ages, 2000 BC–1800 AD*.

RICH, Adrienne, *Of Woman Born: Motherhood as experience and institution*, New York, W.W. Norton, 1976.

RICHARDS, Robert J., *Darwin and the Emergence of Evolutionary Theories of Mind and Behaviour*, London, 1988.

RICHARDSON, Ruth, *Death, Dissection and the Destitute*, London, Routledge & Kegan Paul, 1987.

RIDENBAUGH, Mary Young, *The Biography of Ephraim McDowell, 'The Father of Ovariotomy'*, New York, Webster, 1890. Written by McDowell's granddaughter.

RIDLEY, C.M., *The Vulva*, Churchill, 1988.

RILEY, J., *The Eighteenth Century Campaign to Avoid Disease*, Basingstoke, 1987.

RISSE, G., 'Health and Disease: A history of the concepts', in REICH, W.T., *Encyclopedia of Bioethics*, 2 vols., New York, Free Press, 1978, pp. 579–85.

RISSE, G.B., 'Historicism in Medical History Heinrich Damerow's 'philosophical' historiography in romantic Germany', *Bull. Hist. Med.* 1969, 43, pp.201–11.

RIVINGTON, Walter, *The Medical Profession*, (first Carmichael Prize Essay), 1st edn. 1879, 2nd edn. 1887, Bailliere, Tindall and Cox.

ROBERTS, Shirley, *Sir James Paget: The Rise of Clinical Surgery*, Royal Society of Medicine Services Ltd., 1989.

ROHE, G., 'The Relation of Pelvic Disease and Psychical Disturbances in Women', *American Journal of Obstetrics & Dis. Women & Child.*, 1892, 26, pp. 689–726.

ROOK, A., *The Origins and Growth of Biology*, Harmondsworth, Pelican Books, 1964.

ROSEN, G., 'Disease, Debility and Death,' in DYOSS, H.J., & WOLFF, M. (eds.), *The Victorian City: Images of reality*, 2 vols., London, 1973.

ROSEN, George, *A History of Public Health*, New York, MD Publications, 1958.

ROSENBERG, Charles E., 'The Therapeutic Revolution: Medicine, meaning and social change in nineteenth-century America', in *Perspectives in Biology and Medicine*, 1977, 20, pp. 485–506 and in ROSENBERG, C., & VOGEL, M.J., (eds.), *The Therapeutic Revolution: Essays in the social history of American medicine*, Philadelphia, University of Pennsylvania Press, 1979.

ROSENBERG, Charles E., *The Care of Strangers: The rise of America's hospital system*, New York, Basic Books, 1987.

ROSENBERG, Charles E., 'Factors in the Development of Genetics in the United States: some suggestions', *Journal of the History of Medicine*, 1967, 22, pp. 31–33.

ROSENBERG, Charles E., 'Sexuality, Class and Role in 19th Century America', *American Quarterly*, 1973, 25, pp.131–53.

ROSENBERG, Charles E., *The Cholera Years*, Chicago and London, University of Chicago Press, 1962.

ROSENBERG Charles E., and SMITH-ROSENBERG, Carroll, 'The Female Animal: medical and biological views of woman and her role in 19th century America', *American Quarterly*, 1973, 60, pp.332–356. Reprinted in LEAVITT, *Women and Health in America*.

ROSENBERG, Rosalind, 'In Search of Woman's Nature, 1850–1920,' *Feminist Studies*, 3, Fall, 1975, pp. 141–54.

ROSENBERG, Rosalind, *Beyond Separate Spheres: intellectual roots of modern feminism*, New Haven, Yale University Press, 1982.

ROSSI, Alice, *The Feminist Papers*, New York, Bantam Books, 1973.

ROTHSTEIN, William G., *American Physicians in the Nineteenth Century*, Baltimore, The Johns Hopkins University Press, 1972.

ROUSSEAU, G.S., & PORTER, R. (eds.) *Sexual Underworlds of the Enlightenment*, Manchester, Manchester University Press, 1988, pp. 86–100.

RUSSETT, Cynthia Eagle, *Sexual Science: The Victorian construction of womanhood*, Harvard University Press, 1989.

RUZEK, S.B., *The Women's Health Movement: Feminist alternatives to medical control*, New York, Praeger, 1978.

SAVAGE, G.H., *Insanity and Allied Neurosis*, London, 1884.

SAYERS, Janet, *Biological Politics: Feminist and anti-feminist perspectives*, London, Tavistock Publications, 1982.

SCHARLIEB, Mary, *Reminiscences*, Williams & Norgate, 1924.

SCHATZMAN, Morton, *Soul Murder: Persecution in the family*, London, Allen Lane, 1973.

SCHREINER, Olive, *Women and Labour*, London, 1911

SCOFFERN, John, *The London Surgical Home, or Modern Surgical Psychology*, London, 1867.

SCULLY, Diana, *Men Who Control Women's Health: The miseducation of obstetricians and gynaecologists*, Boston, Houghton Mifflin, 1980.

SCULLY, Diana & BART, Pauline, 'A Funny Thing Happened on the Way to the Orifice: Women in Gynecology Textbooks', *Amer. J. Sociol.* 1973, 78(4), pp. 1045–54. Reprinted in HUBER, Joan (ed.), *Changing Women in a Changing Society*, Chicago, 1973.

SHEPHERD, John A., *Lawson Tait: The rebellious surgeon*, Kansas, Coronado Press, 1980. Includes a full list of his publications.

SHEPHERD, John A., *Spencer Wells: The life and work of a Victorian surgeon*, Livingstone, 1965.

SHORTER, Edward, *Bedside Manners: The troubled history of doctors and their patients*, Simon & Schuster, New York, 1985.

SHORTER, Edward, *A History of Women's Bodies*, New York, Basic Books, 1982.

SHOWALTER, Elaine, *The Female Malady: Women, madness and culture, 1830–1980*, Virago, 1987.

SHOWALTER, Elaine (ed.), *Speaking of Gender*, New York and London, Routledge, 1989.

SHOWALTER, Elaine, *Sexual Anarchy: Gender and Culture at the Fin de Siècle*, New York, Viking, 1990.

SHOWALTER, Elaine & ENGLISH, D. 'Victorian Women and Menstruation', *Victorian Studies*, 1970, 14, pp. 33.

SHRYOCK, H. 'The Advent of Modern Medicine in Philadelphia, 1800-1850,' *Yale J. Biol. Med.* 1941, XIII, pp. 725–731.

SHRYOCK H., 'American Medical Research,' *Past and Present*, New York 1947.

SHRYOCK, H., 'American Indifference to Basic Science During the Nineteenth Century', *Archives Internationales d'Histoire des Sciences*, (1948) no.5.

SHRYOCK, R.H., 'The American Physician in 1846 and in 1946,' *JAMA*, May 31, 1947, CXXXIV, pp. 417ff.

SHRYOCK, R.H., 'Women in American Medicine.' *J Amer Med. Women's Ass.* 1950, V, pp. 371–9.

SHRYOCK, R.H., *The Development of Modern Medicine, An interpretation of the social and scientific factors involved*, University of Wisconsin Press, 1979.

SHRYOCK, Richard, *The History of Nursing*, N.B. Saunders, 1959.

SHRYOCK, Richard, *Medicine in America: Historical essays*, Johns Hopkins press, Baltimore, 1966.

SICHERMAN, B., 'The Uses of Diagnosis: Doctors, patients and neurasthenia, *J. Hist. Med. and Allied Siences*, 1977, 32, pp. 333–65.

SIGERIST, Henry, *Disease and Civilization*, Ithaca, Cornell University Press, 1943.

SIGERIST, Henry, 'The Social History of Medicine,' *Western Journal of Surgery, Obstetrics and Gynecology*, 1940, 48, pp. 715–22.

SIGERIST, Henry, *Great Doctors: A Biographical History of Medicine*, London, George Allen & Unwin, 1933.

SIGERIST, Henry, *On the History of Medicine*, edited by Felix Marti-Ibanez & John Fulton, MD Publications, New York, 1960. This book contains many reprints of Sigerist's articles.

SIGERIST, Henry, *A History of Medicine*, 2 vols., New York, Oxford University Press, 1951.

SIGERIST, Henry, 'The History of Medicine and the History of Science', *Bulletin of the Institute of the History of Medicine*, 1936, 4, pp. 1–13.

SILVERMAN, David, *Communication and Medical Practice*, Calcutta, Fawcett, 1987.

SIMON, Sir John, 'Papers Relating to the Constitution of the Medical Profession, and to the Operation of the Medical Act, 1958', *Rep. Med. Offr. privy Council*, 1869, 12,200 (appendix no.10).

SIMS, J. Marion, *The Story of my Life*, New York, 1884.

SINGER, Charles, *A Short History of Medicine*, 2nd edn., Oxford, 1962.

SKENE, A.J.C., *Treatise on the Diseases of Women*, New York, Appleton, 1889.

SKULTANS, V., *A Study of Women's Ideas Relating to Traditional Feminine Roles, Spiritualism and Reproductive Functions*, PhD Thesis, University of Swansea, 1971.

SKULTANS, V., *English Madness: Ideas on Insanity, 1580–1890*, London, Routledge and Kegan Paul, 1979.

SMITH, F.B., *The People's Health, 1830–1910*, London, Croom Helm, 1979.

SMITH, H.H., *A System of Operative Surgery*, 2nd ed. Philadelphia, 1852, 1856.

SMITH, W.T., 'Lectures on Parturition, and the Principles and Practice of Obstetricy', *Lancet*, 1848, 2, p.119.

SMITH, W.T., 'The Climacteric Disease in Women,' *London Journal of Medicine*, 1848, pp. 601–609.

SMITH-ROSENBERG, C. & ROSENBERG, C., 'The Female Animal: Medical and biological views of woman and her role in nineteenth-century America', *J. Amer. Hist*, 1973 LX, 2, pp. 332–56.

SMITH-ROSENBERG, Carroll, 'From Puberty to Menopause: the cycle of femininity in nineteenth century America', in HARTMAN & BANNER, 1974.

SMITH-ROSENBERG, Carroll, 'The Hysterical Woman: Sex roles and role conflict in nineteenth century America', *Social Research*, 1972, 39, pp. 652–78.

SOFFER, Reba N., 'The Revolution in English Social Thought, 1880-1914', *American Historical Review*, 1970, 75, 1942n17, 1945 (sic) ).

SONTAG, Susan, *Illness as Metaphor*, New York, Farrar, Straus & Giroux, 1978; London, Allen Lane, 1979; Penguin, 1977.

SPEERT, H., *Obsteric and Gynaecologic Milestones: Essays in eponymy*, New York, Macmillan, 1958.

SPENCER, Herbert, *Education: intellectual, moral and physical*, London, Williams & Norgate, 1861.

SPENCER, Herbert, *Principles of Sociology*, 3 vols. London, Williams & Norgate, 1876–82.

SPENCER, Herbert, *The Principles of Ethics*, 2 vols., Williams & Norgate, London 1892–3.

SPENDER, Dale, *Women of Ideas and What Men have done to them: from Aphra Behn to Adrienne Rich*, London, Routledge & Kegan Paul, 1982.

SPRIGGE, S.S., *The Life and Times of Thomas Wakley*, London, Longmans Green, 1897.

STAGE, Sarah, *Female Complaints: Lydia Pinkham and the business of women's medicine*, New York, Norton, 1979.

STANSFELD, James, 'Medical Women', *Nineteenth Century*, July 1877, vol. 1, No. 5 London, pp. 888–901.

STARR, Paul, *The Social Transformations of American Medicine: The rise of a sovereign profession and the making of a vast industry*, New York, Basic Books, 1982.

STATUM, S., & LARSON, D.E., *Patients and Society: Power and authority in medical care*, Ontario, 1981.

STEPAN, N., *The idea of Race in Science: Great Britain, 1800–1960*, London, Macmillan, 1982.

STEVENS, Rosemary, *American Medicine and the Public Interest*, New Haven, Yale University Press, 1971.

STEVENS, Rosemary, *In Sickness and In Wealth: American Hospitals in the Twentieth Century*, New York, Basic Books, 1989.

STEVENS, Rosemary, *Medical Practice in Modern England: The impact of specialization and state medicine*, Yale University Press, 1966.

STEVENSON, Lloyd, 'Science down the Drain,' *Bull. Med. Hist.*, 1955, XXIX, pp. 10–25.

STOCKING, G.W., Jr., *Race, Culture and Evolution Essays in the history of anthropology*, Chicago and London, 1982.

STOCKING, G.W., *Victorian Anthropology*, New York, The Free Press, 1987.

STOLLER, Robert, *Sex and Gender*, London and New York, 1968.

STONE, L., *Family, Sex and Marriage in England 1500–1800*, New York, 1977.

STUDD, John, *Progress in Obstetrics and Gynaecology*, vols. 1–8,

SULEIMAN, Susan Rubin, *The Female Body in Western Culture: Contemporary Perspectives*, Cambridge, Harvard University Press, 1987.

SURGEON-GENERAL'S CATALOGUE.

SUTTON, Sir J. Bland-, *The Story of a Surgeon*. With a preamble by Rudyard Kipling.

SUTTON, Sir J. Bland-, *On Faith and Science in Surgery*, London, Heinemann, 1930.

SZASZ, Thomas, *The Myth of Mental Illness*, New York, Harper & Row, 1961.

TAIT, Lawson, 'Removal of Normal Ovaries', *BMJ*, i, pp. 813–4.

TAIT, Lawson, *BMJ*, 1881, i. 766–7.

TAIT, Lawson, *Two Essays on the Law of Evolution*, Birmingham, 1885.

TAIT, Lawson, *Masturbation, a Clinical Lecture*, Med. News, 1888, 53,2.

TAYLOR, S.T., *Dairy of a Medical Student 1860–1864*, Norwich, 1927.

TEMKIN, Ousei, 'The Role of Surgery in the Rise of Modern Medical Though', *Bulletin of the History of Medicine*, 1951, 25, pp. 248–59.

TEMKIN, Owsei, 'Health and Disease' in WIENER, P., *Dictionary of the History of Ideas*, New York, Scribner's, 1977, Ii, pp. 395–407.

TEMKIN, Owsei, *The Falling Sickness: A history of epilepsy from the Greeks to the beginnings of modern neurology*, Baltimore, The Johns Hopkins Press 1945.Revised Edition 1971.

TEMKIN, Owsei, *The Double Face of Janus and Other Essays in the History of Medicine*, Johns Hopkins University Press, Baltimore and London, 1977.

THOMAS, Keith, *Religion and the Decline of Magic*, London Weidenfeld and Nicolson, 1971.

THOMAS, Keith, 'The Double Standard', *J. Hist. Ideas*, 1959, 20, pp. 195–216.

THOMAS, T.G., *Practical Treatise on the Diseases of Women*, Philadelphia, Lea, 1872.

THOMAS, W., *Diseases of Women*, London, 1884.

TILT, E.J., *The Change of Life in Health and Disease*, London, Churchill, 1887. First edition 1957.

TILT E. J., *A Handbook of Uterine Therapeutics*, London, Churchill, 1863. Fourth edition, New York, William Wood, 1881.

TILT, E.J., *Diseases of Women, and Ovarian Inflammation*, 2nd edn., Churchill, London, 1853.

TILT, E.J., *On Uterine and Ovarian Inflammation; and on the physiology and diseases of menstruation*, 3rd edn., 1862.

TILT, E.J., *The Elements of Health, and Principles of Female Hygiene*, London, Henry G. Bohn, 1852.

TILT, E.J., *On the Preservation of the Health of Women at the Critical Periods of Life*, London, John Churchill, 1851.

TIMES, THE, Quarterly Index.

TOMASELLI S., 'The Enlightenment Debate on Women', *History Workshop*, 1985, 20, pp. 101–124.

VAISEY, D., *The Diary of Thomas Turner*, Oxford, Oxford University Press, 1984.

VAN DE WARKER, E., 'The Fetich of the Ovary', *American J. Obst. and Dis. Wom. and Child.* 54, 1906, p. 369.

VAN INGEN, P., *The New York Academy of Medicine: Its first hundred yers*, New York, 1949.

VAN KEUREN, *Human Science in Victorian Britain*, pp. 116–42.

VAUGHAN, Paul, *Doctors' Commons*, Heinemann, 1959.

VEBLEN, Thorsten, *The Theory of the Leisure Class*, (1948), 1899.

VICINUS, Martha (ed.), *Suffer and Be Still: women in the Victorian age*, Bloomington and London, Indiana University Press, 1972.

VICINUS, Martha, *Independent Women: work and community for single women, 1850–1920*, London, Virago, 1985.

VICINUS, Martha (ed.), *A Widening Sphere: Changing roles of Victorian women*, Bloomington, 1977.

VIGARELLO, Georges, *Concepts of Cleanliness: Changing attitudes in France since the Middle Ages*, Cambridge University Press, 1988.

VOGET, F.W., *A History of Ethnology*, New York, Chicago, San Francisco, 1975.

WADDINGTON, I., 'The Struggle to Reform the Royal Colledge of Physicians, 1767–1771', *Med. Hist.*, 1973, 17:2, p.108.

WADDINGTON, I., 'General Practitioners and Consultants in Early Nineteenth Century England: The sociology of an intra-professional conflict', *Soc. Social. Hist. Med. Bulletin*, 1976, 17, p. 11–12.

WALLACE, Alfred Russel, *The Wonderful Century: its Success and Failures*, New York, 1898.

WALSH, Mary Roth, *Doctors Wanted: No Women need apply: Sexual barriers in the medical profession, 1835–1975*, New Haven, Yale University Press, 1977.

WANGENSTEEN, Owen H., & Sarah D., *The Rise of Surgery, from empiric craft to scientific discipline*, Dawson, 1978.

WARNER, John Harley, *The Therapeutic Perspective: Medical Practice, Knowledge, and Indentity in America, 1820–1885*, Cambridge, Mass. and London, Harvard University Press, 1986.

WARNER, John Harley, 'The Nature Trusting Heresy: American Physicians and the Concept of the Healing Power of Nature in the 1850s and 1860s', *Perspectives in American History*, 1977–8, 11, pp. 291–324.

WATKINS, Dorothy, *The English Revolution in Social Medicine, 1889–1911*, Ph.D. thesis, London, University College, 1984.

WEBSTER, Charles (ed.), *Biology, Medicine and Society 1840–1940*. Cambridge University Pres, 1981.

WEED, Elizabeth (ed.), *Coming to Terms: feminism, theory, politics*, London, Routledge 1989.

WEEKS, Jeffrey, *Sex Politics and Society: The regulation of sexuality since 1800*, London and New York, Longman, 1981.

WELLS, T. Spencer, *On Ovarian and Uterine Tumours: Their diagnosis and treatment*, London, Churchill, 1885.

WELLS T. Spencer, *Diseases of the Ovaries: Their diagnosis and treatment*, 2 vols. London, Churchill, 1865 and 1872.

WELLS, T. Spencer, *Notebook for Cases of Ovarian and Other Abdominal Tumours*, London, Churchill, 1865.

WELLS, T. Spencer, *The Revival of Ovariotomy and its Influence on Modern Surgery*, 1884, 2, pp. 893–6.

WELLS, T. Spencer, 'Abstract of Six Lectures on the Diagnosis and Surgical Treatment of Abdominal Tumours,' *Lancet*, 1878, ii, p. 134.

WELLS, T. Spencer., *Modern Abdominal Surgery:* The Bradshaw Lecture delivered at the Royal College of Surgeons of England, with an appendix on the castration of women, London, 1891, p. 51.

WIGHTMAN, W.P.D., *The Emergence of Scientific Medicine*, Edinburgh, Oliver & Boyd, 1971.

WILLCOCK, J.W., *The Laws Relating to the Medical Profession*, 1830.

WOOD, Ann, 'Fashionable Diseases: Women's complaints and their treatment in 19th. Century America', in HARTMAN & BANNER (eds.), *Clio's Consciousness Raised*, New York, Harper & Row, 1974, and in Leavitt, *Women and Health in America*.

WOOD, George, *Treatise on Therapeutics*, London, 1868.

WOODWARD, J. & RICHARDS, David (eds.) *Health Care and Popular Medicine in Nineteenth Century England: Essays in social medicine* (articles by Inkster and Waddington), London, Croom Helm, 1977.

YOUNG, John Harley, *Caesarian Section: The history and development of the operation from earliest times*, London, H.K. Lewis, 1944.

YOUNG, R., *Darwin's Metaphor, Nature's Place in Victorian Culture*, Cambridge, 1985.

YOUNGSON, A.J., *The Scientific Revolution in Victorian Medicine*, London, Croom Helm, 1979.

# INDEX